Quality and Safety
in Radiation Oncology

D1572878

Quality and Safety in Radiation Oncology

Implementing Tools and Best Practices for Patients, Providers, and Payers

Editors

Adam P. Dicker, MD, PhD

Chair and Professor of Radiation Oncology
Pharmacology and Experimental Therapeutics
Sidney Kimmel Medical College at Thomas Jefferson University
Sidney Kimmel Cancer Center
Philadelphia, Pennsylvania

Tim R. Williams, MD

Medical Director, Radiation Oncology
The Lynn Cancer Institute
Radiation Oncology Department
Boca Raton Regional Hospital
Boca Raton, Florida

Eric C. Ford, PhD

Professor
Department of Radiation Oncology
University of Washington Medical Center
Seattle, Washington

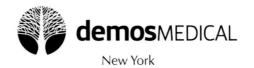

demosMEDICAL

New York

Visit our website at www.demosmedical.com

ISBN: 9781620700747
e-book ISBN: 9781617052460

Acquisitions Editor: David D'Addona
Compositor: S4Carlisle

Medicine is an ever-changing science. Research and clinical experience are continually expanding our knowledge, in particular, our understanding of proper treatment and drug therapy. The authors, editors, and publisher have made every effort to ensure that all information in this book is in accordance with the state of knowledge at the time of production of the book. Nevertheless, the authors, editors, and publisher are not responsible for errors or omissions or for any consequences from application of the information in this book and make no warranty, expressed or implied, with respect to the contents of the publication. Every reader should examine carefully the package inserts accompanying each drug and should carefully check whether the dosage schedules mentioned therein or the contraindications stated by the manufacturer differ from the statements made in this book. Such examination is particularly important with drugs that are either rarely used or have been newly released on the market.

Library of Congress Cataloging-in-Publication Data
Names: Dicker, Adam P., editor. | Williams, Tim R., editor. | Ford, Eric C. (Radiation oncologist), editor.
Title: Quality and safety in radiation oncology: implementing tools and best practices for patients, providers, and payers / editors, Adam P. Dicker, Tim R. Williams, Eric C. Ford.
Description: New York: Demos Medical, [2017] | Includes bibliographical references and index.
Identifiers: LCCN 2016025424 | ISBN 9781620700747 | ISBN 9781617052460 (e-book)
Subjects: | MESH: Neoplasms--radiotherapy | Quality Assurance, Health Care | Radiotherapy--standards | Radiation Oncology
Classification: LCC RC271.R3 | NLM QZ 269 | DDC 616.99/40642--dc23 LC record available at https://lccn.loc.gov/2016025424

Special discounts on bulk quantities of Demos Medical Publishing books are available to corporations, professional associations, pharmaceutical companies, health care organizations, and other qualifying groups. For details, please contact:

Special Sales Department
Demos Medical Publishing
11 West 42nd Street, 15th Floor, New York, NY 10036
Phone: 800-532-8663 or 212-683-0072; Fax: 212-941-7842
E-mail: specialsales@demosmedical.com

Printed in the United States of America by Publishers' Graphics.
16 17 18 19 20 / 5 4 3 2 1

Contents

Contributors

Michael B. Altman, PhD
Assistant Professor
Department of Radiation Oncology
Washington University School of Medicine
St. Louis, Missouri

Aaron Andersen, MS
Physicist
Department of Radiation Oncology
Indiana University School of Medicine
Indianapolis, Indiana

John Banja, PhD
Professor
Center for Ethics
Emory University
Atlanta, Georgia

Alex Bastian, MBA
Vice President
Health, Market Access
GfK Custom Research
San Francisco, California

R. Adam B. Bayliss, PhD
Assistant Professor
Department of Human Oncology
University of Wisconsin
Madison, Wisconsin

James R. Broughman, BS
Medical Student
University of North Carolina School of Medicine
Chapel Hill, North Carolina

Derek Brown, PhD
Associate Professor
Department of Radiation Medicine
   and Applied Sciences
University of California, San Diego
La Jolla, California

Courtney Buckey, PhD
Assistant Professor
Department of Radiation Oncology
Mayo Clinic Arizona
Phoenix, Arizona

Ronald C. Chen, MD, MPH
Associate Professor
Department of Radiation Oncology
University of North Carolina School of Medicine
Chapel Hill, North Carolina

Yohan Cho
Senior Consultant
Market Access
GfK Custom Research
New York, New York

Benjamin Clasie, PhD
Assistant Professor
Department of Radiation Oncology
Francis H. Burr Proton Therapy Center
Massachusetts General Hospital
Harvard Medical School
Boston, Massachusetts

Mary Coffey
Adjunct Associate Professor
Department of Radiation Oncology
Trinity College Dublin School of Medicine
Dublin, Ireland

Heather A. Curry, MD
Director, Radiation Oncology
NantHealth
Philadelphia, Pennsylvania

Indra J. Das, PhD, FACR, FASTRO
Vice Chair, Professor and Director of Medical Physics
Department of Radiation Oncology
New York University Langone Medical Center
Laura and Isaac Perlmutter Cancer Center
New York, New York

Joumana Dekmak, MS, BS, RT (T)
Radiation Therapist Supervisor
Department of Radiation Oncology
University of Michigan Health System
Ann Arbor, Michigan

Dennis R. Delisle, ScD, MHSA, FACHE
Executive Project Director
Thomas Jefferson University and Jefferson Health
Philadelphia, Pennsylvania

Sonja Dieterich, PhD, FAAPM
Associate Professor
Department of Radiation Oncology
University of California, Davis
Sacramento, California

Laura A. Doyle, MS
Clinical Instructor
Department of Radiation Oncology
Sidney Kimmel Cancer Center
Thomas Jefferson University
Philadelphia, Pennsylvania

Suzanne B. Evans, MD, MPH
Associate Professor
Department of Therapeutic Radiology
Yale University School of Medicine
New Haven, Connecticut

Gary Ezzell, PhD
Chair, Medical Physics Division
Associate Professor of Radiation Oncology
Department of Radiation Oncology
Mayo Clinic Arizona
Phoenix, Arizona

David S. Followill, PhD
Imaging and Radiation Oncology Core (IROC)
   Houston/MD Anderson Cancer Center
Houston, Texas

Hiral P. Fontanilla, MD
Department of Radiation Oncology
Princeton Radiation Oncology
Monroe, New Jersey

Eric C. Ford, PhD
Professor
Department of Radiation Oncology
University of Washington Medical Center
Seattle, Washington

Erin F. Gillespie, MD
Resident Physician
Department of Radiation Medicine and Applied Sciences
University of California, San Diego
La Jolla, California

Amy S. Harrison, MS
Medical Physicist, Operations and Safety Director
Department of Radiation Oncology
Sidney Kimmel Cancer Center
Thomas Jefferson University
Philadelphia, Pennsylvania

Ola Holmberg, PhD
Unit Head, Radiation Protection of Patients
Radiation Safety and Monitoring Section
International Atomic Energy Agency
Vienna, Austria

Jennifer L. Johnson, MS, MBA
Senior Medical Physicist and Director for Safety
Department of Radiation Physics
The University of Texas MD Anderson Cancer Center
Houston, Texas

Bernard L. Jones, PhD
Assistant Professor
Department of Radiation Oncology
University of Colorado School of Medicine
Aurora, Colorado

Ajay Kapur, PhD
Director of Medical Physics Research and Education
Department of Radiation Medicine
Hofstra Northwell School of Medicine
Hempstead, New York

Eric E. Klein, PhD
Vice President / Director of Medical Physics
Professor of Radiation Medicine
Northwell Health System
Lake Success, New York

Stephen F. Kry, PhD
Imaging and Radiation Oncology Core (IROC)
   Houston/MD Anderson Cancer Center
Houston, Texas

Kathy Lash, BS, RT (R) (T)
Director of Community Practices
Department of Radiation Oncology
University of Michigan Health System
Ann Arbor, Michigan

H. Harold Li, PhD
Associate Professor
Department of Radiation Oncology
Washington University School of Medicine
St. Louis, Missouri

Yuting Lin, PhD
Fellow
Department of Radiation Oncology
Massachusetts General Hospital
Harvard Medical School
Boston, Massachusetts

Genevieve M. Maquilan, MD
Resident Physician
Department of Radiation Oncology
University of Texas Southwestern Medical Center
Dallas, Texas

James Mechalakos, PhD
Associate Attending Physicist
Department of Medical Physics
Memorial Sloan Kettering Cancer Center
New York, New York

Jeff M. Michalski, MD, MBA
Professor
Department of Radiation Oncology
Washington University School of Medicine
St. Louis, Missouri

Moyed Miften, PhD
Professor and Chief of Physics
Department of Radiation Oncology
University of Colorado School of Medicine
Aurora, Colorado

Kevin L. Moore, PhD, DABR
Associate Professor / Associate Division Director
Department of Radiation Medicine and Applied Sciences
University of California, San Diego
La Jolla, California

Arno J. Mundt, MD
Professor and Chair
Department of Radiation Medicine and Applied Sciences
University of California, San Diego
La Jolla, California

Tom Piotrowski, RN, MSN
Vice President of Clinical Informatics / Executive Director
Clarity PSO
Clarity Group, Inc.
Chicago, Illinois

Louis Potters, MD, FACR, FASTRO
Chairman and Professor
Department of Radiation Medicine
Hofstra Northwell School of Medicine
Hempstead, New York

Sharon Rogers, MHSc, BA
Hospital Ombudsmen
University Health Network
Toronto, Ontario, Canada

Baozhou Sun, PhD
Instructor
Department of Radiation Oncology
Washington University School of Medicine
St. Louis, Missouri

Stephanie Terezakis, MD
Associate Professor
Department of Radiation Oncology and Molecular Radiation Sciences
Johns Hopkins University School of Medicine
Baltimore, Maryland

Bruce R. Thomadsen, PhD
Professor
Department of Medical Physics
University of Wisconsin School of Medicine and Public Health;
Director
Patient Safety Organization
The Center for the Assessment of Radiological Sciences
Madison, Wisconsin

Nicholas A. Thompson, MPH
Communication and Change Enablement Analyst
Thomas Jefferson University and Jefferson Health
Philadelphia, Pennsylvania

Henry K. Tsai, MD
Princeton Radiation Oncology
Monroe, New Jersey

Tim R. Williams, MD
Medical Director, Radiation Oncology
The Lynn Cancer Institute
Radiation Oncology Department
Boca Raton Regional Hospital
Boca Raton, Florida

Brian Winey, PhD
Assistant Professor
Department of Radiation Oncology
Francis H. Burr Proton Therapy Center
Massachusetts General Hospital
Harvard Medical School
Boston, Massachusetts

H. Omar Wooten, PhD
Assistant Professor
Department of Radiation Oncology
Washington University School of Medicine
St. Louis, Missouri

Ying Xiao, PhD
Professor
Department of Radiation Oncology
Perelman School of Medicine
University of Pennsylvania
Philadelphia, Pennsylvania

Yan Yu, PhD, MBA, FAAPM, FASTRO
Vice Chair, Professor and Director of Medical Physics
Department of Radiation Oncology
Sidney Kimmel Cancer Center
Thomas Jefferson University
Philadelphia, Pennsylvania

Preface

This book started as two independent conversations by Tim Williams and me with Rich Winters, formerly the Executive Editor at Demos over 3 years ago. To give context, in 2010, the *New York Times* highlighted medical errors that occurred in the field of radiation oncology. ASTRO created the *Target Safely* campaign at that time and in June 2011, ASTRO's Board of Directors approved a proposal to establish a national radiation oncology-specific incident learning system. A standardized system provides an opportunity for shared learning across all radiation oncology institutions and may be an added value to institutions that track incidents independently. This incident learning system represents a key commitment of *Target Safely,* ASTRO's patient protection plan, designed to improve the safety and quality of radiation oncology. ASTRO partnered with the American Association of Physicists in Medicine (AAPM) to develop RO-ILS: Radiation Oncology Incident Learning System®, the only medical specialty society-sponsored incident learning system for radiation oncology. In part, thanks to Dr. Lawrence Marks, University of North Carolina, I became a member of the Radiation Oncology Healthcare Advisory Council (RO-HAC) for the RO-ILS program. While immersing myself in details of RO-ILS I had the great pleasure working with Dr. Eric Ford, discussing quality and safety initiatives at the institutional and national level.

Given the increasing importance and high profile nature of Quality and Safety for the field of Radiation Oncology, at the Annual ASTRO meeting in 2013 I had discussed the idea of a book on the topic of Quality and Safety with Rich Winters. Rich mentioned that he had a similar conversation with Dr. Tim Williams of the Eugene M. and Christine E. Lynn Cancer Institute at Boca Raton Regional Hospital who was also interested in the subject. Tim was the ASTRO Board Chair in 2010 when the Target Safely initiative was launched. I met with Tim and we discussed our ideas and we both realized that his perspective was different from mine, yet together they would synergize quite well. I suggested we needed a medical physicist who has extensive experience in quality and safety and brought up Dr. Eric Ford, University of Washington, as a partner in the collaborative effort.

This project has been great for bringing together a diverse group of people whose training and backgrounds complement each other, all for the goal of helping patients. The book views Quality and Safety in the context of "Value" and the Institute of Medicine Quality Initiative.

Radiation Oncology is a technically demanding and complex field. It requires a team of individuals working together to deliver high-quality care. We believe by sharing information, as this book does, we can improve the lives of patients worldwide.

Adam P. Dicker, MD, PhD

Acknowledgments

Carolyn, Michal, Josh, Shimshon and Yehuda. Thank you, love you, you're the best!!!!!

I would like to thank the leadership at Thomas Jefferson University who helped us combine sophisticated patient-first, multidisciplinary care with high-impact science for cancer patients.

—*Adam P. Dicker*

I would like to extend my sincere gratitude to the Chapter authors, who devoted much time and effort to deliver an unbelievable work product, our editors at Demos for their guidance and support, and most of all to Adam and Eric, whose patience and understanding with me is the true unsung story of this book.

—*Tim R. Williams*

I would like to thank my many partners in delivering quality care and understanding what it means, Gabrielle Kane, Jing Zeng, Matt Nyflot and the many active team members at University of Washington including Lulu Jordan, Patty Sponseller, Josh Carlson, and many others. I also thank my mentors, colleagues, and friends at Johns Hopkins, Ted DeWeese, Stephanie Terezakis, and Peter Pronovost.

—*Eric C. Ford*

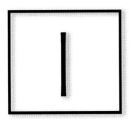

Basic Concepts in Quality, Value, and Safety

Tim R. Williams

1 Introduction to Concepts in Quality, Value, and Safety for Health Care Systems

Tim R. Williams and Alex Bastian

By its very nature, "quality" is a subjective, rather than an objective, concept. Depending on the perspective of the observer, it can mean many different things. Within medicine, and even within the specialty of radiation oncology, it can have many aspects. From the physician's point of view, "quality" could mean the ability to offer the range of services appropriate to his or her skill level, but not above or below. This in itself would imply that one radiation oncologist's "quality" might be filled with "more quality" (or less) than another's. From the point of view of the physicist, quality might be nothing more than the accurate measurement of an accelerator's output or the precise determination of a delivered dose based on an isotope's decay curve. The nurse might see quality as the timeliness of communication with the patient or the appropriate management of side effects. For patients, it could be anything from their belief that the facility is delivering the best treatment for their particular condition to having minimal waiting times, or even simply having access to fresh hot coffee on demand.

To the other stakeholders in a radiation oncology program, "quality" may well be measured in administrative, bureaucratic, financial, or legal terms that have little or nothing to do with patient care or clinical outcomes. In academic centers, "quality" may be determined, at least partially, by the number of articles accepted by peer-reviewed journals. In freestanding, corporate facilities, quality may be standardized into measured or quantifiable work units. For health care payers, quality might translate into a measure of efficiency, where high quality equates to the best possible outcome at the least cost relative to the physicians' peer group. Whatever "quality" is, and from whatever perspective it is assessed, it is generally accepted that more of it is better, and the general goal is to have as much of it as possible.

The concept of quality in the modern sense can be traced to Eli Whitney. It was his idea to standardize the fabrication of parts for firearms so that assembly and repairs could be made easily. Until then each firearm (and all other industrial products, for that matter) was custom made, one at a time. With standardized parts, however, the concept of "quality" emerged as a process to assess the fidelity of the manufacturing process. Higher quality meant a reduction in the number of rejected parts (1). The concept has been developing ever since, and industry is now filled with quality measures, metrics, and assessment tools. The evaluation of quality measures has become an industry in itself, with hundreds of companies offering standardized, recognized quality assessment programs such as Lean, Six Sigma, and Malcolm Baldrige Quality Awards. The airline transport system and the nuclear power industry are often used as prime examples of systems whose quality can be improved by the strict adherence to, and deliberate use of, quality measures. The airline industry, in particular, has developed a very successful, proactive quality/safety culture that has decreased the risk of accidents significantly since 1995 (2).

"Quality" and "value" are close cousins, and there can be considerable overlap in their assessment. Whereas quality is a multidimensional concept, depending on the perspective of the analyst, value is more commonly considered as health care translated into economic terms. It is very common in the health care policy literature to evaluate medicine as if it were a market, and governed by market forces.

Any basic market requires two things: a buyer and a seller. It is the economic philosophy governing each market, however, that defines the form and protocol from which any transactions between these two parties may occur. In most liberal capitalist markets, it is the rational pursuit of self-interest—by both the buyer and the seller—that ultimately defines value (3). The definitions of value may be highly personal, reflecting the importance of perspective and an understanding of stakeholder preferences that are required to define value. In normal markets, it is these very same perspectives that will impact how the relevant actors, or stakeholders, will define their decision criteria and value thresholds for buying and selling of health care goods and services. The business of medicine, however, is not a *normal* market.

MEDICINE IS NOT A NORMAL MARKET

Medicine is not a normal market because of several structural, political, and ethical features. It is highly regulated, data-poor, and the consequences—in humanistic and economic terms—are grave, with the agency relationship adding further complexity to the normal interactions between a buyer and seller. Because of these issues, health policymakers have found varying means of addressing these challenges, albeit none without limitations, using unique methods of value assessment for health care goods and services.

The regulatory environment in most health markets imposes specific demands on any seller (i.e., the manufacturer) that wishes to sell their medical technology. This includes requirements for clinical trials to demonstrate safety and efficacy with a high degree of certainty in a health technology's stated purpose, providing a high level of reproducibility and predictability. Most regulators have chosen to focus on aspects related to the evaluation of the quality, safety, and efficacy of medicinal products for human use. This regulation is intended primarily to establish that they perform according to their intended purpose and cause no unreasonable harm to users (3,4). Importantly, regulators and governments also often place patent protection rights onto innovators, allowing temporary or intermittent monopoly rights for these technologies. Each of these features has an important impact on the health marketplace that differs greatly from pure open markets such as those for automobiles, Internet technologies, or consumer goods.

Most products or services also serve a purpose—providing an expressed *utility* for the consumer of such a good. In the health marketplace, this is often expressed through the clinical trial program or eventual outcomes that are seen within the real-world use of such a good. Clinical trial and real-world data often correlate poorly, and variable outcomes may be experienced because of patient heterogeneity and the often weak link between surrogate endpoints with real-world outcomes. The utility or benefit gained, thus, is difficult to determine at the moment of the purchase decision for most consumers. Unlike with many other industries, the belief that one may achieve a utility from a product is largely unknown a priori. As each individual's response to any medical technology may vary, it is difficult to determine with certainty the

level of benefit to be gained, particularly at the time the value judgment must be made. This ambiguity becomes extremely important as the majority of physicians and health consumers often face difficult trade-offs when deciding on any given treatment option.

The grave consequences that patients and health policymakers face include those relating to longevity, quality of life, and resource sustainability. Furthermore, these factors may vary significantly based on patient characteristics. One example of the extremes might be elderly patients who may prefer quality of life to additional years of life if they are already in their mid-90s, compared with younger patients who may be willing to temporarily compromise quality of life if they are ensured additional years of life. As neither of these groups knows with absolute certainty the true impact of the health technology on either of these measures, they will have to grapple with the hope and promise that one course of action may have on their lives. In radiology, this may be illustrated in the case of younger patients with head and neck cancer, where quality-of-life benefits may have a meaningful effect over the years among long-term survivors. Late complications such as dysphagia, xerostomia, and osteonecrosis are typical in this setting. Minimizing the occurrence and severity of these complications can improve the survivorship experience of patients, decrease the cost associated with long-term management of these morbidities, and mitigate the loss of productivity in these patients (4,5). Individual goals, perceived benefits and toxicities, and time horizon are important considerations for any health consumer.

The financial impact of any health good or service also has a critical impact on the associated cost perceptions that must be balanced by any perceived benefits. Although this may be very personal (e.g., a small copay), it may also be very unidimensional (e.g., only for inpatient care delivered) or multidimensional (e.g., total cost of care, including health technologies). Considerations of costs may include direct medical/nonmedical, indirect, and intangible costs. *Direct costs* refer to immediate, first-degree transactions for health technologies or services as well as nonmedical costs (e.g., drugs, treatment, travel or home services). *Indirect costs* may include second-degree costs such as loss of productivity by patients and their caregivers as a result of illness or treatment. *Intangible costs* refer to the psychosocial consequences and are often further removed from the immediate health transaction. As described earlier, the concept of value considers these various costs with the benefits gained. This will often vary significantly depending on the perspective taken and set of values prioritized by any given health stakeholder.

Policymakers deal with the provision and financing of care at various degrees for their citizens. Primarily funded through finite means with set budgets measured on an annual basis, the pressure to provide funding for health care means that health care may become the primary expenditure in most developed countries (5).

The trade-offs between use of funding for health goods and services must be weighed against other commitments to items such as education, infrastructure, public sanitation, and a variety of other societal goods. An example of this in the United States might be the manner in which state Medicaid programs grapple with annual budgets in the face of additional pressures on public funding. This too, however, is often explicitly linked to the prevailing economic philosophy of the government. Large increases in funding for new technologies may require additional unplanned expenditures or trade-offs in the use of funds earmarked for use on other causes. Providing vaccines at the expense of building new roads is an example of when policymakers must decide to allocate resources to either a health technology or other nonhealth public services such as new roads or school textbooks.

The role of the policymaker or societal stakeholder brings us to a final, but critically important, feature within health markets that differs from a more traditional market for goods and services: the agency relationship. The relationship between payer, provider, and patient in the health care market is often characterized as a principal–agent, or "agency relationship." The principal (the patient) appoints an agent (a health provider) to advise the principal in making decisions about treatment or to make decisions on the principal's behalf—which are all paid for by a public or private payer (the insurance company or government) in most markets. The provider is expected to be a perfect agent, combining professional knowledge with the patient's preferences to determine a choice that the patient would make on the basis of that information. In few markets, the buyer (i.e., The Patient) will be different from the decision maker (i.e., The Physician), who is also different from the person paying for the good (i.e., The Payer). The interests of each of these actors may influence the perception of "value" or willingness and ability to pay for a health good or service. But it is within the agency relationship that we begin to note that a particular level of expertise is required to assimilate and interpret the volumes of medical literature that may exist for any intervention. This may require multidisciplinary involvement from a variety of stakeholders, further confounding simple definitions of value within any given setting. One basic way to examine the interests of multiple parties involved in any health decision is to analyze their interests, good and bad, to determine where clear value exists or is absent, and where more scrutiny or discussion is warranted. The accompanying figure is an example of where the best interests, or value perceptions, are aligned or misaligned when compared with the interests of society at large, or the health system.

Those situations where the best interests (or highest value) are served for the patient as well as society or the system represent clear win-win settings where value prevails. Alternatively, those situations where any course of action may not be in the best interests (or negative value) of the patient and society, are also easy to align. Examples of

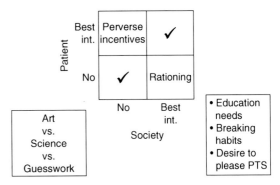

Aligning patient and societal best interests.

these situations are clearly seen in the "Choosing Wisely" campaign, which plucks the low-hanging fruit of aligned interests. One example is the recommendation not to perform PET, CT, or radionuclide bone scans in the staging of early prostate cancer at low risk for metastasis (6). This recommendation was based on a lack of evidence that it improved the detection of disease or survival, clearly highlighting the lack of benefit for patients. One step further, it was also based on the fact that unnecessary imaging can lead to harm through unnecessary invasive procedures, overtreatment, unnecessary radiation exposure, and misdiagnosis. The most difficult decisions relating to value are those where the interests of one stakeholder may not align with the best interests of another. This is the case where something that is in the best interests of the system—such as limiting or rationing care—may not be in the personal interests of the patient—such as receiving salvage therapy even when there is little hope of long-term survival.

The agency relationship reveals some important distinctions when considering costs and benefits for any given health technology. Use of newer radiation techniques provides a useful example of these distinctions. For example:

- Three-dimensional conformal radiotherapy (3D-CRT) allows for more targeted visualization of organs during the treatment planning process, thereby allowing optimization of beams to improve the therapeutic ratio during treatment.

- The development of intensity-modulated radiation therapy (IMRT), through which radiation dose distributions could be manipulated to minimize dose to surrounding normal structures, represents another important technique for clinicians.

- Proton beam therapy (PBT) is another modality that harnesses protons to arrive at an even more conformal radiotherapy plan. Ideally, this conformation will spare normal tissues from receiving doses of radiotherapy.

- The next generation of PBT—intensity-modulated proton therapy (IMPT)—could theoretically further improve the conformality of treatment.

Although these improvements are well perceived by the medical community, these achievements may be less recognized by other health stakeholders. While payers, for example, may value the benefits of these conformational therapies in terms of mortality, morbidity, or quality of life, these therapies come with significant costs. These costs are a function of both an increase in labor to apply these newer technologies and an increase in expense for the technology itself. For example, IMRT requires more time from the clinician, dosimetrist, and physicist, and the treatment mandates rigorous quality assurance procedures and advanced delivery technologies. PBT not only accrues these increased costs but also requires an extremely large up-front capital investment (7). These costs should not, however, be confused with the cost that may be borne by the payers, which is typically reimbursement for delivery of these services. Yet for the clinical stakeholders, the costs of delivering the technology are of central importance. It should be noted that in countries such as the United States, Switzerland, or a variety of the emerging markets, patients are likely required to cover a portion of costs, so their perspective must be considered when determining the value of these radiation therapies.

The varying perspectives of each stakeholder are critical when assessing value, with each defining the context and individual priorities from which the judgment is made. Patients, for example, often seek care based on a unique and personalized approach that fits their needs. The view of the physician may align in most cases with the needs of the patient, but also might have conflicts related to the desire to provide prudent restraint or based on a deeper understanding of the medical literature and the treatment setting. The use of pain medications or antibiotics, for example, provides an apt illustration of the challenges that patients may present when desiring too much or inappropriate care. In these cases, the prudent judgment and action of the physician is good for the patient—even if it runs counter to the individual patient's wishes in the moment. The health system, however, may sometimes have slightly different perceptions of value from an individual patient or physician. A patient told to go into the emergency room may negatively affect the system's quality measures. Such incentives impact only the health system rather than the individual doctor or patient. Additionally, reimbursement for common procedures in a health system may, in fact, be less than what it costs to deliver a given procedure. When facing these challenges, health systems may act in their own self-interest to eliminate perceived waste or poor economic consequences—including Pharmacy and Therapeutics (P&T) reviews for pharmaceutical goods or the institution of protocols for medical services. Finally, an all-encompassing societal view reflects what was described earlier, representing a more utilitarian balance to the provision of health resources among other public goods and services. How these final decisions are often made is based on the intersecting interests of all stakeholders involved, including the incentive structures that may exist to reinforce the pursuit of self-interest. Somewhere, between the intersection of the perspectives from the multitude of stakeholders—including the patients, their families and caregivers, the physicians and their multidisciplinary providers, the health system, its payers, and society as represented by policymakers—the concept of value in health care takes shape.

Within the varying perspectives of individual stakeholders, the benchmarks and time frame also influence the definition of value. The benchmarks signal whether the concept of value is anchored in comparison with something else or must truly be an independent judgment. Markets in the European Union, for example, have focused on incremental or additional benefit compared with currently available therapies. Though feasible for health technologies for which a current standard of care exists, it is more challenging for new therapy areas where no alternatives may be appropriate for comparison. The demands for such comparisons also frame the way in which assessments of value may be carried out and how cost should be viewed in relation to the perceived benefits. For example, the role of IMRT as the standard-of-care radiotherapeutic modality for head and neck cancer is well established, yet its incremental therapeutic value and cost-effectiveness compared with older radiation techniques are not well established in the clinical literature. It is unlikely that randomized trials will be performed on IMRT versus more conventional techniques, and thus analyses of its value and cost-effectiveness primarily hinge on the clear xerostomia benefits, potentially improved global quality-of-life improvements, and questionable survival gains that may be independently observed or compared with historical, cohort controls (8).

The time frame is important in defining value because, as we have already noted, it sets the confines within which the health technology has to demonstrate its benefit and cost. An example of how this varies might be best illustrated by comparing the time horizon that a typical U.S. state Medicaid program might have (e.g., an annual budget) with the Veteran's Affairs (VA) system or Medicare program (e.g., until death). The longer time horizon, generally, the longer the visibility into downstream benefits or cost savings that could be achieved by integration of a new health technology or service. However, it is the longer time horizon that also leads to generally weaker certainty of outcomes and, thus, predictability of these being achieved at the time of the treatment decision.

DEFINING VALUE

Incorporating the perspectives of various stakeholders, value might be calculated in the following manner:

Value = importance of certainty × probability of outcome × (benefits ÷ costs) − alternative value [if comparisons/alternatives exist]

The closer one gets to a value of "1," the more value one would attribute to any health technology or service. When analyzing this equation, it becomes easier to disaggregate the various elements that may color the various perspectives of stakeholders involved in defining value.

In studies of behavioral economics, the application of the term *cognitive dissonance* also comes into the vernacular when discussing value. The idea that one may consider value after the purchase decision is of importance when considering value in health care. From the patients' perspective, this may relate to their experience going through treatment, suffering side effects, or bearing the financial consequences. For the health system, such a concept may exist in the legacy systems that are purchased and, long after the purchase decision, may have an impact on the value perceptions by a variety of stakeholders. An expensive but early electronic medical records system, for example, might have been perceived as high value before implementation, but deemed exceedingly costly after installation, education, and maintenance. Another example may be the cost outlays on expanding a new division or department with the newest, latest technology. Forgoing other strategic purchases or activities might have a short-term impact, but the long-term impact of a need to pay for and amortize such equipment will have various consequences that influence the discussion of value. From the physician's perspective, for example, a trusted drug is withdrawn from the market in view of previously unknown toxicities. During the recent recall of such a medication, the authors stated, "Physicians and the public deserve to be in a position to make informed choices about risks and benefits, and the disclosure and dissemination of information about potential risk immediately after its recognition is absolutely essential. Our study provides insight into what should have been known about the risks of rofecoxib. . . . If we are to detect harms early and protect the public's health, while ensuring the availability of new, clinically effective therapeutics, a system must be established that makes full use of all existing evidence" (9). In this way, the certainty and evolution of clinical outcomes and knowledge become critically important for clinicians when making decisions or attributing value to a health technology or service.

Radiation oncology, in particular, has the particular challenge in a traditionally data-poor environment. This is primarily a result of the U.S. Food and Drug Administration (FDA) requirements that new devices used to deliver radiation therapy perform the function reliably as they are intended to do, not in terms of demonstration of patient outcomes (10). Thus, there is limited information on the relative effectiveness or expected outcomes during value assessment for most radiotherapy. Quality, control of process, avoidance or elimination of errors, and risk management protocols become particularly important considerations when assessing value in this setting.

Patient Safety

In the American health care sector, the adoption of the concept of quality and the derivation of its postulated benefits, at least in the context of medical decision making, has been slow. Value, defined as the relationship between costs and outcomes, is also an evolving concept. At least in general terms, however, it has been acknowledged that medical care is not as safe as it should be. The highly respected Institute of Medicine (IOM) provided the watershed moment that brought the concept of safety into the mainstream of health care with the publication, in 1999, of its report *To Err is Human: Building a Safer Health System.* The IOM review included two studies of hospital admissions, one from New York using data from 1984, and the other from Colorado and Utah, based on 1992 data. As was widely reported at the time, 2.9% and 3.7%, respectively, of patients experienced an adverse event. The proportion of adverse events attributable to errors (and thus thought to be avoidable) was 58% and 53%, respectively. Without comment on its statistical merit, the IOM extrapolated this data over the entire 33.6 million hospital admissions in 1997, and derived the now famous conclusion that as many as 98,000 deaths per year were attributable to medical errors. (They did have a lower estimate of 44,000 deaths, but this smaller number received only passing attention.) Thus, it became dogma that preventable hospital errors were the eighth leading cause of death in the country, and quality, value,

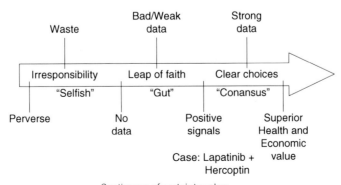

Continuum of certainty value

and safety came to be defined in the context of error prevention (11).

A similar study in Canada, interestingly, concluded that avoidable errors were associated with between 9,000 and 24,000 deaths from their national experience of 2.5 million annual hospitalizations. Extrapolated out to the same number of hospitalizations in the United States from the IOM study (33.6 million), one would conclude that the Canadian system would have caused more than 300,000 unnecessary deaths, over three times the IOM estimate for the United States (12).

Other studies have shown that error reporting systems used in hospitals may be inaccurate, with the number of actual events being much larger than estimated, with an event of any type occurring in up to one-third of all hospital admissions (13). An extensive Office of the Inspector General (OIG) report in 2012 also concluded that, as currently used, the hospital incident reporting system was not capturing most adverse events that were occurring. In interviews with 189 hospitals, the OIG found that 86% of adverse events were not being reported. Of those that were reported, from a sample of 40 adverse events, only five resulted in a policy change (14).

The problem of safety was refocused on with a different lens in 2003 when a major study from Rand calculated that, not even considering adverse events, patients were receiving only about 55% of their recommended care. In measuring the quality of care, 30 clinical areas representing the leading causes of death were examined. A staff of medical experts developed quality indicators through a consensus-based process of reviewing the available quality guidelines and the relevant medical literature. A total of 12 metropolitan areas were studied, and the performance was remarkably similar across all geographic areas. Performance ranged from a low of 51% in Little Rock to a high of 59% in Seattle. Quality varied substantially according to the conditions studied, ranging from 11% for alcohol dependence to 65% for hypertension. Impressively, poor compliance with consensus-based, recommended care was unaffected by race, gender, or financial status. Equally interesting was the finding that an individual's insurance status also did not affect quality of care. Fifty-four percent of individuals with no insurance received recommended care, the same as those enrolled in private insurance plans. Only 55% of Medicaid and 57% of Medicare patients received recommended care (15). Such low rates of patients receiving recommended care are also seen in other health care systems, for example, in England (16).

Just as adverse events are associated with poor outcomes, so too is not receiving recommended care. In one study evaluating the quality of care delivered to elderly patients, after 3 years 28% of patients that received 44% of recommended care had died, while only 18% of patients had died if they received 62% of recommended care (17).

If the process of caring for the sick can be regarded as a "system," by most outcomes measures (i.e., adverse events, receiving recommended therapy, etc.) the system is underperforming. It would be expected, then, that lessons learned from making other systems safer could result in improved outcomes. There are numerous industries that have derived benefit from a critical and methodical evaluation of their processes and flow patterns. The nuclear power industry, NASA, car manufacturing, mining operations, and the power grid are all examples of systems that have improved their quality and safety through these programs. The two major quality improvement platforms that are commonly used in industry are Lean and Six Sigma.

Lean is best described as more of a cultural shift than a mathematical analysis of failure patterns. The central theme traces its origins back to W. Edwards Deming, who developed the concept of "Plan–Do–Study–Act" (18). Over its evolution, with respect to health care, Lean has been defined as "an organization's cultural commitment to applying the scientific method to designing, performing, and continuously improving the work delivered by teams of people, leading to better value for patients and other stakeholders" (19). Lean basically creates a "system of principles" that leads to a cultural shift in both people and processes that simultaneously improves both efficiency and outcomes. It is based on the deployment and acceptance of six principles. Principle One creates an atmosphere of continuous improvement. Principle Two instills a culture of value creation by using repeated "Value Stream" maps to identify and correct inefficiency and waste in program processes. The Third Principle creates a "Unity of Purpose" based on input from all stakeholders to develop precisely defined and accountable goals and plans for their establishment. This is commonly described as defining a "True North." Principle Four establishes a management system that values and respects the effort of the employees who do the work of the department. The Fifth Principle describes the process as visual, in the sense that there are easily and readily accessible flow maps and process diagrams to describe the value stream, areas of change, and desired outcomes. Lastly, the Sixth Principle describes the process as "Flexible Regimentation." This has been defined as a system or standard process that includes ongoing efforts to make incremental improvements (20).

The other quality improvement platform in common use is Six Sigma. Contrary to Lean, Six Sigma is a statistical platform based on the manufacturing concept of limiting defects to one in 3.4 million opportunities. It was initially developed at the Motorola Corporation in the 1980s. The Six Sigma process is based on a five-step process of quality improvement: Define, Measure, Analyze, Improve, and Control. The process is highly driven by statistics. Specially trained experts, identified as Black Belts or Green Belts, manage it. They generally serve as advisors to the facility, embedding a flexible and customizable data-driven process into the organization (21).

Both of these quality improvement platforms have been increasingly used over the past 10 to 15 years, and many health care programs have benefited from them.

The concept of safety in health care has been translated in many different ways and with many different methods. It is increasingly used in "product improvement" with Lean and Six Sigma programs, with the definition of the product to be improved left up to the individual program's priorities. Despite all the issues associated with the objectification of concepts as subjective as quality, value, and safety, and the many different manifestations, definitions, and perceptions to which they are subjected, to a radiation oncologist these concepts, ultimately, are best defined as the process that brings about the best possible patient outcome.

REFERENCES

1. Carrigan M. Quality management: an overview. In: Pawlicki T, Dunscombe PB, Mundt AJ, et al, eds. *Quality and Safety in Radiotherapy*. Boca Raton, FL: CRC Press;2012:12.

2. Logan TJ. Error prevention as developed in airlines. *Int J Radiat Oncol Biol Phys*. 2008;71(1):S178–S181.

3. U.S. Food and Drug Administration. How drugs are developed and approved. 2015. www.fda.gov/Drugs/DevelopmentApprovalProcess/HowDrugsareDevelopedandApproved/default.htm.

4. Mendenhall WM, Amdur RJ, Palta JR. Intensity-modulated radiotherapy in the standard management of head and neck cancer: promises and pitfalls. *J Clin Oncol*. 2006;24(17):2618–2623.

5. European Medicines Agency. Mission statement. 2015. www.ema.europa.eu/ema/index.jsp?curl=pages/about_us/general/general_content_000106.jsp&mid=WC0b01ac0580028a44.

6. American Society of Clinical Oncology, The American Board of Internal Medicine. Choosing wisely: five things physicians and patients should question. 2013. www.choosingwisely.org/wp-content/uploads/2015/02/ASCO-Choosing-Wisely-List.pdf.

7. Rosenthal DI, Lewin JS, Eisbruch A. Prevention and treatment of dysphagia and aspiration after chemoradiation for head and neck cancer. *J Clin Oncol*. 2006;24(17):2636–2643.

8. Chen AM, Farwell DG, Luu Q, et al. Intensity-modulated radiotherapy is associated with improved global quality of life among long-term survivors of head-and-neck cancer. *Int J Radiat Oncol Biol Phys*. 2012;84(1):170–175.

9. Ross JS, Madigan D, Hill KP, et al. Pooled analysis of rofecoxib placebo-controlled clinical trial data. *Arch Intern Med*. 2009;169(21):1976–1985.

10. American Society of Clinical Oncology. Reimbursement for cancer treatment: coverage of off-label drug indications. *J Clin Oncol*. 2006;24(19):3206–3208.

11. Weinstein MC, Statson WB. Foundations of cost-effectiveness analysis for health and medical practices. *N Engl J Med*. 1997;296:716–721.

12. Baker GR, Norton PG, Flintoft V, et al. The Canadian Adverse Events Study: the incidence of adverse events among hospital patients in Canada. *CMAJ*. 2004;170(11):1678–1686.

13. Classen DC, Resar R, Griffin F, et al. "Global trigger tool" shows that adverse events in hospitals may be ten times greater than previously measured. *Health Aff*. 2011;30(4):581–589.

14. Office of the Inspector General, Department of Health and Human Services. *Hospital Incident Reporting Systems Do Not Capture Most Patient Harm*. Washington, DC: US Department of Health and Human Services, Office of the Inspector General; 2012 (January). Report no. OEI-06-09-00091.

15. Asch SM, Kerr EA, Keesey J, et al. Who is at greatest risk for receiving poor quality health care. *N Engl J Med*. 2006;354(11):1147–1156.

16. Marshall M, Roland M, Campbell SM, et al. *Measuring General Practice: A Demonstration Project to Develop and Test a Set of Primary Care Clinical Quality Indicators*. Santa Monica, CA: Rand Corporation; 2003.

17. Higashi T, Shekelle PG, Adams JL, et al. Quality of care is associated with survival in vulnerable older patients. *Ann Intern Med*. 2005;143(4):274–281.

18. Moen R, Norman C. Evolution of the PDCS cycle. http://pkpinc.com/files/NA01MoenNorman-Fullpaper.pdf.

19. Womack J, Jones D. *Lean Thinking: Banish Waste and Create Wealth in Your Corporation*. 2nd ed. New York, NY: Free Press; 2003.

20. Toussaint J, Berry L. The promise of Lean in health care. *Mayo Clin Proc*. 2013;88(1):74–82.

21. Bandyopadhyay J, Coppens K. Six Sigma approach to healthcare quality and productivity management. *Int J Qual Prod Manag*. 2005;5(1):V1–V12.

2 Defining Value, American Style

Alex Bastian, Yohan Cho, and Tim R. Williams

The concept of "value-based health care" in the U.S. health care market was, for many years, not considered applicable. Recent initiatives and policy changes, particularly those related to the Affordable Care Act (ACA), have started to shift the U.S. health care market from "volume-based" to "value-based" care. For the U.S. Department of Health and Human Services (HHS), the shift from the quantity of services performed in the fee-for-service (FFS) model to a more patient-centered health outcomes and quality-of-care model aims to lower costs while improving outcomes (1). New incentives and market experiments have taken the form of Accountable Care Organizations (ACOs) and other shared savings programs, taking a significant step in addressing this challenge. As recently as March of 2016, the Centers for Medicare and Medicaid Services (CMS) has proposed new models seeking to bundle care (2) and reform Part B reimbursement of drugs (3) in order to improve quality of care and deliver better value for Medicare beneficiaries. The goal of these experiments is to reduce the number of overall therapies and procedures while encouraging the use of high-value therapies for the right patients. For that reason, the ability to determine the clinical value of health technologies is becoming a higher priority in the United States.

Unlike the European countries outlined in Chapter 3, the United States does not have a single authoritative body that is assigned to assess the value of new health technologies. Further complicating this, the U.S. health care market is a multipayer system with a heterogeneous mix of both private and public payers, who often have differing capabilities in regard to their goals of successfully delivering health care. For example, Kaiser Permanente, a highly integrated payer–provider network organization, may desire to reduce the total cost of care over the patient's entire lifetime, whereas a state Medicaid program may be forced to focus on reducing costs in the short term because annual budget constraints are typically a major consideration depending on the benefits such as drugs, mental health care, or other health services—which may be partially or completely outsourced to another entity. In this way, an organization such as Kaiser Permanente may find more value in a technology that is more expensive up front (e.g., preventative use of cholesterol medications or treatment of low-risk hepatitis C virus (HCV) patients), but that may result in significant cost reductions down the road (e.g., avoidance of a heart attack or need for a liver transplant). In contrast, for a budget-constrained state Medicaid program, long-term cost savings may be of secondary concern to being able to provide health care to all the eligible Medicaid patients on a limited annual budget. While the definition of "value" certainly differs *between* stakeholders such as patients, physicians, and payers, it may also vary considerably *within* each of these stakeholder groups, particularly for payers in the United States. As a result, numerous organizations have established their own approaches to attempt to assess the value of health technologies.

Value in radiation oncology
Dr. Robert Zimmerman, Associate Medical Director, Radiation Oncologist, AIM Specialty Health

In recent years, significant advances in cancer treatment have resulted in longer survival and better quality of life for more than 500,000 Americans diagnosed with the disease annually. Cancer mortality has decreased by 20% from its peak (4). But not all of the cancer news is good. An exponential rise in cancer-related health care expenditures threatens to bankrupt our health care system. The price of drugs and the rapid adoption of costly radiation modalities lacking clinical study both contribute to this problem. Insurance payers play an important role in assuring that high-value radiation treatments remain available for everyone while keeping premiums and out-of-pocket costs affordable.

(Continued)

Payers in the United States face a dual mandate: providing access to the most effective cancer treatments and doing so at a reasonable cost. Cost should only be considered if care is not compromised. When a novel treatment demonstrates a significantly better outcome, payers logically conclude that it is appropriate and medically necessary. *Clinically significant* improvements have to be differentiated from clinically insignificant but *statistically significant* findings. And, even when a specific modality has been shown to improve outcomes for one disease or patient population, its use for other conditions or groups must be considered separately. More commonly, a new treatment either demonstrates parity with or has not been compared with conventional treatment in a scientific fashion, leaving no justification for coverage when the cost is greatly increased.

The use of proton beam therapy (PBT) is illustrative of many of the payer considerations outlined here. PBT is an extremely conformal way to deliver radiation and allowed for high-dose treatment to prostate and brain tumors adjacent to critical normal tissues decades before today's computer technology allowed for similar dose distributions with x-rays. Over time, however, linear accelerators have become more sophisticated and are now able to safely deliver the same doses as protons for these diseases while providing equivalent cure rates and complications. Given that protons are significantly more expensive than x-ray based treatments, payers have begun to reevaluate the value this modality provides. Most payers still consider PBT medically necessary for pediatric patients, in whom even low doses of radiation can affect growth and development, but no longer cover protons for the treatment of prostate cancer. Coverage of PBT for other indications will have to be based on randomized clinical trials or other forms of comparative effectiveness research that clearly demonstrate their superiority. Alternatively, the cost of PBT must decrease to the point where its value is equal to or better than that of other radiation options.

Because the FDA 510(k) approval process for radiation devices requires only demonstration of "substantial equivalence" to an approved device in terms of safety and effectiveness, new radiation technologies are often widely adopted before they have undergone rigorous testing in clinical trials. Relevant examples include the approval of IMRT software based on physics testing and using diagnostic CT scanners as the predicate approved device (5) and the approval of the MammoSite balloon catheter based on nonrandomized feasibility testing of the device in only 43 patients without long-term follow-up (6). In both examples, radiation oncologists were quick to begin treating with the new devices. Emerging technology and Current Procedural Terminology (CPT) codes were soon adopted and assigned lofty reimbursements. This provided significant incentives to use these modalities despite a lack of clinical equivalency, much less superiority, compared with conventional treatments. Once adopted, the treatments are heavily marketed to patients who are then unlikely to participate in the clinical trials needed to justify their higher cost.

Recently, payers are looking beyond radiation modality and beginning to examine the appropriate number of treatments or fractions for a given disease. For both early stage breast cancer and bone metastases, there are multiple randomized, controlled, clinical trials showing the benefit of fewer fractions. In breast cancer, the abbreviated treatment controlled the cancer as well as prolonged therapy, but resulted in fewer acute and late side effects. For bone metastases, a single treatment provides equally effective relief as two weeks or more of treatment. For both, there are fewer trips to the clinic and greatly reduced direct and indirect financial burden. Providers have been slow to adopt these strategies, with a recent study showing that only 34.5% of suitable patients received short-course radiation for early breast cancer (7). The reasons for this slow uptake of the less toxic treatment are not fully understood, but the fact that providers are paid based on the number of fractions surely plays a role.

Cost aside, more is not always better. IMRT delivers low-dose radiation to a much larger volume than conventional treatment, with unknown long-term effects. Seven weeks of breast radiation is no more effective than 3 to 4 weeks and is more toxic. Radiation therapy should be held to the same standard as other medical interventions. All stakeholders benefit from adopting a framework for considering the appropriateness of advanced radiation treatments based on both efficacy and value.

CENTERS FOR MEDICARE AND MEDICAID SERVICES: COVERAGE ADVISORY GROUP

The CMS is the federal agency that administers the social health insurance programs such as Medicare for the elderly. One of CMS's responsibilities includes issuing national coverage determinations (NCDs) for health technologies carried out and issued by a Clinical Advisory Group (CAG). NCDs decisions are binding Medicare coverage decisions. In some cases, CMS may request formal Health Technology Assessment Programs (HTAs) to be conducted by independent agencies and committees such as the Agency for Healthcare Research and Quality (AHRQ) and the Medicare Evidence Development & Coverage Advisory Committee (MEDCAC). Back in 1989, Medicare attempted to formalize the use of cost-effectiveness within its set of evaluation criteria for new medical technologies (8), but the proposal was withdrawn after facing significant controversy. As summarized best by Neumann et al (9), there are a variety of reasons, ranging from cultural to political, behind this:

> The reasons for Medicare's resistance to the use of cost-effectiveness analysis are many and include Americans' affinity for new medical technology, a distaste for explicit limit setting, a sense of entitlement with regard to Medicare funds, the perception that in a vast and wealthy country, health care resources are not really constrained, a political system in which interest groups wield enormous influence, and a splintered and pluralistic health care system in the United States, in which no single payer is responsible for allocating resources for health care. Other reasons include widespread mistrust of the making of medical decisions by organizations, rather than by individual physicians and patients, concern about the transparency of the decision making process, and mistrust of the methods used in cost-effectiveness analysis.

Today, CMS has clearly outlined its role when making coverage decisions and during its review of medical technologies. "When making national coverage decisions, CMS evaluates relevant clinical evidence to determine whether or not the evidence is of sufficient quality to support a finding that an item or service falling within a benefit category is *reasonable* and *necessary* for the diagnosis or treatment of illness or injury or to improve the functioning of a malformed body member. The critical appraisal of evidence enables us to determine to what degree we are confident that: (a) the specific assessment questions can be answered conclusively; and (b) the interventions will improve health outcomes for patients." An improved health outcome is one of several considerations in determining whether an item or service is 'reasonable and necessary'" (10) *regardless of cost*. Although AHRQ and MEDCAC

conduct the HTAs, they only provide an advisory role, with final determinations on NCDs being made by CMS.

Not all technologies are formally assessed by CMS. In fact, CMS will look for advice from AHRQ when there is "conflicting or complex medical and scientific literature available, or when CMS believes an independent analysis of all relevant literature will assist us in determining whether an item of service is reasonable or necessary" (11). CMS may refer a topic to MEDCAC on the basis of a variety of circumstances, including:

- Significant controversy among experts,
- Methodological flaws of studies,
- Lack of research,
- Conflicting results of published studies,
- Request for greater public input,
- Controversial use of technology among the public,
- Dissemination of technology would have a major impact on Medicare program, or
- Decisions informed by broad societal perspective of factors not directly related to scientific review of evidence but nevertheless relevant to the decision.

In 2010 (updated in 2013), AHRQ carried out a technology assessment for CMS regarding "Radiation Therapy for Localized Prostate Cancer." This assessment sought to answer the following key questions:

1. What are the benefits and harms of radiation therapy for clinically localized prostate cancer compared with no treatment or no initial treatment in terms of clinical outcomes?

2. What are the benefits and harms of different forms of radiation therapy for clinically localized prostate cancer in terms of clinical outcomes?

3. How do specific patient characteristics (e.g., age, race/ethnicity, presence or absence of comorbidities, preferences) affect the outcomes of these different forms of radiation therapy?

AHRQ used available literature, including randomized controlled trials and nonrandomized direct comparisons of adult male patients with clinically localized disease, that reported clinical outcomes (12). When looking at the available information to answer the assessment's key questions, the AHRQ qualified the evidence as being "insufficient." As a result, the assessment concluded that the definitive benefits of radiation treatments compared with no treatment or no initial treatment for localized prostate cancer could not be determined because of insufficient data. Comparative effectiveness between different forms of radiation treatments was also deemed to be inconclusive. In regard to radiation therapy for localized prostate cancer, CMS has currently not issued a NCD.

MEDICAID

Medicaid is a joint federal and state program that helps with medical costs for patients with limited income and resources (13). Implementation of Medicaid differs from state to state; however, most states administer Medicaid through their own programs or through MCOs.[1] Much of the funding for Medicaid is the responsibility of each state, creating stress among state legislators on how to adequately and appropriately fund the program. In general, costs in the Medicaid program are controlled by adjusting (downward) payments to providers, or reducing the number of people eligible for benefits. With the recent expansion of eligibility requirements for Medicaid, coupled with the overall increases in health care costs, the majority of states have been experiencing mounting pressure to provide care to more patients with limited resources and federal support. The certainty for future sustainability remains a critical factor for many state Medicaid programs. Faced with these pressures, many states have explored HTA initiatives in an attempt to manage overall health care costs while still providing high-quality care to patients who need it the most. Most states have implemented or encouraged the formation of Pharmacy and Therapeutics (P&T) committees to evaluate the inclusion of technologies for reimbursement. The mix of considerations in each state will vary considerably and is often ratified by the state's department of health.

EARLY HISTORY OF VALUE IN MEDICAID: THE OREGON EXPERIMENT

In the 1980s, the costs of the Oregon Medicaid program were increasing unsustainably year after year. In 1987, as part of an overall strategy to control the growth in spending, the Oregon legislature voted to discontinue funding bone marrow transplants. Previously, starting in 1983, requests for funding were approved on a case-by-case basis. By 1985, changes mandated by the U.S. Congress required the state to fund all requests that fell under the program. Then, in 1987, the cost of covering transplants increased to $2.2 million from $1 million the previous year. It fell to the Human Resources Subcommittee to resolve the shortfall. They opted to move transplant funding from the regular budget to another list, one that included other requests for special social programs, including those for the mentally ill, juvenile delinquents, the elderly, and head trauma victims. The subcommittee had funding requests for $43 million, and only $20 million in available funds.

Ultimately, there was no money for transplants, and they were removed from the list of covered services. The next transplant patient to request coverage was Coby Howard, a 7-year-old boy with leukemia. The mother was unemployed and uninsured. Medicaid officials denied the service. In the local community, an extensive effort was made to complete a private fund-raising campaign. The cost was $100,000. They were $30,000 short when the child died on December 7, 1987. National media attention was drawn to the case.

At the time, there were five other patients who needed transplants. Their applications had also been denied. In January of 1988, Representative Tom Mason introduced a motion in the Legislative Emergency Board to approve $220,000 to fund the transplants. State Senator Kitzhaber opposed the motion. The motion to approve the funding failed on a tie vote (14). As one of the legislators voting against the funding, Senator Kitzhaber was later quoted as saying, "We cannot keep people alive forever. That is part of life . . . . [W]hat we can do with our limited money is to try to reduce the number of deaths . . . to save as many people as we can save" (15). Thus, in Oregon, a great social experiment was performed. The Oregon Basic Health Services Act was designed both to provide universal access and to control costs. To do this, the state government would create a rationing system that would rank medical services from most to least important, determine how much the state could afford each year, and "draw the line" excluding services that fell below the calculated financial threshold. The access and compensation aspects of value would be resolved, and "value" would be determined by a strict rationing plan.

The legislation proposed to carry this reform was S.B. 27, and its central theme was to sacrifice benefits in order to increase the number of covered lives. At the time, there were some 400,000 citizens who were not covered by either the Medicaid program or private insurance. Covering them would cost a considerable sum, and there was no clear picture of what the benefits package would look like. Many stakeholders, including senior citizens, providers, payers, and minority groups, all advocated a defined list of covered services in exchange for support for the reform bill. An 11-member Health Services Commission sponsored public hearings, town meetings, and phone surveys to ensure input from the public. In May 1990, what emerged from the process was a list, ordered by priority, of the quality and value of 1,600 medical procedures. It would define the benefits package, but only in the sense that a line would be drawn each year, and in relation to how much money was available. The program would not cover whatever fell below the line. The list was far from perfect,[2] including a number of

---

[1]More than half of all Medicaid beneficiaries nationally receive most or all of their care from risk-based managed care organizations (MCOs) that contract with state Medicaid programs to deliver comprehensive Medicaid services to enrollees (http://kff.org/data-collection/medicaid-managed-care-market-tracker/)

[2]For example, ranking tooth-capping above surgery for ectopic pregnancy, and temporomandibular joint splints above an appendectomy. Also, crooked teeth were ranked higher than early treatment for Hodgkin's disease, and treatment for thumb-sucking was ranked higher than hospitalization for child starvation.

intuitively wrong rank-order anomalies (16). But, at least in theory, by explicitly rationing services, coverage for Medicaid beneficiaries could be expanded so that more people could be covered.

The initial list had numerous critics. Even Commission Chair Harvey Klevit, himself, was quoted as saying that the first time he saw the list he threw it in the trash can (17). An Alternative Methodology Subcommittee was created to review and rework the original formula, and by February of 1991, they had created a "Prioritized Health Services List." The list had been simplified to only about 800 services. There were 17 major categories, and bone marrow transplants were no longer ranked at the bottom (18).

Ready for deployment, the plan now needed a waiver from the federal government. Initially, it failed. In 1992, the plan was rejected on the grounds that it violated the Americans with Disabilities Act (ADA). The rationale for the rejection was the recognition that the quality-of-life measures were based on the preferences of healthy individuals and did not include those of the disabled. Also, restoring a disabled individual to a "normal" disabled state could be undervalued compared with returning one to a "healthy" state. Ultimately, a third list emerged that, after yet another modification that gave more weight to the judgments of the commissioners, was granted a waiver in 1993. The plan did include all Oregon residents up to 100% of the poverty line (universal coverage) and secured higher reimbursement for managed care plans. It was implemented in 1994.

At least from an enrollment standpoint, the program was an overnight success. Twice as many people enrolled as expected, and the state budget had to be revised. Dr. Kitzhaber, now the state governor, was quoted as saying, "The debate is not over the list anymore. The debate is how we are going to pay for it" (19). Ultimately, as the years passed, the plan developed a fairly generous benefit package, the effort to prioritize services fell victim to benefit expansion, and the threshold line kept getting moved lower and lower. Examples of expansion included coverage for dental care, full drug coverage, mental health and chemical dependency programs, and the integration of the elderly and disabled citizens that were below the poverty line (20). Oregon's expenditures for its rationed services–based Medicaid program increased 39% in the first 3 years. Nationally, the average increase was 30%.

Because of the generosity of the benefits package, few services ended up actually being rationed. Patient satisfaction was generally as good as that reported with other state Medicaid programs, and one study found that only 10% of patients in the plan did not receive care because their treatment was "below the line" (21). The main exclusions were for self-limited conditions or treatments that were regarded as marginal or ineffective (for example, treatment of chronic low back pain).

There was also some evidence that physicians manipulated the system by changing a diagnosis to move a condition to a covered service, provided an uncovered service at the time of a visit covered for another purpose, coded comorbid conditions instead of the noncovered condition, or simply provided the service anyway despite the lack of coverage (22–24).

As the years went by and the experiment in rationing matured, it was emulated by no other state. Despite the efforts of health policy experts and proponents of defining quality as rationing, the overall expenditures, insured lives, covered services, and outcomes appear essentially the same for Oregon compared with the rest of the country. More recently, Oregon embarked on another experiment, this time with Medicaid eligibility. In 2008, the state decided to increase enrollment not by economic or social criteria, as there were already too many potential beneficiaries in all categories and subgroups. Rather, a simple lottery system would be used. This established, for all practical purposes, a randomized trial comparing the health care outcomes of lottery winners and losers. At the time, there were 90,000 people on the waiting list, and 29,835 citizens were invited to apply for the Medicaid program. The 2-year follow-up on a series of 6,387 adults who were in the program was compared with 5,842 who were not selected. The study showed no significant improvements in measured physical outcomes between the two groups over the study period. It did show an increased use of health care services, increased rates of detection of type 2 diabetes, lower reported rates of depression, and decreased financial difficulties (26). Thus, a person's health outcome was essentially the same regardless of whether or not he or she participated in the Medicaid system.

Perhaps the lesson in Oregon's long association with innovative health care reform, at least as it relates to quality and value, is that despite the sweeping nature of the attempts, the overall quality of care seems to remain more or less the same. Defining quality in terms of services offered (or not offered) by rationing care, or allowing citizens access to the insurance system via lottery, seems to have little impact on the overall holistic well-being and general health of the population. Fundamentally, there may well be other social forces at work, subtly guiding and controlling the process of policy deployment, beyond those within the mainstream political and administrative control.

WASHINGTON HEALTH TECHNOLOGY ASSESSMENT PROGRAM

Established by state law in 2006, the Washington Health Technology Assessment Program (WA-HTA) conducts health technology assessments that result in coverage determinations that are binding on three state government agencies purchasing health care, including Medicaid, the Health Care Authority, and the Department of Labor and Industries. The WA-HTA conducts approximately 10 HTAs each year focusing on safety, efficacy, and cost-effectiveness (25). In February 2014, the WA-HTA conducted an HTA for proton beam therapy (PBT) in partnership with the Institute for Clinical and Economic Review (ICER), an independent nonprofit health care research organization. The assessment sought to determine the net health benefit (NHB) of PBT across various cancers and patient types as well as the cost and expected budget impact. The resulting coverage determination was that PBT would be "covered benefit with conditions." PBT is covered only for specific patient types where the NHB was deemed to be "superior" (e.g., ocular cancers, pediatric cancers) and not for all other conditions. In contrast to Medicare's technology assessment of radiation therapy in prostate cancer, WA-HTA resulted in actionable decisions, limiting the coverage of a radiation therapy to patients for whom it was deemed to provide the highest "value."

PATIENT-CENTERED OUTCOMES RESEARCH INSTITUTE

The PCORI is an independent nonprofit, nongovernmental organization authorized by Congress in 2010 as part of the ACA. PCORI's mandate is to improve the quality and relevance of evidence available to help patients, caregivers, clinicians, employers, insurers, and policymakers make informed decisions. Specifically, PCORI funds comparative clinical effectiveness research (CER), as well as supporting work that hopes to improve the methods used to conduct such studies (27). The research funded by PCORI aims to evaluate and compare the health outcomes and clinical effectiveness, risks, and benefits of two or more treatments, services, and other aspects of health and health care (28). Interestingly, the concept of cost has been explicitly forbidden within any of PCORI's activities. The ACA specifically forbids the use of cost per quality-adjusted life-year (QALY) "as a threshold." And while the exact intent and implications of this language are unclear in the long term, it could be interpreted that PCORI, or its contractors or grantees, could still calculate cost-per-QALY ratios as long as they are not compared with a threshold (e.g., $100,000 per QALY) or used to make a recommendation based on such a threshold (29). Comparisons of cost-per-QALY ratios across interventions could still be useful to decision makers even without the invocation of an explicit threshold. As the Executive Director of PCORI, Joe Selby, stated in 2011, "You can take it to the bank that PCORI will never do a cost-effectiveness analysis." While plenty of support and funding has been directed to PCORI, the role and impact of this organization is still being determined. David B. Nash, MD, MBA, editor in chief of four national journals,[3] commented on PCORI (30):

> It's too early to tell the progress of the Patient-Centered Outcomes Research Institute, or PCORI. Certainly, they got a lot of funding support. They've moved into beautiful new offices, they have all full-time staff now. They brought people from all over the country, from Kaiser, from Aetna, and elsewhere. They have a national advisory board. But it will be two to five years before we have any feedback as to the work that was accomplished under the grant award system. . . . NICE is a wonderful British idea for making sure that if we are going to put a drug or device on a national formulary it has good cost-benefit and cost-effectiveness ratios. Nothing like that exists in the United States. The FDA is basically safety and efficacy, and that's where the conversation stops. In the current state of events, no way will PCORI become NICE. It might become NICE-lite, but as we know from the Affordable Care Act passage, the Republican party insisted that PCORI's work not be tied to any aspect of reimbursement. It's a statutory prohibition against linking PCORI to any aspect of payment, most especially for pharmaceuticals.
>
> Here's where we're headed: We will see the FDA asking more questions about whether we really need that 10th beta blocker and that 14th ACE inhibitor—good questions that they ought to ask—but it will be a long time before we are even ready for NICE-lite. If there's going to be a NICE lite, PCORI will probably fill part of that void. (30)

PCORI serves as an example of the push for "value-based" health care existing in the United States; however, the limitations and challenges these newly created bodies face is having actionable impact on the provision of health care.

MANAGED CARE ORGANIZATIONS—BLUE CROSS BLUE SHIELD ASSOCIATION TEC

For most people with health insurance in the United States, health care is financed and delivered through private managed care organizations (MCOs). The Blue Cross Blue Shield Association (BCBSA) is a national federation of

---

[3]*American Journal of Medical Quality*, *Population Health Management*, *American Health and Drug Benefits*, and *P&T* .

36 independent nonprofit insurance companies that provide health care coverage *throughout* the United States (31). Since 1985, BCBSA has assessed technologies through its Technology Evaluation Center (TEC), recently renamed the Center for Clinical Effectiveness (CCE). The CCE produces a number of clinical resources, including the *Medical Policy Reference Manual* and Specialty Pharmacy Reports, as well as individual TEC assessments. Each TEC assessment is a comprehensive evaluation of the clinical effectiveness and appropriateness of a given

---

Value of radiation oncology: the US payer perspective
Ed Pezalla, VP, National Medical Director for Pharmacy Policy and Strategy, Aetna

Across the world, payers, providers, and health policymakers are concerned with the value of health care products and services. This concern with value is manifested in different ways depending on the health system, payment arrangements, and the resources of each country. Value is a function of both the cost and the quality of health care, and in many countries, this function is expressed as the cost of a quality-adjusted life-year (QALY), and thresholds may be applied for the upper limit to be paid for one QALY.

In the United States, private and public payers do not generally use cost per QALY thresholds in determining coverage or payment policies. Instead, value is considered within the broad context of available interventions and desirable patient outcomes. This is not to say that cost is not also important. It is not a good or rational use of resources to pay more for an intervention that does not improve outcomes over the standard of care. Outcomes are defined in both clinical terms (survival, disease progression, safety, and cure) and humanistic terms (symptom alleviation, better quality of life).

Most payers face the question of value when considering a new treatment, or a new application for an existing treatment modality. The decision-making process is not too difficult if the new intervention provides better outcomes for the same price, or the same outcomes for a lower price. Of course, *worse* outcomes are not considered. However, important issues arise when both the price and the outcomes go in the same direction: upwards. Using these quantitative methods, it is difficult to know how much is too much, or too little, to pay for an incremental improvement. Because incremental improvements are often rather small, health plans generally will not tolerate significantly higher costs and will seek to limit the intervention to those with the most need. This would include patients who cannot tolerate the side effects of the standard therapy or who are in a group that will clearly benefit from the new intervention.

Value considerations are important in many aspects of health care, including radiation oncology. Generally, U.S. payers consider value within context, rather than agnostically; oncology care is not compared with that for patients with other conditions and, within oncology, comparisons are not made between different tumor areas. The contextual approach avoids concerns regarding equity in the use of resources between different patient groups and demographics. Resources are allocated according to need and the cost of care within a specific context or setting.

The practical application of this is that radiation oncology is set into the context of oncology care. The first consideration is for appropriate use according to the medical evidence and accepted guidelines. Choosing radiation therapy is generally a matter of following an accepted protocol and must be discussed by the physician and patient as part of the overall care plan. They should take into account the patient's ability to tolerate therapy and the potential results versus other treatment options. Health plans become involved and apply criteria for evidence and value in some cases. That is, plans generally want for the right patient to receive radiation therapy. The choice of provider for the intervention is also important in that there can be marked differences in cost between sites for the same intervention, a clear case where the outcome is the same but for a lower cost. Finally, the type of radiation therapy covered may depend on whether there is a less expensive alternative that will provide the same outcome and level of patient safety.

In summary, radiation oncology is evaluated within the oncology context and is generally covered based on proven clinical efficacy. Cost and value play a role in determining the site of care and the modality of radiation treatment.

medical procedure, device, or drug. The aim of these reports is to provide health care decision makers with timely, rigorous, and credible information on clinical effectiveness. In addition to informing clinical policies set by BCBSA, TEC assessments serve a wide range of customers in both the private and the public sectors, including Kaiser Permanente and the CMS.[4] TEC assessments are scientific opinions, provided solely for informational purposes. BCBSA specifically mentions that TEC assessments are "not meant to advocate, require, encourage, or discourage any particular treatment, procedure, or service; or the payment or nonpayment of the technology or technologies evaluated" (10). The purpose of these assessments is to attempt to define the value of health technologies to understand where and when these therapies will have the highest impact on clinical outcomes.

OTHER INSTITUTIONS

As the idea of defining value of health technologies takes hold in the United States, several nonpayer organizations have begun to roll out their own frameworks for defining value. In June 2015, the American Society of Clinical Oncology (ASCO) introduced its conceptual value framework in the *Journal of Clinical Oncology* (32). The Value in Cancer Care Task Force was charged with developing a framework for comparing the relative clinical benefit, toxicity, and cost of treatment in the medical oncology setting. At the clinical level, the goal of the ASCO framework is to provide a standardized approach to assist physicians and patients in assessing the value of a new drug treatment for cancer as compared with one or several prevailing standards of care. Using this framework, it is possible to provide medical oncologists with the information and physician-guided tools necessary to assess the relative value of cancer therapies as an element of shared decision making with their patients. At the societal level, the assumption underlying this effort is that the cost of a given intervention should bear a relationship to the beneficial impact it has on the patients who receive that treatment. The ASCO framework evaluates drugs by individual trials outputting a value score based on the NHB. This

score represents the total sum of clinical benefit (as expressed by median overall survival, progression-free survival, hazard ratio, response rate, and adverse event rates) and bonus points (e.g., doubling of survival at twice the median survival, palliation of symptoms, etc.). Cost details are also provided separately from the NHB score on a monthly basis (for advanced disease) or total cost per course of therapy basis (for adjuvant disease). How physicians, patients, payers, and other stakeholders will use the ASCO framework in making decisions still remains to be determined.

The American Society for Therapeutic Radiology and Oncology (ASTRO) currently assesses emerging technologies through a task force within its Evaluation Subcommittee to evaluate emerging technologies. The Emerging Technology Committee (ETC) explicitly states that its primary role is to "provide technology assessments regarding emerging technologies to various stakeholders within and outside the society. It is not the role of the committee to develop or defend code definitions, valuation recommendations, or other payment policy development functions." While not binding to any stakeholder groups, this is a systematic, structured analysis of technologies. This process involves a thorough analysis of the technology as well as potential future development that might be anticipated for clinical application or implementation. Factors such as required set-up and delivery time are considered, along with capital expenses and cost per unit, and technical features such as applicators and treatment sites are detailed. The impact of the new technology is also considered, outlined in terms of the product marketing and competitive environment, including similar products and price comparisons (33). While educational in nature, the ultimate impact of these assessments is not well understood.

ICER is a nonprofit organization that evaluates evidence on the value of medical tests, treatments, and delivery system innovations. It develops analyses on effectiveness and costs and prepares reports to attempt to translate clinical evidence into decisions for clinical practice and policymaking (34). Among ICER's initiatives are the New England and Midwest Comparative Effectiveness Public Advisory Councils (CEPAC) and the California Technology Assessment Forum (CTAF). These public deliberative bodies represent a platform from which ICER aims to advance collaborative efforts to analyze scientific evidence on what works best, to foster dialogue about the evidence on effectiveness and value with the public, and to translate this evidence into action. ICER evaluates comparative clinical effectiveness through a rating scale that examines the level of certainty (high to low) and net health benefit (negative to substantial) on a matrix (35):

---

[4]CMS may reference external technology assessments, even if not requested specifically on behalf of the CMS for its activities. This may be included in the evidence reviewed for creation of policy or coverage requirements (e.g., with evidence development). Such was the case of CMS's decision memo to require coverage with evidence development (CED) for Positron Emission Tomography (FDG) for Solid Tumors. In this memo, CMS acknowledges a 2010 Special Report from the Blue Cross Blue Shield Technology Evaluation Center (BCBS/TEC) (www.cms.gov/medicare-coverage-database/details/nca-decision-memo.aspx?NCAId=263).

Comparative clinical effectiveness

Based on the final analysis, scores for any technology could be the following:

I. A = "Superior" —high certainty of a substantial (moderate–large) net health benefit

II. B = "Incremental"—high certainty of a small net health benefit

III. C = "Comparable"—high certainty of a comparable net health benefit

IV. D="Negative"—high certainty of an inferior net health benefit

V. B+ ="Incremental or better"—moderate certainty of a small net health benefit, with high certainty of at least incremental net health benefit

VI. C+ ="Comparable or better"—moderate certainty of a comparable net health benefit, with high certainty of at least comparable net health benefit

VII. P/I = "Promising but inconclusive"—moderate certainty of a small or substantial net health benefit, small (but nonzero) likelihood of a negative net health benefit

VIII. I = "Insufficient"—either moderate certainty that the best point estimate of comparative net health benefit is comparable or inferior, or any situation in which the level of certainty in the evidence is low

Although independent, ICER has a desire to improve the reliability and transparency of value determinations made by insurers in the United States, an outcome that seeks to produce greater consistency across insurers, provide greater certainty for manufacturers, and enhance the legitimacy of medical policy decisions with patients and the public. At least one large managed care organization, Express Scripts, has come out in support of ICER's efforts: "ICER's new program will make a huge difference by providing what is sorely needed: an independent, trusted source of information about new drugs. I believe many payers and policy makers will find this information of critical importance as they evaluate the new drugs, and we look forward to using it to help us improve the ability of patients to get access to new, innovative drugs at a price the system can afford" (36). Under a program announced in 2015, ICER reports will support all health care stakeholders and policymakers in discussions about the value, while also providing a transparent, objective basis for price negotiations and coverage decisions. The first studies for agents in oncology (lung cancer and multiple myeloma) were released in 2016.

Not to be absent from the discussion on value in U.S. cancer care, the National Comprehensive Cancer Network (NCCN) has created its own value framework, the Evidence Blocks. NCCN's goal is to provide this information for the use of health care providers and patients in order to make more informed choices related to treatments, the supporting evidence, and—importantly—cost. The essence of this initiative is to provide a visual means of expressing value within the NCCN Clinical Practice Guidelines. Limiting its utility, this framework is focused on systemic drug therapies and has not yet provided any Evidence Blocks for radiation therapy or surgical treatments (37).

Each therapy is provided with a rating on five distinct elements, based on the sum of evidence and consensus ratings by a panel of NCCN committee members. The five features included in this evaluation are the Efficacy and Safety of regimens, Quality and quantity of evidence, Consistency of evidence, and Affordability.

To develop the NCCN Evidence Blocks, NCCN panel members score each measure using a standardized scale from "1" to "5," with "1" being the least favorable and "5" the most favorable rating. For efficacy and safety, panel members use their knowledge of the published data and their clinical experience with the treatments in the real world. Quality and consistency of the data are rated using the panel members' knowledge of the data supporting the treatment. Finally, affordability is rated using the panel members' knowledge of the overall cost of the regimen. This process is based on perception rather than any structured analysis of the data, and thus is highly variable and imprecise.

Resulting data are analyzed, and final scores are based on an average of ratings from the panel members, rounding to the closest whole number. These scores are then used to populate a matrix that constitutes the "Evidence Block" for the drug in any particular treatment setting. Each column in the Evidence Block corresponds to an outcome characteristic, from left to right including: efficacy (E), safety (S), quality and quantity of evidence (Q), consistency of evidence (C), and affordability (A). The rows of the block are shaded in from bottom to top, representing the corresponding score for each measure.

The efficacy rating is the "extent to which an intervention is helpful in prolonging life, arresting disease progression, or reducing symptoms of a medical condition." The scale used to measure efficacy ranges from 5, "highly effective," to 1, "palliative only." Highly effective scores are given when a long-term survival advantage or potential cure is a likely outcome to be expected. A palliative treatment will largely impact symptomatology only, not survival or disease control.

Safety refers to the assessment of the relative likelihood of side effects from an intervention, with fewer side effects being scored more favorably. The scale used to measure safety also ranges from 5, "atypical occurrence of meaningful toxicity," to 1, "highly toxic." The most advantageous scores are reserved for those drugs that rarely have a negative impact on activities of daily living (ADLs). A toxic therapy is one that is severe or life threatening and may, at times, be fatal. Such a therapy also has a regular, pronounced impact on ADLs. For significant chronic or long-term toxicities, the score may be decreased to reflect the magnitude or persistence of this attribute for a patient.

Two features—the Quality and Consistency of evidence—were traditionally categorized by NCCN in guidelines on a single, blended scale prior to the introduction of the Evidence Blocks:

I. Category 1: Based on high-level evidence, there is uniform NCCN consensus that the intervention is appropriate

II. Category 2A: Based on lower-level evidence, there is uniform NCCN consensus that the intervention is appropriate

III. Category 2B: Based on lower-level evidence, there is NCCN consensus that the intervention is appropriate

IV. Category 3: Based upon any level of evidence, there is major NCCN disagreement that the intervention is appropriate

While the category levels still exist in the updated guidelines, the new Evidence Block framework provides a more nuanced view by splitting these categories into two separate features: Quality and Consistency. For both of these factors, five levels are further broken out in detail. To determine a score, panel members may weigh the depth of the evidence, such as the numbers of trials that address this issue and their design. The scale used to measure quality of evidence ranges from "little or no evidence" (score = 1) to a setting with "multiple well-designed randomized trials and/or meta-analyses" (score = 5). *Consistency of evidence* refers to the degree to which the clinical trials addressing an intervention have consistent results. The scale used to measure *consistency of evidence* ranges from "anecdotal experience" (score = 1) to a trial-set containing "multiple trials, all with similar outcomes" (score = 5).

The affordability measurement is intended to represent "an estimate of overall total cost of a therapy, including but not limited to acquisition, administration, in-patient versus out-patient care, supportive care, infusions, toxicity monitoring, antiemetics and growth factors, and hospitalization" (38). The span of ratings represents different levels of affordability of the regimen or single agent. A less expensive intervention is rated more highly than more expensive ones. This attribute, even more than the other elements, is debased from any underlying data to substantiate or quantify actual cost or "affordability." With the stated goal of utility to the patient, the affordability will also likely be something much more personal for patients, considering factors other than ratings of panelist perceptions of total costs, but instead the copay or cost sharing of any regimen—including medical costs for care—will be associated with their treatment. In this sense, the NCCN framework mixes user perspectives, and only time will tell the utility of this value experiment.

UNITED STATES QUALITY-ADJUSTED LIFE-YEAR THRESHOLD ESTIMATES

Despite the number of initiatives being undertaken by a variety of U.S. stakeholders to define *value*, no consensus has been achieved on a single metric toward measuring value. Considering interventions as diverse as medical procedures, regulations from the Consumer Product Safety Commission, the Occupational Safety and Health Administration, the Environmental Protection Agency (EPA), and others, it has been reported that the value of a life-year saved, depending on the action taken, can vary from $0 (NHTSA, install windshields with adhesive bonding) to $99,000,000,000 (establish EPA chloroform emission standards at 48 private pulp mills) (39). QALY is a metric used by a number of cost-effectiveness institutions, including NICE in the UK, for measuring and comparing the health effects of various interventions. In the United States, the use of QALY and estimated thresholds that represent a meaningful clinical benefit has been contentious and not without debate. The ACA, for example, specifically forbids the use of cost per QALY "as a threshold" by PCORI in its assessments (30). The ASCO framework explicitly does not use QALY because of "limitations associated with the approach," such as individuals having different preferences for a health state within cancer care (32).

However, several attempts have been made to quantify an acceptable incremental cost-effectiveness ratio (ICER) threshold in the U.S. context. The World Health Organization (WHO) estimated the appropriate boundary for any nation to be approximately three times (40) the gross domestic product (GDP) per capita. Based on 2014 estimates of GDP (US$54,630) (41), the estimated ICER would be $163,890 in the United States, a far cry from the acceptable threshold in the UK (£20,000–£30,000) and other markets. An international study of willingness-to-pay (WTP) for one additional QALY gained, by Shiroiwa et al (42), estimated a value of approximately $62,000 per QALY in the United States. These studies relied upon societal or health economist views of acceptable thresholds, but other methods of estimation have also been conducted.

As early as 1982, authors relied upon what was called the "dialysis standard," which equated to the approximate cost of expenditures related to tertiary medical care (43). Adjusted to the year 2007, this was approximately $197,000 per QALY. Braithwaite et al (44) analyzed two different approaches and determined that "[b]ecause the gains in life expectancy since 1950 have been bought at an estimated average cost of $183,000 per year of life expectancy gained, on average Americans must be willing to pay at least that much for a year of life." Upon sensitivity analysis, this estimate ranged from less than $100,000 up to $264,000 based on various characteristics. More recently, similar estimates were discussed by Ramers-Verhoeven et al (45), although they acknowledged the importance of perspective in determining this threshold. Further commentary by Neumann et al (46) reflected this sentiment perfectly:

Whose preferences should be used? Leaders in the field have often argued that preferences for QALY estimates should be based on members of the general public, reasoning that societal resource allocation decisions should reflect "community" values. Others have argued for using patients' preferences on the grounds that the values of people who have experienced the condition under investigation are most relevant. People with an illness tend to value their health state, even if diminished, more favorably than those who have not experienced the illness. The general explanation for the discrepancy is that patients adapt to their condition. The source of preference weights remains a contentious issue.

Several authors have taken a slightly different approach to estimating this threshold, instead asking various stakeholders to define thresholds. Ubel et al (47) asked oncologists in the United States and Canada how much benefit, in additional months of life expectancy, a new technology would need to provide to justify its cost and warrant its use. When asked what treatment cost per life-year gained represented "good value for money," approximately 70% selected an ICER of $100,000 or less. But when oncologists were randomly presented with hypothetical new drugs for metastatic cancer that cost either $50,000 or $125,000 *more* than standard chemotherapy costing $25,000, the median increase in life expectancy stipulated by oncologists to justify using the $75,000 drug was 6 months, translating into approximately $100,000 per life-year gained. The median survival benefit oncologists selected to support use of the more expensive drug also was 6 months, but in this case the calculated cost per life-year gained was almost $250,000. Similarly, Nadler et al (48) asked a small sample of academic medical oncologists to estimate the cost and effectiveness of a hypothetical new technology to justify a price. The implied cost-effectiveness thresholds, derived from the scenarios, averaged roughly $300,000 per QALY. One final analysis took an interesting view: that of the patient. In their study of how cancer patients valued "hope," Lakdawalla et al (49) found that almost three-quarters (77%) of patients with melanoma, breast cancer, or other solid tumors preferred hopeful gambles to safe bets. Their conclusion was that technology assessments, which could determine access to cancer therapies, "may be missing an important source of value to patients and should either incorporate hope into the value of therapies or set a higher threshold for an acceptable cost-effectiveness ratio in the end-of-life context" (49). Indeed, some patients were willing to pay up to $500,000 for a hopeful therapy. While none of these offers a perfect estimate of what a threshold might look like in the United States, they offer a glimpse of the range and varying perspectives across stakeholders.

One study used QALY to assess the value of radiation oncology treatments. Kohler et al (50) looked at the value of IMRT from the Medicare perspective, with health states divided into two levels of xerostomia and dysphagia (e.g., high dysphagia/high xerostomia, and thus four total levels) and transition probabilities informed by patient-level data from PARSPORT. The authors found that IMRT was less cost effective in the first 2 years of treatment (ICER $101,100 (USD)/QALY), but was clearly the higher-value treatment in the long term (ICER $34,523 (USD)/QALY). Since the standard time horizon for these cost-effectiveness studies is the entire lifetime, this study does ultimately parallel the results of an analysis in Canada, albeit with a less impressive ICER. Interestingly, although the absolute difference in treatment costs was greater in the U.S. data (approximately $9,000 USD vs. approximately $2,500 CAD), the Canadian study assumed significantly higher utility improvement from intensity-modulated radiation therapy (IMRT), which largely accounted for the more robust ICER (50, 51). In any case, although different health care systems may have different payment thresholds for a given technology, both studies—one from a nationalized health care system and the other from the United States—support head and neck IMRT as the cost-effective treatment option for head and neck cancer.

As far back as 1996, the U.S. Public Health Service (PHS) convened a panel of experts to examine the use of cost effectiveness in health and medicine. This panel was comprised of nonfederal experts in cost effectiveness, clinical medicine, ethics, and health outcomes measurement. The conclusions of this process, after 2.5 years of discussion, related to the very same considerations still being debated in the United States: (a) components belonging in the numerator and denominator of a cost-effectiveness (C/E) ratio; (b) measuring resource use in the numerator of a C/E ratio; (c) valuing health consequences in the denominator of a C/E ratio; (d) estimating effectiveness of interventions; (e) incorporating time preference and discounting; and (f) handling uncertainty. They also stated that recommendations are subject to the "rule of reason," balancing the burden engendered by a practice with its importance in the larger context (52). Today, decades later, we are no closer to answering these questions in the U.S. context than we were decades ago.

SUMMARY

Without a single authoritative body to assess the value of health technologies, much ambiguity still exists in what is considered valuable and what is not in the United States.

A standardized approach to assessing value as well as a metric and threshold for measuring it are still lacking in the United States, leaving questions as to how best to utilize health technologies. Yet this set of challenges, in some way, also reflects the varying considerations that should be made in any effort to assess value in health care. Although there has been a shift to value-based models, questions remain on how to define value and the utility it holds to the variety of stakeholders whose lives are touched by decisions in the delivery of care and the use of new technologies.

These considerations include the span of benefits and costs that any stakeholder might evaluate, as well as the time horizon for capturing these attributes. Fragmentation in the U.S. health system means that different viewpoints will likely provide conflicting assessments of value based on their preferences, vested interests, and role within the health care delivery system. The certainty and transparency of information is also a vexing problem, as the clinical trial and regulatory approval systems are inadequate to answer some of the most difficult questions related to the establishment of value. The opacity pervades our system, particularly related to costs, preventing a more holistic view from arising that could align stakeholders on cost or benefit claims. As we enter a new age in medical technology, the way in which stakeholders evolve to capture real-world outcomes, costs of care, and predictability in response will have tremendous utility for those that desire to evaluate the quality and value of any health technology.

Single-payer systems do not solve the problem of value assessment in health care; they only reduce the complexity and diverse tapestry of individual actors, or stakeholders, with interest in having their views, preferences, and desires reflected in the evaluation of benefits and costs. As shown by the varied and complex manners in which value is defined today across the world, the process of defining the concept is often not a difficult challenge for stakeholders. Translating that perception into a price that one must pay in the health care marketplace in most markets is a challenge. This is only made more difficult by the variety of influences discussed in this chapter, which all stakeholders work to navigate on a daily basis.

REFERENCES

1. Leonard D. The health care paradigm shift: moving from volume to value. 2015. http://morningconsult.com/opinions/the-health-care-paradigm-shift-moving-from-volume-to-value.

2. Centers for Medicare & Medicaid Services. Oncology care model. 2015. https://innovation.cms.gov/initiatives/oncology-care.

3. Centers for Medicare & Medicaid Services. CMS proposes to test new Medicare Part B prescription drug models to improve quality of care and deliver better value for Medicare beneficiaries. 2016. www.cms.gov/Newsroom/MediaReleaseDatabase/Fact-sheets/2016-Fact-sheets-items/2016-03-08.html.

4. Masters GA, Krilov L, Bailey HH, et al. Clinical cancer advances 2015: annual report on progress against cancer from the American Society of Clinical Oncology [published online ahead of print January 20, 2015]. *J Clin Oncol.* doi:10.1200/JCO.2014.59.9746.

5. Summary of safety and effectiveness. (1996, April 9). www.accessdata.fda.gov/cdrh_docs/pdf/K940663.pdf.

6. Kuerer HM, Pawlik TM, Strom EA. Intracavitary balloon brachytherapy for breast cancer: surgical considerations. in regard to Keisch M, Vicini F, Kuske RR, et al., IJROBP 2003;55:289–293. *Int J Radiat Oncol Biol Phys.* 2003;57(3):900–902.

7. Bekelman JE, Sylwestrzak G, Barron J, et al. Uptake and costs of hypofractionated vs conventional whole breast radiation after breast conserving surgery in the United States, 2008–2013. *JAMA.* 2014;312(23):2542–2550. doi:10.1001/jama.2014.16616.

8. U.S. Department of Health and Human Services, Centers for Medicare & Medicaid Services. Medicare program: criteria and procedures for making medical services coverage decisions that relate to health care technology. *Fed Regist.* 1989;54(30):4302–4318.

9. Neumann PJ, Rosen AB, Weinstein MC. Medicare and cost-effectiveness analysis. *N Engl J Med.* 2005;353(14):1516–1522.

10. Blue Cross Blue Shield Association. Technology evaluation center (TEC). 2015. http://web.southcarolinablues.com/employers/understandingyourcoverage/resources/technologyevaluationcenter.aspx.

11. U.S. Department of Health and Human Services, Centers for Medicare & Medicaid Services. Medicare program: revised process for making Medicare national coverage determinations. *Fed Regist.* 2003;68(187):55634–55641. www.gpo.gov/fdsys/pkg/FR-2003-09-26/pdf/03-24361.pdf.

12. Agency for Healthcare Research and Quality. Comparative evaluation of radiation treatments for clinically localized prostate cancer: an update. 2010 (August 13). www.cms.gov/Medicare/Coverage/CoverageGenInfo/downloads/id69ta.pdf.

13. U.S. Department of Health and Human Services, Centers for Medicare & Medicaid Services. Medicaid. www.medicare.gov/your-medicare-costs/help-paying-costs/medicaid/medicaid.html.

14. Fox DM, Leicher HM. Rationing care in Oregon: the new accountability. *Health Aff.* 1991;10(2):7–27.

15. Beggs CE. Oregon cuts off funds for transplants. *Associated Press.* May 23, 1988.

16. Tengs TO, Meyer G, Siegel JE, et al. Oregon's Medicaid rankings and cost effectiveness: is there a relationship? *Med Decis Making.* 1996;16:99–107.

17. Morell V. Oregon puts bold health plan on ice. *Science.* 1990;3:468.

18. Brown LD. The national politics of Oregon's rationing plan. *Health Aff.* 1991;10(2):28–51.

19. Woodward S. Philosophy collides with finance. *Bus Health.* 1995;13(5):5156.

20. Leichter HM. Oregon's bold experiment: what ever happened to rationing? *J Health Polit Policy Law.* 1999;24(1):147–160.

21. Mitchell JB, Haber SG, Khatutsky G, et al. Impact of Oregon's health plan on access and satisfaction of adults with low income. *Health Serv Res.* 2002;37(1):11–32.

22. Kilborn PT. Oregon falters on a new path to healthcare. *New York Times.* January 3, 1999:A1.

23. Bodenheimer T. The Oregon health plan: lessons for a nation. *N Engl J Med.* 1997;337(9):651–655.

24. Mitchell JB, Bentley F. Impact of Oregon's priority list on Medicaid beneficiaries. *Med Care Res Rev.* 2000;57(2):216–234.

25. Oregon Health & Science University, Center for Evidence-based Policy Medicaid Evidence-based Decisions Project. Health technology assessment: rapid review. 2011. www.ohsu.edu/xd/research/centers-institutes/evidence-based-policy-center/evidence/med/upload/Health-Technology-Assessment_Public_RR_Final_08_18_2011-2.pdf.

26. Baicker K, Taubman SL, Allen HL, et al. The Oregon experiment—effects of Medicaid on clinical outcomes. *N Engl J Med.* 2013;368:1713–1722.

27. Patient-Centered Outcomes Research Institute. About us. 2014 (October 6). www.pcori.org/about-us.

28. Barksdale DJ, Newhouse R, Miller JA. The Patient-Centered Outcomes Research Institute (PCORI): information for academic nursing. *Nurs Outlook.* 2014;62(3):192–200.

29. Neumann PJ, Weinstein MC. Legislating against use of cost-effectiveness information. *N Engl J Med.* 2010;363(16):1495–1497.

30. Nash DB, Marcille J, Sherritze S. A conversation with David B. Nash, MD, MBA: game changers for population health. *Manag Care.* 2014;23(1):19–23.

31. Blue Cross Blue Shield Association. About Blue Cross Blue Shield Association. 2015. www.bcbs.com/about-the-association.

32. Schnipper LE, Davidson NE, Wollins DS. American Society of Clinical Oncology statement: a

conceptual framework to assess the value of cancer treatment options. *J Clin Oncol.* 2015;33(26).

33. Park CC, Bevan A, Podgorsak MB, et al. Emerging technology committee: report on electronic brachytherapy. 2008 (May 23). www.astro.org/uploadedfiles/main_site/clinical_practice/best_practices/etcebt.pdf.

34. Institute for Clinical and Economic Review. About ICER. (n.d.). www.icer-review.org/about.

35. Institute for Clinical and Economic Review. Methodology: ICER integrated evidence rating. 2013. www.icer-review.org/wp-content/uploads/2013/04/ICER-Rating-System-Apr-2013-Update-FINAL.pdf.

36. Institute for Clinical and Economic Review. ICER launches new drug assessment program with $5.2 million award from the Laura and John Arnold foundation. 2015 (July 21). www.icer-review.org/icer-ljaf-drug-assessment-announcement.

37. The National Comprehensive Cancer Network (NCCN) Organization. NCCN Clinical Practice Guidelines in Oncology (NCCN Guidelines®) with NCCN Evidence Blocks™. www.nccn.org/evidenceblocks/default.aspx.

38. The National Comprehensive Cancer Network (NCCN) Organization Website. NCCN Clinical Practice Guidelines in Oncology (NCCN Guidelines®) with NCCN Evidence Blocks™ frequently asked questions. www.nccn.org/evidenceblocks/pdf/EvidenceBlocksFAQ.pdf.

39. Tengs TO, Adams ME, Pliskin JS, et al. Five-hundred life-saving interventions and their cost-effectiveness. *Risk Anal.* 1995;15(3):369–390.

40. World Health Organization. *The World Health Report 2002: Reducing Risks, Promoting Healthy Life.* Geneva, Switzerland: World Health Organization; 2002.

41. The World Bank Group. Data catalog: GDP per capita (current US$). 2015. http://data.worldbank.org/indicator/NY.GDP.PCAP.CD.

42. Shiroiwa T, Sung YK, Fukuda T, et al. International survey on willingness-to-pay (WTP) for one additional QALY gained: what is the threshold of cost effectiveness? *Health Econ.* 2010;19(4):422–437.

43. Kaplan R, Bush J. Health-related quality of life measurement for evaluation research and policy analysis. *Health Psychol.* 1982;1(1):61–80.

44. Braithwaite RS, Meltzer DO, King JT, et al. What does the value of modern medicine say about the $50,000 per quality-adjusted life-year decision rule? *Med Care.* 2008;46(4):349–356.

45. Ramers-Verhoeven CW, Geipel GL, Howie M. New insights into public perceptions of cancer. *ecancermedicalscience.* 2013;7:349. doi:10.3332/ecancer.2013.349. http://www.ncbi.nlm.nih.gov/pmc/articles/PMC3766630.

46. Neumann PJ, Greenberg D. Is the United States ready for QALYs? *Health Aff.* 2009;28(5):1366–1371.

47. Ubel PA, Berry SR, Nadler E. In a survey, marked inconsistency in how oncologists judged value of high-cost cancer drugs in relation to gains in survival. *Health Aff.* 2012;31(4):709–717.

48. Nadler E, Eckert B, Neumann PJ. Do oncologists believe new cancer drugs offer good value? *Oncologist.* 2006;11(2):90–95.

49. Lakdawalla DN, Romley JA, Sanchez Y. How cancer patients value hope and the implications for cost-effectiveness assessments of high-cost cancer therapies. *Health Aff.* 2012;31(4):676–682.

50. Kohler RE, Sheets NC, Wheeler SB, et al. Two-year and lifetime cost-effectiveness of intensity modulated radiation therapy versus 3-dimensional conformal radiation therapy for head-and-neck cancer. *Int J Radiat Oncol Biol Phys.* 2013;87(4):683–689.

51. Yong JH, Beca J, O'Sullivan B, et al. Cost-effectiveness of intensity-modulated radiotherapy in oropharyngeal cancer. *Clin Oncol (R Coll Radiol).* 2012;24(7):532–538.

52. Weinstein MC, Siegel JE, Gold MR, et al. Recommendations of the panel on cost-effectiveness in health and medicine. *JAMA.* 1996;276(15):1253–1258.

3 Defining Value in European Health Care Systems

Alex Bastian, Yohan Cho, and Tim R. Williams

In the United Kingdom, three assessment bodies exist for new technologies. The UK is made up of England, Scotland, Wales, and Northern Ireland, and each of these territories has its own approach to health technology assessment (HTA). The most prominent of the HTA bodies is the National Institute for Health and Care Excellence, or NICE, in England. Positive recommendations by NICE following a technology appraisal are legally binding, and health authorities in England and Wales are obliged to provide funding and resources for their implementation. NICE and the National Coordinating Centre for Health Technology Assessment (NCCHTA) are the key national HTA organizations for England, Wales, and Northern Ireland. NICE, originally established in 1999, is a special health authority legislated in 2013 as a nondepartmental public body that acts independently of the government to reduce variation in the availability and quality of National Health Service (NHS) treatments and care (1). As defined in its charter, NICE's focus is on improving the quality of care while ensuring careful and targeted use of finite resources. NICE guidance and advice set out an evidence-based case for investment and disinvestment, intended to guide commissioners and providers of health and social care in making the best use of their money while delivering high-quality care for patients and service users (2). NICE guidance has many forms, each of which has a different status within the NHS, public health, and social care settings.

In contrast to the methods of health care evaluation in other countries, NICE does not evaluate all interventions as they reach the market. NICE has published guidelines on how interventions for review are selected, such as whether the technology is likely to (a) result in a significant health benefit, (b) result in a significant impact on other health-related government policies (e.g., reduction in health inequalities), (c) have a significant impact on NHS resources (financial or other), or (d) enable the

Institute to add value by issuing national guidance[1] (3). Using a horizon scanning approach and applying these criteria, NICE proposes its future work program, but the final decision on which technologies will be referred for assessment is made by health ministers. The health technology assessment from NICE considers evidence on the health effects, costs, and cost-effectiveness of a health technology. The principal source of evidence for the assessment of a single technology is the content in the manufacturer's submission, which is primarily dictated by a prescriptive template supplied by NICE. Cost-effectiveness analysis used by NICE is an assessment of whether the expected health gain from the use of a new technology exceeds the health likely to be forgone as other NHS activities are displaced to accommodate the additional costs of the new technology.

When NICE was chartered in 1999, it was the result of the convergence of political, economic, and social forces. The Labor Party had come to power at the same time that increases in health care costs and issues with access were emerging, and the new science of evidence-based medicine was growing (4). In health care, one of the issues with quality has always been regional variation in services for the same condition, and the inability to track positive outcomes with intensity of services. There are simply physicians who use more resources than others to achieve the same results, and an increasingly limited health care budget and a tradition of centralized control of the health care economy. In effect, in England, quality becomes what NICE says it is. This makes NICE very powerful.

One result of NICE's activities has been the emergence of a rough "standard" for acceptance of a new technology,

---

[1] For example, whether the absence of guidance is likely to arouse significant controversy, mixed interpretation, or significance judgments of the available evidence on clinical and cost-effectiveness for the technology.

based on a metric called the QALY, or "Quality Adjusted Life-Year." While no explicit threshold has been established, in general, £30,000/QALY appears to be something of a soft ceiling (5). NICE regularly uses QALYs as a basis for its decisions (6), as do other European nations, Canada, and Australia (7).

The QALY is a common unit of measurement of quality, at least in the context of equilibrating the relationship between quality and value. In the most general terms, the QALY is a calculation used to relate health, or the improvement of health, across a population. There is a fundamental assumption that such a quantity is accurately (or actually) measurable, a point of considerable interest to those associated with its calculation and use. It is important to note that, at least initially, the QALY was not intended to be used in individual patient decision making. Rather, the QALY is a considered a valuation of health benefit (8).

In its pure mathematical form, a QALY can be represented as:

$$\text{QALY}_{conv} = \sum_{t=1\ldots T} \sum_{s=1\ldots S} p_{st}\, V(H_{st})\, (1+r)^{t-1}$$

where p_{st} is the probability that an individual will occupy a particular health state at time t, $V(H_{st})$ is the "value" measure assigned to the individual being in a particular health state at time t, $(1 + r)^{t-1}$ is a "discount factor" designed to bring $V(H_{st})$ into present value terms (with r being a selected discount rate reflecting time preference for health outcomes), s is the number of discrete health states that may be occupied, and T is the time horizon for relevant decision making (9).

The QALY has assumed a stature, acceptance, and utility among health care economists that belie its underlying controversy. The QALY calculation is filled with assumptions, conceptual issues, and methodological concerns. Fundamentally, the assessment assumes that people enjoy (or endure) different health states at different times, and each individual health state has a quantifiable value. Thus, "health" can become an objective, measurable quantity rather than a holistic, subjective attribute. By simple assumption, death has a value of 0 and perfect health a value of 1. Significantly, the value scale must be calibrated so that a change from 0.2 to 0.4 is a gain equally valuable as a change from 0.6 to 0.8.

Of all of the ambiguity surrounding the calculation of a QALY, none is more controversial than the calculation of the $V(H_{st})$ or the value of a particular health state. Good health is, to say the least, a multidimensional notion, and depends on more than physiological or functional capacity. All physicians have seen this personally in their clinics. There are as many different valuations of overall health as there are patients, none being measured by the same personal yardstick. It falls to psychometrics, selection of the survey parameters, and statistics to refine these variables. This value/health parameter is generally called the Health-Related Quality of Life (HRQoL). There are

six generally accepted survey instruments to calculate this important parameter.

One of the most commonly used traces its origin to Europe, and is called the EuroQol EQ-5D, for convenience shortened to the EQ-5D. It measures five basic dimensions of health: mobility, self-care, usual activities, pain/discomfort, and anxiety/depression. Each of these dimensions is subdivided into "no difficulty," "moderate difficulty," and "extreme difficulty," numbered from 1 to 3 respectively. Thus, scoring each state individually between 1 and 3 yields 203 possible combinations, ranging from a person who had no health problems for any of the five states, a score of 11111, to the worst possible state, 33333 (10). One advantage of the instrument is that it is easy to administer. By phone survey, it can easily be completed in less than 15 minutes. In exchange for simplicity, it assumes that each surveyed individual has the same, or at least similar, comprehension of the nature and relative severity of the variable aspects of each parameter. For example, the entire subjective universe of pain and discomfort is distilled into only three states. There is also some uncertainty over the use of the instrument across different countries and cultures (11).

Another instrument that can be used to measure quality of life is the Health Utilities Index Mark 2 (HUI2) and Mark 3 (HUI3). The two HUI systems are technically independent of each other, although they are complementary. Taken together, they can describe almost 1 million unique health states. Obviously more complex than the EQ-5D instrument, the HUI Mark 2 classification scheme has seven attributes, including sensation, mobility, emotion, cognition, self-care, pain, and fertility. Fertility was initially included because the HUI was developed to assess infancy and childhood issues. It has been dropped in more recent versions. Each of the HUI2 parameters has three to five levels, and ultimately can describe some 24,000 separately identifiable health states. The HUI3 system has eight attributes. They include vision, hearing, speech, ambulation, dexterity, emotion, cognition, and pain. Each of these has five or six levels, and therefore yields 972,000 possible health states (12). Most versions of the survey include 31 questions, but the actual number can vary depending on the overall scope and goals of the interviewer.

The Quality of Well Being Index (QWBI) is another assessment tool designed to comprehensively measure health-related quality of life. A paper questionnaire, it was developed in the 1970s. It was difficult to administer and required a trained interviewer because of the branching and probing nature of the questions. Later versions have been modified to a self-administered instrument, which can now be completed in about 15 minutes. It does have some advantages, including an assessment of symptoms in addition to generic areas of functioning. Also, when scored, it uses an accepted correction factor, population-derived preference weights.

The assessment consists of the measurement of overall well-being over the past 3 days with respect to physical activity, social activities, mobility, and symptom/problem complexes. Each dimension has up to five function levels, and each function level has a weight ranging from 0 to −0.1. Each of these dimensions is then given an additional weighting from a table of symptom and problem complexes scale. These weights are also all negative, ranging from 0 to −0.727. The overall final QWBI ranges from 1 to 0. Thus, it is possible to have a value below 0, or a state "worse than death" (for example, a persistent vegetative state). The scaling weights have been extensively evaluated and validated and are considered generally reliable. The accuracy of the QWBI assessment is dependent on this scaling validity, which still remains somewhat controversial, and the skill level of the interviewer, who must have considerable training (13).

The SF-6D HRQoL tool is a simplified, modified version of the larger, well-known SF-36. The SF-36 consists of 36 questions, reduced to 6 in the SF-6D. They include physical functioning (one to six levels), role limitations (four levels), social functioning (five levels), pain (six levels), mental health (five levels), and vitality (five levels). A relatively simple survey, it can be completed in 10 to 15 minutes. On the basis of the number of possible combinations, some 18,000 different health care states can be independently identified (14).

A final measurement system commonly used in QALY calculations is the Health and Activities Limitations Index (HALex). This survey is derived from the National Health Interview Survey, and is a generic measure of health, incorporating information about the individual's perception of health and activity. It is a simple self-administered survey that yields a single, composite score. It can be used to assess QALYs when adjusted for life expectancy (15).

Any of these assessment tools can be used to calculate QALYs, and in different contexts all of them are. Unfortunately, they do not yield the same values. Each instrument has its own limitations and assumptions. As Fryback (16) has reported, from a survey of 3,844 respondents, the six HRQoL indexes showed "similar but not identical trends in population norms." As a result, depending on which assessment tool was used to measure "Health" and "Value," different results for quality can be obtained. This ambiguity could possibly produce a different conclusion regarding the use of the QALY when applied to social or economic policy, or, more significantly, if used for medical decision making for an individual patient.

The QALY also has limitations based on subjective concepts of fairness and equanimity. Because, at least in the mathematical sense, one QALY is as good as another, they convey no sense of distributional utility. For example, it has been pointed out that the QALY gained by a healthy individual from the relief of erectile dysfunction would likely not be considered equal to a QALY gained by a person who received life-extending dialysis for end-stage renal disease. As noted in Chapter 2, Oregon's Medicaid program decision in the 1980s to deny coverage for childhood bone marrow transplants and divert these resources to increase the number of covered lives was estimated to increase basic benefits for 1,500 citizens at the expense of 34 transplant candidates. At the QALYs mathematical and statistical end game, it has been suggested that there is no number of cured sore throats that could equal the value of saving a life (17).

The QALY also fails to measure, if it can be measured at all, differences in subgroup preference for specific health care outcomes. Using QALYs as a surrogate for sound medical judgment in decision making can actually undermine the quality of a good doctor–patient relationship. Physicians have the ethical responsibility to provide the most appropriate care to obtain the best possible outcome. Defining quality in terms of QALYs may compromise decision making, rather than informing and aiding it (18).

There exists no specific standardization in the economic, social, medical, or political literature of the value of a specific intervention or the benefits derived from an improvement in quality.

The cost-effectiveness threshold represents an estimate of the health forgone as services are displaced, and is largely a value judgment for what represents the most effective use of NHS resources. It can be defined as an economic study design in which consequences of different interventions are measured using a single outcome, usually in "natural" units (for example, life-years gained, deaths avoided, heart attacks avoided, or cases detected) (19). Currently, the threshold used by NICE has little empirical basis (20), but is in the range of £20,000 to £30,000[2] (21) per QALY. This range is followed by appraisal committees, and NICE has stated that "[this range] represents a reasonable compromise between ensuring everyone has fair and equitable access to the NHS and enabling access to new and innovative treatments" (21,22). NICE is not without its critics. Its very first recommendation, not to cover the antiviral zanamivir in the face of the 1999 to 2000 flu season, was based on a population-based analysis which concluded that the overall costs were not justified after considering the anticipated benefits. This decision was heavily criticized and was ultimately reversed (24). The three treatments that were not approved were prophylactic removal of wisdom teeth, laparoscopic surgery for colorectal cancer, and autologous cartilage transplantation for knee

---

[2] The major step was the 2004 *Guide to the Methods of Technological Appraisal* that provided these details, although the definition of the £20,000 to £30,000 threshold range may be considered loose and open to interpretation. Although the 2004 guide was one of the first official references to the threshold, Sir Michael Rawlins did state at the 2001 NICE Annual General Meeting that the Institute would "need to be very clear in its reasons for supporting technologies with cost-effectiveness ratios higher than £30,000 per QALY."

joints (4). In oncology, NICE was heavily criticized for its reluctance to endorse trastuzumab for the treatment of breast cancer, another decision that was later reversed (24). Additionally, NICE was compelled to revisit a decision on the use of imatinib for the treatment of chronic myelogenous leukemia (CML). While NICE initially recommended the drug for use only in the accelerated phase of CML, the indication was ultimately broadened for patients in the chronic phase as well (25).

NICE does recognize limitations to the focus on cost/QALY for making value judgments:

> And we need to think carefully about what's being valued. Concentrating only on QALYs means we are in danger of losing sight of other things that people, health systems and the government value very highly. This includes encouraging an innovative UK research base, or perhaps valuing more highly specific treatments that may be the only option for people with certain conditions. These aspects are not captured by the QALY, which is [one reason] why our committee has never used QALYs as the sole determinant in their decisions (22).

Perhaps recognizing these limitations with the threshold set for all health technologies[3] in all care settings, in 2009 NICE introduced new criteria and increased the threshold—up to £80,000 per year of life gained (26) for end-of-life[4] treatments based on altered willingness-to-pay in this setting. As described elsewhere, a variety of factors may be considered in NICE's assessment of a new technology, including (20):

- Uncertainty (e.g., of the incremental cost-effectiveness ratio (ICER) or variables in the model)
- Severity, burden, or characteristics of the illness/disease (e.g., end-of-life treatment)
- Special population characteristics (e.g., disabled, disadvantaged, children)
- Availability of comparators—or lack thereof
- Stakeholder opinions (e.g., patients, physicians, public/political priorities)
- Anticipated length of benefit
- Innovation

- Societal costs and benefits
- Size of the population
- Availability of resources

Through the multitude of features outlined here, the concept of value begins to come forward to the English health system. It is the assessments conducted and evaluated by NICE and other stakeholders in the UK that define this value from the cost-effectiveness perspective.

In addition to the technology appraisals that base recommendations on cost-effectiveness, NICE also provides guidance through the Highly Specialized Technologies (HST) program, which, unlike the technology appraisals, does not base recommendations on cost per QALY. The HST evaluations are recommendations on the use of new and existing highly specialized medicines and treatments within the NHS in England, considering drugs only for very rare conditions (27). The process for evaluation is similar to technology appraisals; however, recommendations are not based on predetermined ICER thresholds. Rather, value is determined through a multi-criteria approach that includes clinical evidence such as the "impact of the technology," and cost evidence such as "value for money." Being a relatively new guidance (only one published assessment at the time of writing), there is limited experience in understanding the details of this approach. However, a number of technologies (currently only drug therapies) are undergoing this process, which will give future insight into the process and have an impact on treatment decisions.

FRANCE: HAUTE AUTORITÉ DE SANTÉ

The French National Authority for Health (HAS) was set up by the French government in August 2004 to bring together under a single roof a number of activities designed to improve the quality of patient care and to guarantee equity within the health care system. HAS activities are diverse and range from assessment of drugs, medical devices, and procedures to publication of guidelines to accreditation of health care organizations and certification of doctors. All are based on rigorously acquired scientific expertise, and training in quality issues and information provision are key components of its efforts. HAS, in itself, is not a government agency, but rather an independent public body with financial autonomy that is mandated by law to carry out specific functions. It liaises closely, however, with government health agencies, national health insurance funds, research organizations, unions of health care professionals, and patients' representatives to ensure adequate expertise but also alignment *throughout* the centralized bureaucracy of the French system (28).

HAS carries out its initiatives through six specialized committees. Two committees, the Transparency Committee (TC) and the National Committee for the Evaluation of

---

[3] The NICE cost per QALY threshold was established in 1999 and has never been altered or increased.

[4] End-of-life criteria are applied in the following circumstances and when all the criteria are satisfied: (a) for patients with a short life expectancy, normally less than 24 months; (b) sufficient evidence to indicate that the treatment offers an extension to life, normally of at least an additional 3 months, compared with current NHS treatment; and (c) is licensed or otherwise indicated for small patient populations.

Medical Devices and Health Technologies (CNEDiMTS), carry out evaluations for drugs and medical devices/medical procedures, respectively, to determine the value of the technologies. For both of these committees, the value of a health technology is measured by the clinical benefit compared with products and procedures treating the same indication. In regard to CNEDiMTS, the French assessment of value for medical devices is a two-step process; the first step determines the actual benefit (AB), and the second determines the added clinical value (ACV). In determining the AB, CNEDiMTS defines the assessment as (29):

The actual benefit is evaluated, for each of the indications of the product or service, and, when appropriate, per group of the population, as a function of the two following criteria:

- The significance of the product or service as regards, on the one hand, its therapeutic or diagnostic effect or compensation for a disability as well as undesirable effects or risks linked to its use; on the other hand, the role of the product or service in therapeutic or diagnostic strategy or compensation for a disability, taking account of other available therapeutic or diagnostic methods or means to compensate for the disability;

- Its expected public health benefit, in particular its impact on the health of the population, in terms of mortality, morbidity and quality of life, its ability to fulfill a therapeutic or diagnostic need or to compensate for a disability, its impact on the health service and its impact on public health policies and programmes.

If the actual benefit is deemed insufficient, there is no funding for the product, and the process stops. For medical devices and health technologies that demonstrate a sufficient actual benefit and recommendation for funding, the second assessment is conducted to determine the ACV. The ACV assessment is "in relation to a comparable product, procedure, or service or a group of comparable well-defined procedures, products or services, considered to be the gold standard according to available scientific data and regardless of whether this gold standard is, or not, reimbursed." This ACV classifies the assessment as:

- Major (I)
- Substantial (II)
- Moderate (III)
- Minor (IV)
- Absent (V)

Once the ACV has been determined for the medical device or health technology, and guidance for the use of this product has been set by CNEDiMTS, the reimbursement tariff is negotiated between the manufacturer and the Economic Committee and Health Products (CEPS), a governmental committee, to determine the commercial conditions for the product (29).

For medical/surgical procedures, the process is much longer and complex and can take up to 5 years, whereas the process for medical devices typically takes 3 to 4 months. First, the procedure has to be selected from among others to be added on the HAS work program (i.e., not all procedures are assessed). For the procedure to be selected, a dossier including all available data on the procedure and its potential benefit has to be submitted to the HAS by a health care professionals organization (e.g., French Association of Urology). The CNEDiMTS then votes to define which medical procedures will be selected. This has shown to be challenging, as only 3 to 5 medical/surgical procedures (among 30–40) are selected to be assessed each year. Once selected, HAS works in collaboration with a multidisciplinary working group to assess the procedure. The conclusions of this assessment are presented to CNEDiMTS members for them to vote on the procedure's AB. When a procedure demonstrates sufficient AB and is recommended for funding, the funding process and conditions are then to be worked out and approved by L' Union Nationale des Caisses d'Assurance Maladie (UNCAM), the French public health care organizational system that coordinates between the major national health insurance funds (known as sickness funds in France).

In regard to radiotherapy, few assessments have been carried out through this process. One assessment (30) stands out in the French system: high-intensity focused ultrasound (HIFU) for the treatment of localized prostate cancer. The assessment conducted by the now defunct Committee for Assessment of Medical and Surgical Procedures (merged with CNEDiMTS in 2010) was first carried out in 2003, but declared the need for further clinical research and longer follow-up with patients. In 2009, at the request of the French Association of Urology (AFU), a reassessment began to update the payer's viewpoint on the use of HIFU. In this assessment the HAS evaluated the clinical effectiveness of HIFU as applied for primary treatment of low- and intermediate-risk localized prostate cancer (T1-T2 NxMO) in patients older than 70 years, and for local recurrence of prostate cancer after radiotherapy failure. This assessment examined the incremental benefit in terms of mortality, morbidity, and posttherapeutic complications from these alternatives. The assessment included an in-depth literature search and analysis of scientific data—both published and unpublished—in consultation with a multidisciplinary working group composed of French urologists, radiotherapists, medical oncologists, and other physicians. The primary conclusion was that no strong evidence exists for rating one treatment as being more beneficial than another when comparing HIFU with radical prostatectomy, radical external beam (conformal) with internal (brachytherapy) radiotherapy.

Owing to the poor quality of evidence[5] and short follow-up, the committee was unable to conclude that HIFU provided sufficient advantages to counterbalance the complication and uncertainty of results in the long term compared with standard treatment options such as watchful waiting or hormonal treatment. The committee requested further research into the measures of benefit of HIFU in terms of survival, long-term survival, long-term adverse effects, and quality of life as demonstrated through controlled clinical trials or observational studies with sufficient follow-up to measure these effects. As a result, HIFU is not an approved medical procedure in France, as the evidence was viewed to be insufficient in determining the benefit or risk of the therapy for prostate cancer. Furthermore, HAS states, "it is unlikely that this conclusion would be changed in the near future due to the lack of ongoing of planned studies."

Although a standardized process for defining value exists in France, it is still heavily dependent on the available data and information. While a new technology or procedure may have great promise, the quality and breadth of the evidence ultimately determine its value in the French health care system.

GERMANY: GEMEINSAMER BUNDESAUSSCHUSS

Assessments of value are a new concept in the German marketplace, only established by the German Parliament in 2011 through the Act on the Reform of the Market for Medicinal Products (AMNOG). Earlier, Germany was regarded as a "free pricing" marketplace, allowing manufacturers to set prices for their technology without review or restraint. This legislation completely revised pricing regulations for newly authorized pharmaceuticals and their reimbursement by statutory health insurance providers. It assigned key responsibility to the Federal Joint Committee (G-BA) and the Institute for Quality and Efficiency in Health Care (IQWiG) to conduct benefit assessments of newly authorized pharmaceuticals in accordance with the German Social Code, Book Five (SGB V), section 35a (31). Health care companies were thereafter required to submit a dossier on product benefit when launched into the German market or when they are authorized for new indications. The conclusion of an assessment takes the form of a resolution, published immediately, that includes the G-BA's decision on the pricing procedure for the new medicine. Within 6 months, if additional benefit is proven, the Central Federal Association of Health Insurance Funds (GKV-Spitzenverband) and the pharmaceutical company negotiate the reimbursement price paid by the statutory health insurance funds. This takes the form of a rebate on the retail price originally set by the company—thereby

translating into the value-based price in accordance with the magnitude of additional benefit (31). This benefit is assigned in comparison with an appropriate comparator defined by the committee, in each subpopulation or "slice" representing a relevant patient group within that label setting. In conducting their assessment, IQWiG and the G-BA rely upon only "patient-relevant" endpoints with gradations of certainty, ranging from Proof, Indication, or Hint of benefit. The extent of this additional benefit is evaluated in relation to the severity of the disease and is expressed as:

1. Major additional benefit
2. Considerable additional benefit
3. Minor additional benefit
4. Unquantifiable additional benefit
5. No additional benefit
6. Less benefit than the appropriate comparator

Achieving a benefit rating in the top four categories (1, 2, 3, or 4 in the preceding list) results in subsequent price negotiations between the technology manufacturer and the GKV-Spitzenverband, often resulting in a premium to the current comparator therapies. A rating of "no additional benefit" results in protracted negotiations and limitation of pricing discussions to the appropriate comparator benchmark, and may result in the technology being placed into a reference price group. If found to have "less benefit" than the comparator, the technology may require additional studies or be restricted in, or excluded from, reimbursement. In the German system, value is defined by the additional benefit provided by therapies. Subsequent negotiation of a final price—or rebate/discount—is based in large part on this assessment.

Upon receiving the rating of additional benefit for relevant subpopulations in any given treatment setting, a new technology will enter price negotiations with the GKV-Spitzenverband. This negotiation is based on a variety of features, including the outcome from the benefit assessment from the G-BA and the current net prices of any appropriate comparators in Germany and other European countries. Additional features may be considered in determining the final price of a technology, including cost-benefit analysis; cost-offset data; budget impact; any data available on treatment reality or product benefit that were not included in the initial benefit rating; and data on compliance, persistence, or other patient-relevant outcomes (32). Finally, if no agreement can be reached, pharmacoeconomic evidence and arbitration may ensue. However, if the central price negotiation with GKV-Spitzenverband concludes successfully, the manufacturer may still negotiate selective contracts with individual sickness funds (KKs), modifying or complementing the collective price negotiation scheme (e.g., budget capping or risk

---

[5] The committee examined 21 case-series, relating to approximately 2,500 selected patients with short-term follow-up.

sharing). This deliberate and iterative process in the German system reflects the varying criteria in defining value, while aligning around the concept of "additional benefit" for new technologies.

ITALY: AGENZIA ITALIANA DEL FARMACO

In Italy, regional provision of health care is of primary concern because of the decentralized nature of the political and administrative health functions. The initial entry into the Italian marketplace, however, occurs at a national level. Two centralized bodies at the national level handle Italy's HTA activities: the Italian Medicine Agency (Agenzia Italiana del Farmaco—AIFA) that focuses on pharmaceuticals, and the National Agency for Regional Health Services (Agenzia Nazionale per I Servizi Sanitari Regionali—AGENAS) for medicine/technology including medical devices.

AIFA was established in 2003 and assesses and approves drugs to be added for reimbursement on the National Pharmaceutical Formulary (Prontuario Farmaceutico Nazionale—PFN). A committee within AIFA, the Technical and Scientific Committee (Comitato Scientifico e Tecnico), is responsible for the assessment of new drugs and for conducting any HTA activities for pharmaceuticals. Newly approved drugs marketed in Italy are assigned to one of three classes for reimbursement purposes by AIFA:

- Class A—Essential medicines and those that treat chronic disease for full reimbursement

- Class H—Drugs that are only reimbursed for hospital use

- Class C—Not reimbursed through national health insurance funds and must be paid for by patients unless included by regional health departments in reimbursement schemes

The A, H, C classification system used by AIFA is reimbursement focused and does not take into account the effectiveness of the drugs (33). Other activities conducted by AIFA include HTA assessments that look at clinical efficacy, cost-effectiveness, and budget-impact analyses. Clinical efficacy in Italy is measured through the "therapeutic innovation" of the product, using a specific algorithm that compares the new drug with existing therapies. This system informs pricing of the drug, including allowing for the possibility of innovative products to achieve a premium price, acknowledging recognized value to the Italian system. The final price is negotiated between the manufacturer and AIFA's Pricing and Reimbursement Committee (Comitato Prezzi e Rimborso—CPR), which takes into account assessments for cost-effectiveness and risk-benefit, as well as the economic impact on the National Healthcare System (Servizio sanitario nazionale—SSN), daily cost of therapy compared with products of similar efficacy, achievable market share estimates, and comparisons of price and consumption with other European countries.

AGENAS was formally established in 2007 to take on several responsibilities, including:

- Supporting the national priority-setting process at the national and regional levels

- Producing HTA reports for the Ministry of Health

- Providing technical and operational support for the development of HTA programs in the Italian regions (34)

The responsibility of conducting HTAs for medical devices falls under AGENAS, which evaluates:

- Clinical effectiveness of the technology on the basis of a systematic review of clinical studies

- Contextual analysis to understand how the technology is currently used

- Economic analysis that incorporates a systematic review of the economic evidence, cost analysis, reimbursement of the technology, and a budget-impact analysis

- Patients' views to understand their perspectives, expectations, and desires relating to the technology

The conclusions of the assessments are used to formulate recommendations on the adoption and use of the technology, aimed to be used across the individual Italian regions.

A recently released HTA report on selective internal radiation therapy (SIRT) in colorectal liver metastases provides an example of this process being conducted for radiotherapies. The objective of the report was to assess the effectiveness, acceptability, costs, and organizational aspects of SIRT for the treatment of liver metastases from colorectal cancer (CRC) (35). AGENAS utilized systematic literature reviews and questionnaires with treatment centers in assessing the clinical effectiveness, context analysis, and economic analysis, as well as a review of studies that measured quality of life to understand the patient's views. The assessment was not without limitations, as the clinical effectiveness was based on one open-label, randomized trial carried out on 46 patients, in regard to which AGENAS commented that the study was "small and its generalizability is unclear" (36). This study also did not provide sufficient data for the cost-effectiveness analysis, as it provided weak survival data and did not have available QALYs. AGENAS concluded that the evidence on the effectiveness of the use of SIRT in this setting was very limited, but noted that several large studies were still ongoing. Considering the stage of the disease for patients eligible for treatment with this technology, the cost of the SIRT and the uncertainty surrounding its effects, AGENAS recommended that "the adoption of the SIRT treatment would be advisable in few selected cases, to concentrated in few qualified high specialized centers" (36).

While at the national level the HTA activities are centralized through AIFA and AGENAS, the Italian health care system as a whole is decentralized, with regions and autonomous provinces implementing the results of the national HTA activities at their own discretion. In fact, only five regions—Veneto, Emilia-Romagna, Lombardy, Piedmont, and Tuscany—have included HTA in their health care decision-making processes (34). Each region also makes individual decisions that can impact pricing, particularly with pharmaceuticals, which can result in price differences across the country.

Each region in Italy makes decisions based on considerations related to budget impact and cost–utility trade-offs. Other considerations also may include:

- Use and cost of current interventions (actual)
- Use and cost of new interventions (anticipated)
- Target population
  - Current alternative interventions
  - New intervention and market effects
  - Off-label uses of the new intervention
    - Cost of the current or new intervention mix
- Impact on other costs
  - Condition-related costs
  - Indirect costs
- Time horizon
- Time dependencies and discounting
- Choice of computing framework
- Uncertainty and scenario analysis
- Validation

These considerations may vary by region, reflecting the unique perspective and context in such decisions. Thus, the ultimate emphasis on any of the modeling considerations depends on the regional institutions and stakeholders involved in the decision-making process. The decentralized health care structure affects the consistency in defining value for health technologies across Italy. As the current structure allows a high degree of local-level autonomy, the perception of the value of a new product will likely differ from north to south or east to west.

REFERENCES

1. National Institute for Health and Care Excellence. Who we are. 2014. www.nice.org.uk/about/who-we-are.

2. National Institute for Health and Care Excellence. NICE charter. 2013. www.nice.org.uk/Media/Default/About/Who-we-are/NICE_Charter.pdf.

3. International Society for Pharmacoeconomics and Outcomes Research. Pharmaceutical HTA and reimbursement processes—United Kingdom. 2008. www.ispor.org/HTARoadmaps/UK.asp.

4. Raferty J. NICE: faster access to modern treatment? Analysis of guidance on health technologies. *Brit Med J.* 2001;323:1300–1303.

5. Towse A, Pritchard C. Does NICE have a threshold? An external view. In: Towse A, Pritchard N, Devlin N, eds. *Cost Effectiveness Thresholds: Economic and Ethical Issues.* London, UK: King's Fund and Office of Health Economics; 2002.

6. National Institute for Health and Care Excellence. www.nice.org.uk.

7. O'Donnell J, Pham S, Pashos C, et al. Health technology assessment: lessons learned from around the world. *Value Health.* 2009;12(Suppl 2):S1–S5.

8. Weinstein MC, Statson WB. Foundations of cost-effectiveness analysis for health and medical practices. *New Eng J Med.* 1997;296:716–721.

9. Lipscomb J, Drummond M, Fryback D, et al. Retaining and enhancing the QALY. *Value Health.* 2009;12(Suppl 1):S18–S25.

10. Shaw JW, Johnson JA, Coons SJ, et al. US Valuation of the EQ-5D health states, development and testing of the D1 valuation model. *Med Care.* 2005;43(3):203–217.

11. Busschbach JJ, Weijnen T, Nieuwenhuizen M, et al. A comparison of EQ-5D time trade-off values obtained in Germany, the United Kingdom, and Spain. In: Brooks R, Rabin R, de Charro R, eds. *The Measurement and Valuation of Health States Using EQ-5D: A European Perspective.* Berlin, Germany: Springer; 2003.

12. Horsman J, Furlong W, Feeny D, et al. The health utilities index (HUI): concepts, measurement, properties, and applications. *Health Qual Life Outcomes.* 2003;1:54. www.hqlo.com/content/1/1/54.

13. McDowell I. *Measuring Health: A Guide to Rating Scales and Questionnaires.* 3rd ed. London, UK: Oxford University Press; 2006:675–683.

14. Brazier J, Roberts J, Tsuchiya A, et al. A comparison of the EQ-5D and SF-6D across seven patient groups. *Health Econ.* 2004;13:873–884.

15. Erickson P. Evaluation of a population-based measure of quality of life: the health and activity limitation index (HALex). *Qual Life Res.* 1998;7:101–114.

16. Fryback,D.,et al, US Norms for Six Generic Health Related Quality of Life Indexes from the National Health Measurement Study, Medical Care 45:12, 1162–1179, 2007.

17. Kamm FM. To whom? *Hastings Cent Rep.* 1994;24(4):29–32.

18. Nord E. An alternative to QALYs: the saved young life equivalent (save). *Brit Med J.* 1992;305(6858):875–877.

19. Phillips C. *What Is Cost-Effectiveness?* London, UK: Hayward Medical Communications; 2009. http:// www.medicine.ox.ac.uk/bandolier/painres/download/ whatis/Cost-effect.pdf.

20. Claxton K, Martin S, Soares M, et al. Methods for estimation of the NICE cost-effectiveness threshold. *Health Technol Assess.* 2015;19(14).

21. Claxton K, Martin S, Soares M, et al. Appendix 1: Systematic review of the literature on the cost-effectiveness threshold. In: *Methods for the Estimation of the National Institute for Health and Care Excellence Cost-Effectiveness Threshold.* Southampton, UK: NIHR Journals Library—Health Technology Assessment; 2015.

22. Dillon A. Carrying NICE over the threshold. 2015. www.nice.org.uk/news/blog/ carrying-nice-over-the-threshold.

23. Appleby J, Devlin N, Parkin D. NICE's cost effectiveness threshold. *Brit Med J.* 2007;335(7616):358–359.

24. Powell M. Latest decision on zanamivir will not end postcode prescribing. *Brit Med J.* 2001;322:489.

25. Burke K. No cash to implement NICE, health authorities tell MP's. *Brit Med J.* 2002;324:258.

26. Mayor S. NICE estimates that its recommendations have cost the NHS £575M. *Brit Med J.* 2002;325:924.

27. Bosley S, Sparrow A. Johnson lifts NHS ban on top-up treatment. *The Guardian.* November 4, 2008. www.theguardian.com/politics/2008/nov/04/ nhs-health-cancer-topup-treatment.

28. National Institute for Health and Care Excellence. NICE highly specialised technologies guidance. 2014. www.nice.org.uk/about/ what-we-do/our-programmes/nice-guidance/ nice-highly-specialised-technologies-guidance.

29. International Society for Pharmacoeconomics and Outcomes Research. Pharmaceutical HTA and reimbursement processes—France. 2009. www.ispor .org/HTARoadmaps/France.asp.

30. Haute Autorité de Santé. Medical device assessment in France. 2009. www.has-sante.fr/portail/ upload/docs/application/pdf/2010-03/guide_dm_ gb_050310.pdf.

31. Haute Autorité de Santé. High intensity focalized ultrasound for the treatment of localized prostate cancer. 2010. http://www.has-sante.fr/portail/ upload/docs/application/pdf/2011-12/summary_ hifu.pdf.

32. Federal Joint Committee (Gemeinsamer Bundesausschuss). The benefit assessment of pharmaceuticals in accordance with the German Social Code, Book Five (SGB V), section 35a. www.english .g-ba.de/benefitassessment/information.

33. Bouslouk M, Pirk O, Fricke F. Additional patient related benefits are the key to price negotiation in Germany—practical experience with benefit dossiers and the assessment process. 2012. www .ispor.org/congresses/berlin1112/presentations/ W17_All%20Slides.pdf.

34. The Economist Intelligence Unit. Value-based health assessment in Italy: a decentralised model. 2015. www.economistinsights.com/sites/default/ files/Value-based%20Health%20Assessment%20 in%20Italy.pdf.

35. The International Network of Agencies for Health Technology Assessment. AGENAS—The National Agency for Regional Health Services. 2015. http:// www.inahta.org/members/agenas.

36. Chiarolla E, Paone S, Lo Scalzo A, et al. HTA report: selective internal radiation therapy (SIRT) in colorectal liver metastases. 2013. www.salute.gov .it/imgs/C_17_pagineAree_1202_listaFile_item-Name_0_file.pdf.

37. Ferre F, de Belvis AG, Valerio L. Italy: health system review. *Health Syst Transit.* 2014;16(4):30.

4 Systems Engineering and Process Control

Ajay Kapur and Louis Potters

INTRODUCTION

Quality control and assurance of treatment equipment have been at the core of efforts to ensure safe and effective care for patients since the inception of radiation medicine. Radiation medicine today is thus, not surprisingly, one of the safest forms of modern medicine. However, injuries due to erroneous care are as old as the field itself, starting with those sustained by some of its pioneers. The quality of care is crucially dependent on the performance of the entire system of radiation medicine that drives its technology. As the system evolves in complexity with its intent toward greater precision in patient care, so does the opportunity for new forms of error. Serious accidents that have occurred serve as learning opportunities to understand our systemic failures more deeply and to proactively engineer safety in new ways. Over the past two decades, there has been a substantial rise in the perceived need for, as well as use of, systems engineering and Six Sigma methodologies for the improvement of quality in a wide range of industries, including health care.

This chapter provides an overview of the foundational aspects of these approaches for potential adoption by radiation medicine. The context of systems complexity and existing frameworks for quality are described first, followed by illustrations of how systems engineering and Six Sigma thinking can potentially augment those frameworks in controlling the flow of clinical processes that deliver care.

COMPLEXITY AND THE NEED FOR SYSTEMS THINKING

Health care is replete with examples of errors culminating in adverse events that compromise the quality and value of care (1). The characteristic of human fallibility (*To Err Is Human*) is often linked with safety events across industries. Historically, there has been an overarching tendency to place culpability on individuals when errors occur. Apart from reckless behavior on the part of the *individual* worker, the majority of adverse events are attributable instead to error-provoking conditions prevalent at the *system* level, particularly those with complex interactions (2–10), for which a normal rate of accidents may be expected (11).

Systems are collections of interconnected components (people, multifunctional teams, processes, equipment, material, software) that interact within a broader environment to meet common goals (12–14). A complex system is characterized by nonlinear interactions that yield new emergent properties not exhibited by the components themselves (15,16). In such systems, error-provoking conditions tend to fall into recurrent self-organizing patterns; more rare events are observed than would be expected from a normal bell curve (fat-tailed behavior), and small changes in initial conditions can potentially trigger large effects (butterfly effect) (16–18). Examples include our immune system, tropical rain forests, and the Internet.

Health care systems, particularly those with rapidly evolving technologies and human interactions such as radiation medicine, exhibit characteristics of complex systems (19–21). New life cycles for technologies potentially come with subsequent adaptations in those interactions. Although risks in radiation medicine are low compared with other health care systems (19) and compared with the risk of death from cancer itself (22), tragic accidents do occur (23–27). Accidents in radiation medicine due to software bugs are often quoted as being among the worst errors that have occurred (4,28). Thus, safety risk mitigation efforts in these systems should embrace the science of complexity and a systems approach, rather than a reductionist one that focuses mainly on components, particularly in the current era of increasing complexity (29–33). Complexity scientists suggest a direction for steering risk mitigation, namely, to identify recurrent risk patterns, as already described, and to enhance control over critically associated lever points (16). Similarly, Reason (4–6), in his Swiss cheese model of error propagation, focuses on addressing recurrent patterns involving active and latent error-creating conditions as the targets for error reduction.

As the complexity of the humans who operate such systems may not match that of the systems themselves (8), these strategies to extract lever points would be well served by augmenting existing health care quality and safety frameworks with systems-engineering approaches deployed in hazardous industries (34–37). Attempts to measurably improve the quality of care could benefit from corporate Six Sigma and Lean approaches that aggressively seek to minimize defects and reduce inefficiencies, respectively (38–43). Trends for adoption of such approaches have begun to emerge in health care (44–48), as well as in radiation medicine, in recent years (49–54).

CURRENT FRAMEWORKS FOR QUALITY

The Institute of Medicine framework for quality

The Institute of Medicine (IOM) defines health care quality as "the *degree* to which *health care services* for individuals and populations increase the likelihood *of desired health outcomes* and are consistent with *current professional knowledge*" (55). Six aims for achieving quality have been indicated, namely, that care is safe, effective, timely, efficient, equitable, and patient centered (56). To assess quality, these aims are associated with quality indicators from professional practice standards, quantifiable using quality measures with evidence-based links to outcomes. This definition and broad framework have been widely adopted in health care (57) and in radiation medicine (58). Although most existing measures pertain to safety and effectiveness aims (59), general guidelines for devising indicators and measures have been suggested for the broader context of health care (60,61) and for radiation medicine (62,63). The definition, aims, indicators, and measures thus provide the current framework for defining, assessing, and improving quality.

The Donabedian framework for quality assessment

The IOM framework is rooted in the conceptual work of Avedis Donabedian (64–66), a physician and public health professional who identified seven pillars of quality: efficacy, efficiency, optimality, acceptability, legitimacy, equity, and cost. He stated that the underlying links between three dimensions of systems—namely, structures, processes, and outcomes—must be understood as a precursor of quality assessment, the assumption being that good structures yield good processes, which in turn yield good outcomes (Figure 4.1, inner wheel). Structures relate to the core set-up of the system, including organizational hierarchies, budgets, treatment delivery platforms and techniques, case mixes, policies, accreditation status, peer review, and health care provider credentials. Processes refer to the technical and interpersonal actions and encounters taken by the health care providers in specifying and delivering care to patients. Outcomes refer to the net effect of these processes on the overall health status and quality of life of individual patients and populations relative to presenting conditions. These dimensions are clearly reflected in the IOM definition of quality as well as the six aims.

The Donabedian framework has significantly impacted radiation medicine standards. Patterns of care studies in radiation medicine were based on it (62). Structure, process, and outcome dimensions constituted 64%, 26%, and 10% of 454 standards, respectively, from eight radiation medicine standard setting groups globally (67). Their uneven distribution is perhaps related to the difficulties in collecting scientifically acceptable data. Assessment of outcomes is challenging, as they may not be realized immediately, and cofactors such as multidisciplinary specialty care, sample sizes, evolving technologies, and patient characteristics complicate risk adjustment models (62,63). Structural aspects upstream of processes are easiest to glean, with some, such as volumes, linked to outcomes, and are deployed by accreditation organizations (63). Process measures are easier for health care providers to relate to, as they are proximal to errors, can be relatively easily benchmarked using policies and medical records, require less follow-up, and provide direct feedback, but they must be linked to outcomes (63). As no single process represents the totality of care provided, multiple process measures are considered. Further, not all poor processes lead to poor outcomes (60). Understanding of the causal links between the dimensions is thus confounded by the nonlinear nature of interactions in complex systems. These considerations underscore the difficulties with using any of these measures independently as surrogates for quality. Deviations from radiotherapy treatment protocols in clinical trials built on firm structural and process bases, however, have been linked with poorer patient outcomes (68). Thus, all dimensions should be collectively considered along with an understanding of the causes of deviation and variation to assess quality in an environment of "watchful concern" (69).

Incident reporting and Codman principles

In the context of watchful concern, reporting systems serve as a feedback mechanism for registering unexpected outcomes, deviations from protocols, or unsafe conditions that lead or nearly lead to unintended outcomes (1,70–73). Errors may embrace all aspects of care indicated in the six IOM aims. It is important for error reporting to encompass the Donabedian dimensions to extract underlying causal links attributed to their genesis and propagation (Figure 4.1). This transforms incident reporting systems into incident learning systems (ILS). Systems that deploy such a framework in a responsive and nonpunitive way allow growth and dissemination of knowledge with successful risk mitigation, exemplified in high-reliability industries (74). The need for reporting was perceived a century ago by a surgeon, an early pioneer of the use of x-rays, and a founder of the American College of

Surgeons, Ernest Amory Codman (75). Codman took the first steps in systematically documenting and publicizing errors in processes and their links with end outcomes through years of follow-up with his patients at his private hospital (76). His visionary endeavors were, however, professionally stymied because of the prevailing culture opposing transparency at the time. The culture of enhanced safety today has enabled the recent launch of a national radiation oncology-ILS (RO-ILS) built on a consensus of recommendations and sponsored by major professional societies in radiation medicine (72,73).

The Deming cycle and the framework for quality improvement

The rationale for assessing quality is to be able to improve it in a measurable way. Efforts may be reactive, that is, based on addressing observed errors; or proactive, where improvements are sought even if basic performance goals have been met. One of the most widely used frameworks for quality improvement stems from the foundational efforts of electrical engineer and mathematical physicist William Edwards Deming (77–79) in the area of statistical variations and process control. Inspired by physicist and statistician Walter Andrew Shewhart's (80) concepts of statistical process control, Deming realized the potential for using the same concepts in management. His focus on appreciating systems and component interactions, understanding and controlling variation, epistemology, and human psychology enabled a substantial transformation of Japanese product quality and culminated in the Plan–Do–See–Act (PDSA) cycle for iterative quality improvement. The cycle is separated into four phases to minimize the buildup effect of interactions that would otherwise confound cause analyses, thus inherently incorporating complex systems into its design. It is conceptually rooted in the scientific method of hypothesis building, experimentation, and evaluation put forth by Sir Francis Bacon (81). "Plan" refers to setting objectives and processes to meet outcomes; "Do" refers to implementing and executing the plan along with collecting data for analysis; "See" refers to analyzing the data for variability and deviations from expected outcomes; "Act" refers to replanning if the analyses did not reflect improvement from the baseline. The cycle spirals outward continuously, each loop representing a potential improvement in quality, and thereby potentially new standards within the structure–process–outcome dimensions as technologies continue to evolve (Figure 4.1, outer circle).

A call for systems engineering and Six Sigma

Current frameworks for quality assessment and improvement in health care are clearly rooted in firm scientific principles. The challenges of providing reliable, valid, and generalizable indicators and measures notwithstanding, specific

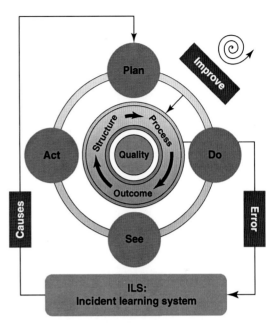

FIGURE 4.1 Frameworks for quality assessment, reporting, and improvement.

examples bear testimony to their effectiveness. Examples include substantial reduction of central venous catheter bloodstream infections, and deaths caused by anesthesia during surgery by deployment of interventions based on concrete evidence and measures into routine clinical practice. Yet demonstrable improvements in the broader context of health care are not apparent more than a decade after the grassroots realization of their utility and the need for them (82–84). The *implementation* of quality frameworks at the level of the individual clinic may not have commensurate rigor or uniformity in practice as their conceptual origins. It is here, however, where errors occur. Practical methods to effectively and efficiently *engineer* their translation into clinical practice are therefore needed to bridge the gap and cross the quality chasm. Herein lies the potential opportunity for systems engineering and Six Sigma.

SYSTEMS ENGINEERING AND SIX SIGMA METHODOLOGIES

Overview

The International Council on Systems Engineering (INCOSE) defines systems engineering as "an *interdisciplinary* approach and means to enable the realization of successful systems" (35). The Apollo program and the International Space Station are examples of the applications of systems engineering. Tracing its roots to the 1930s (37), systems engineering focuses on the system as a whole through all life cycles with particular emphasis on communication, uncertainty, and complexity in the interaction of its components (including humans). It enables the translation of qualitative customer requirements into quantitative product/ process specifications through up-front discovery, learning, diagnosis, and dialog. By discovering problems upfront as well as stratifying failure modes with the greatest risk, it enhances the reliability of the system to meet the customer requirements in a proactive manner.

Six Sigma methods (introduced by Motorola in the 1980s) are statistically driven methods that aim to achieve high-quality process performance relative to customer expectations. Quantitatively, the aim is to minimize defect rates to fewer than 3.4 per million opportunities. The sigma level is a measure of the ability of a process to achieve a desired mean value, centered within a tolerance range such that the variability in the process itself (standard deviation) is much smaller than the difference between the mean value and tolerance limits. A defective process is one that falls outsides the tolerance range. Thus, a Six Sigma process is one where the standard deviation is one-sixth of that difference and corresponds to a long-term defect-free rate of 99.99966%. Over multiple opportunities, such processes are more robust to variation and therefore more reliable (Figure 4.2). Reaching this level of defect-free performance requires a comprehensive system understanding of the factors that affect the process, including variations, along with strategies to enhance process control. This is achieved using dedicated phased approaches similar to the PDSA cycle (44).

Systems engineering and Six Sigma methodologies emerged when traditional approaches to quality management were deemed inadequate to meet different but related needs. Rising complexity within systems, particularly in the aerospace and defense industries, affected *reliability*, thus leading to the rapid growth of systems engineering (35).

In contrast, fierce market competition among companies called for aggressive reduction of composite product *defects and variability,* thus leading to Six Sigma approaches (44). Although levels of complexity were arguably different in these industries, the common element was the need to focus on performance improvement of the system in a holistic manner and to seek novel methods to address the challenges. The two approaches thus have more similarities than differences, with many convergent tools and methods used by multidisciplinary teams in both. One key takeaway is that these methodologies and tools designed with complex systems in mind were instrumental in achieving and sustaining the level of change needed.

In the context of parallels in health care, the same drivers are relevant to the aims of the IOM quality framework. Although health care represents a very different customer—the patient—and comes with its unique challenges, there is value in exploring the feasibility of using or adapting some of these methodologies and tools given our unmet needs in quality improvement described earlier (38). In the following sections, the basic principles of select methodologies and tools from systems engineering and Six Sigma methodologies are discussed in the context of application to radiation medicine.

Quality function deployment

Quality function deployment (QFD) is a top-down iterative systems engineering approach to quality developed in Japan in 1966 to include the voice of the customer along with that of the multifunctional company stakeholders through the cascade of product design stages down to parts requirements, manufacturing processes, and quality

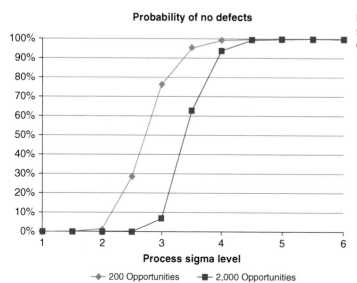

FIGURE 4.2 Illustration of the effect of sigma level on defect rates over multiple opportunities.

control (85). Management, technical, and business elements are considered together; correlations between key enabling factors are made transparent; and prioritization of efforts is established to ensure quality efforts are directed at key control parameters (KCP) and key noise parameters (KNP).

The process starts with obtaining key customer requirements, also known as critical-to-quality characteristics (CTQs), or "Ys" (Figure 4.3). The relative importance of each CTQ is ranked by the customer, and corresponding competitive benchmarks obtained by the team. Next, technical product characteristics, also known as "Xs," required for each of the CTQs are established. The magnitude of correlation (high, medium, low or numerical ranks) between each X and all Ys, along with the direction (increase, decrease), determines their overall relationships. The Xs are pareto sorted in the order of their overall impact on all Ys using the weighted rank sum. Thus, the Xs most important for all the Ys may be extracted. Force-field analysis between the Xs identifies whether interactions between them are inimical or conducive to one another. This completes the first "House of Quality." The Xs from this house then become the Ys for the next house of quality, where product characteristics are correlated with parts requirements; and iteratively to manufacturing process and quality control requirements. Moving from one house to the next engages different functional teams. Completing the QFD thus provides a comprehensive view of how all components of the system are linked with CTQs in a quantifiable way.

CTQ flow-down or flow-up maps provide effective visual means to assess the overall complexities therein. Findings may be used in subsequent Six Sigma or Lean projects for further quality improvement on the KCPs to reduce variability, reduce defect rates, or improve efficiencies in processes.

The QFD tool may be adapted to health care in many ways to better integrate the patient perspective (86). As described previously, the QFD iteratively links CTQs with structural and process elements within a manufacturing system, although it may be applied to services as well. Specific aims of the IOM could potentially be considered CTQs in this context. Such a study focused on the patient-centered aim has been conducted in a radiology department to determine how effectively existing practice guidelines address patient needs, although the voice of the patient was extrapolated from secondary sources (87). In radiation medicine, QFDs have been conducted to select and prioritize Lean Six Sigma projects (88), or initiatives for risk reduction (53). Alternatively, this approach may be used to incorporate the voice of our patients directly in terms of satisfaction with the services provided in radiation medicine (patient-centered aim).

Retrospective and prospective error analysis

Mitigation of risk in radiation medicine is primarily centered on the safety aim of the IOM framework.

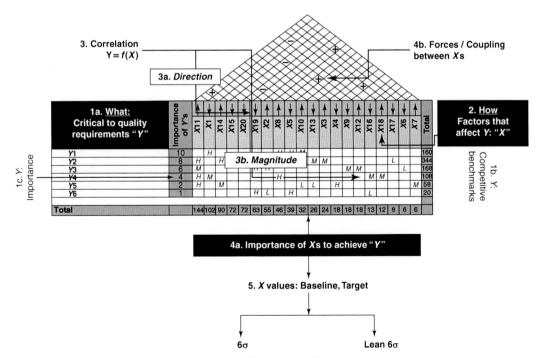

FIGURE 4.3 Schematic diagram illustrating quality function deployment.

Analysis may focus on errors that have occurred or that may be predicted, so a combined approach is optimal for surveillance (89,90). Root cause analyses (RCAs) and failure mode and effects analyses (FMEAs) are relevant systems and safety engineering tools that are also deployed in Six Sigma projects for retrospective and prospective surveillance, respectively (58). Successful implementation of these tools requires a multidisciplinary team approach.

RCA is usually done when errors are reported in an ILS. The goal is to identify contributory factors that lead to unsafe conditions, near misses, or incidents that reach the patient (72,73). The underlying taxonomy provides a comprehensive systems perspective in the form of a fishbone diagram so as to steer mitigation toward all relevant aspects, including people, methods, machines, materials, measurements, and environment (91). The taxonomy deployed in RO-ILS for radiation medicine is based on similar principles (Figure 4.4) (58).

FMEA is usually performed when new technologies are deployed or changes to existing processes occur such that sufficient experience with these changes has not been accrued by the department. It requires the detailed description of the process as a starting point. Team members identify steps in the process where errors *may*

occur, how they may appear, what causes them, and what existing controls may mitigate them. Three risk factors are assigned on an ordinal scale corresponding to potential severity of errors, their likelihood of occurrence, and their likelihood of detection if they do occur (Figure 4.5). The product of these three risk factors represents the composite risk, the risk priority number (RPN). Methods to further mitigate failure modes are brainstormed in decreasing order of the RPN and implemented accordingly. FMEA exercises have been conducted in various radiation medicine departments (90,92) as well as at the professional society level (93).

Six Sigma Design–Measure–Analyze–Improve–Control for quality improvement

Design–Measure–Analyze–Improve–Control (DMAIC) is a data-driven Six Sigma approach used to improve existing processes using various tools in five sequential phases (44). The first three phases concentrate on understanding the problem, and the last two on solving it. A key requirement for DMAIC is that relevant performance characteristics be measurable. The scope of the problem must be well defined and narrow for DMAIC to work

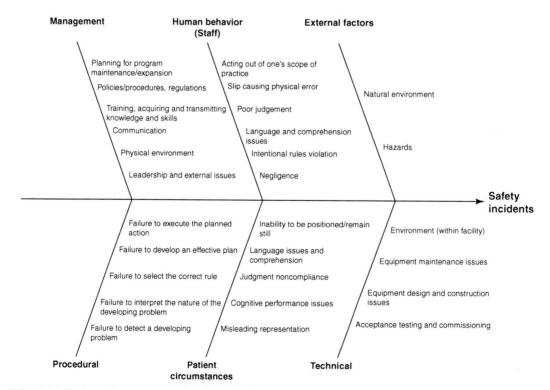

FIGURE 4.4 Fishbone diagram representing the top-level contributory factors from the AAPM consensus guidelines leading to safety incidents. (*Source*: From Ref. (58). Ford EC, Santos LF, Pawlicki T, et al. Consensus recommendations for incident learning database structures in radiation oncology. *Med Phys*. 2012;39:7272–7290.)

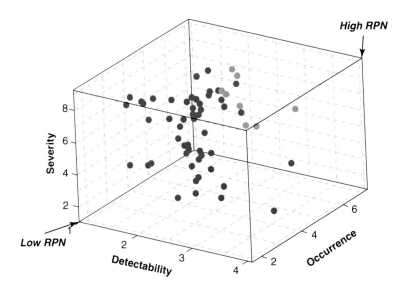

FIGURE 4.5 Risk stratification for sample failure modes for the radiation safety process map. (*Source*: From Ref. (90). Kapur A, Goode G, Riehl C, et al. Incident learning and failure-mode-and-effects-analysis guided safety initiatives in radiation medicine. *Front Oncol*. 2013;3:305.)

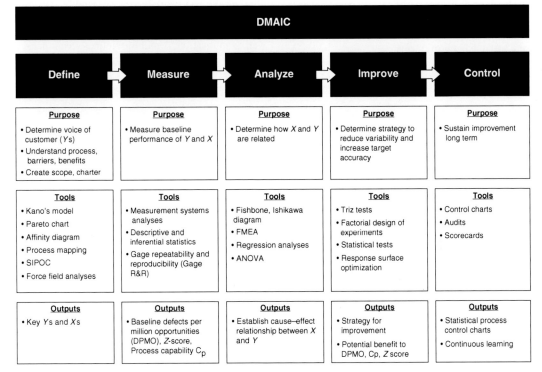

FIGURE 4.6 The five phases of DMAIC.

efficiently. The phases must be completed in the correct order, and all necessary steps within must be completed. Given that process measures described in the previous section tend to be used more often than outcomes measures, and that relevant data may be comparatively easier to access, DMAIC may potentially be used to address process-related problems for all six aims identified in the IOM framework. It has been used successfully in many health care settings (44) and more recently in radiation medicine with a focus on safety (53).

The purpose, possible tools to use, and relevant outputs of each of the phases are described in Figure 4.6

We illustrate the approach here with an example where there is a need to reduce the turnaround time between consultation appointments and treatment start dates (IOM aim: timeliness). In the define phase, CTQ or "Y" would be turnaround time. Process mapping and supplier–input–process–output–customer (SIPOC) tools (Figure 4.7) could be used to map the various steps (Xs) taken in between the two appointments. The scope could be limited to specific types of treatment sites, e.g., head and neck. In the measure phase, Ys and times for Xs could be potentially measured for a sample of patients by extracting data from the electronic medical records if available. The descriptive statistics tool could be used for baseline statistics (mean, standard deviation). Defect rates for the various Xs could be calculated on the basis of the number of slip days and hence the process sigma level. In the analyze phase, regression analysis could be used to identify which Xs take the most time and have higher variability, and reasons for that explored. Thus, in the improve phase, strategies to minimize variation and slip days could be developed and piloted, and defect rates and sigma levels recalculated. Statistical tests could be used to demonstrate improvements if any. Finally, in the control phase, control charts and audits could be maintained to ensure sustained improvements.

Lean Six Sigma and Kaizen

Whereas Six Sigma methodologies focus on reducing defects and process variability, Lean methodologies focus on improving performance by identifying and eliminating wasteful or non–value-added steps. Non–value-added steps reduce process efficiency and can potentially cause higher defect rates. Similarly, high defect rates can potentially add wasteful steps. Thus, Lean Six Sigma combines the two approaches to accomplish both goals by incorporating Lean tools within the DMAIC phases (44,94).

Although the potential for addressing difficult problems with Six Sigma or Lean Six Sigma approaches is high, time and resource allocation to these projects in a busy clinical practice may be challenging. An alternative, the kaizen approach (44), may be more practical to implement in the clinic, with a turnaround time of a week or so. Here, the focus is on creating a departmental mindset for continual improvement, fixing narrower-scope or smaller problems within the department instead of with multidisciplinary focus groups. The culture of continual small improvements by engaged staff members potentially culminates in greater productivity over the long term, as well as innovation. A multidisciplinary team maps out

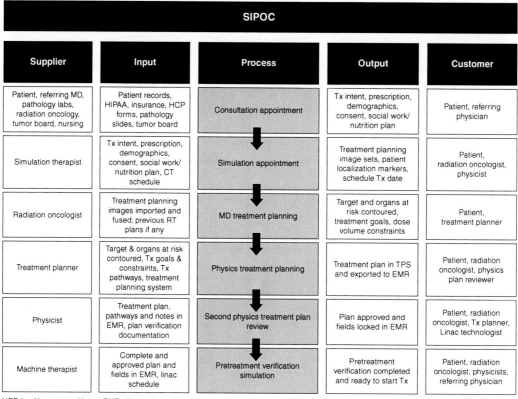

HCP, health care practitioner; EMR, electronic medical record; RT, radition therapy; TPS, treatment planning system; Tx, treatment

FIGURE 4.7 Sample SIPOC approach used in the define phase of DMAIC.

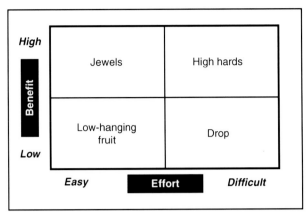

the process from the ground up. The process map is then evaluated by using value-stream mapping to identify steps that do not add value. In addition, wasteful activities are identified using the Muda tool (transport, inventory, motion, waiting, overproduction, overprocessing, defects) and then cast into a 2 × 2 matrix to segregate those that would require little effort to fix but that would yield high benefits (Figure 4.8). Improvement strategies are implemented, evaluated, and then sustained if successful. Usually, this approach leads to quick improvements, yet have statistical rigor. Such approaches have started to be used in radiation medicine (88,95,96).

SUMMARY

Systems engineering and Six Sigma methodologies have the potential to enhance quality in radiation medicine and serve as the foundation for enhancing outcomes across the board. While initial trends for the use of select approaches, such as QFD, RCA, FMEA, DMAIC, and Lean have demonstrated feasibility as well as success, the opportunity yet unexplored is vast. However, the principles for providing quality radiation medicine are not unique to any one facility; therefore, the process improvements achieved through the approaches discussed can be translated and incorporated by others, enhancing the value of the field.

REFERENCES

1. Kohn LT, Corrigan JM, Donaldson MS, eds. *To Err Is Human: Building a Safer Health System*. Washington, DC: Committee on Quality of Health Care in America, Institute of Medicine, National Academy Press; 2000:6.

2. Brennan TA, Leape LL, Laird NM, et al. Incidence of adverse events and negligence in hospitalized patients: results of the Harvard Medical Practice Study I. *N Engl J Med*. 1991;324(6):370–376.

3. Leape LL, Brennan TA, Laird NM, et al. The nature of adverse events in hospitalized patients: results of the Harvard Medical Practice Study II. *N Engl J Med*. 1991;324(6):377–384.

4. Reason J. Understanding adverse events: human factors. *Qual Health Care*. 1995;4:80–89.

5. Reason J. Achieving a safe culture: theory and practice. *Work & Stress*. 1998;12(3):293–306.

6. Reason J. Human error: models and management. *BMJ*. 2000;320:768–770.

7. Weick KE. Organizational culture as a source of high reliability. *Calif Management Rev*. 1987;29:112–127.

8. Weick KE, Sutcliffe KM, Obstfeld D. Organizing for high reliability: process of collective mindfulness. In: Sutton RS, Staw BM, eds. *Research in Organizational Behavior*. Stanford, CA: Jai Press; 1999:81–123.

9. van Beuzekom M, Boer F, Akerboom S, et al. Patient safety: latent risk factors. *Br J Anaesth*. 2010;105(1):52–59.

10. Marx D. Discipline: the role of rule violations. *Ground Effects*. 1996;2:1–4.

11. Perrow C. *Normal Accidents: Living With High-Risk Technologies*. Princeton, NJ: Princeton University Press; 1984.

12. Von Bertalanffy L. An outline of general systems theory. *British J Philos Sci*. 1950;1:134–165.

13. Rechtin E. *Systems Architecting: Creating and Building Complex Systems*. Englewood Cliffs, NJ: Prentice Hall; 1991.

14. Rivera AJ, Karsh BT. Human factors and systems engineering approach to patient safety for radiotherapy. *Int J Radiat Oncol Biol Phys*. 2008;71(Suppl 1):S174–S177.

15. Ablowitz R. The theory of emergence. *Philos Sci.* 1939;6(1):1–16.

16. Holland JH. Studying complex adaptive systems. *J Syst Sci Complexity.* 2006;19(1):1–8.

17. Karkuszewski ZP, Jarzynski C, Zurek WH. Quantum chaotic environments, the butterfly effect, and decoherence. *Phys Rev Lett.* 2002;89(17):170405.

18. Vogt PK, Hart JR, Yates JR III. A butterfly effect in cancer. *Mol Cell Oncol.* 2015;3(1):e1029063.

19. World Health Organization. *Radiotherapy Risk Profile.* Geneva, Switzerland: World Health Organization; 2008. www.who.int/patientsafety/activities/technical/radiotherapy_risk_profile.pdf.

20. Donaldson SR. *Towards Safer Radiotherapy.* London, UK: The Royal College of Radiologists; 2008.

21. International Atomic Energy Agency (IAEA). Lessons learned from accidents in radiotherapy. Vienna, Austria: IAEA, 2000. (Safety Reports Series 17).

22. Munro AJ. Hidden danger, obvious opportunity: error and risk in the management of cancer. *Br J Radiol.* 2007;80:955–966.

23. Bogdanich W. The radiation boom series: radiation offers new cures, and ways to do harm. *New York Times.* January 24, 2010:A1.

24. Bogdanich W. The radiation boom series: as technology surges, radiation safeguards lag. *New York Times.* January 27, 2010:A1.

25. Bogdanich W, Rebelo K. The radiation boom series: they check the medical equipment, but who is checking up on them? *New York Times.* January 27, 2010:A19.

26. Bogdanich W. Safety features planned for radiation machines. *New York Times.* June 10, 2010:A19.

27. Bogdanich W, Rebelo K. The radiation boom series: a pinpoint beam strays invisibly, harming instead of healing. *New York Times.* December 29, 2010:A1.

28. Garfinkel S. History's worst software bugs. *Wired News.* November 8, 2005.

29. Hawking S. I think the next century will be the century of complexity. *San José Mercury News, Morning Final Edition.* January 23, 2000.

30. Fraass BA, Lash KL, Matrone GM, et al. The impact of treatment complexity and computer-control delivery technology on treatment delivery errors. *Int J Radiat Oncol Biol Phys.* 1998;42:651–659.

31. Marks LB, Light KL, Hubbs JL, et al. The impact of advanced technologies on treatment deviations in radiation treatment delivery. *Int J Radiat Oncol Biol Phys.* 2007;69:1579–1586.

32. Amols HI. New technologies in radiation therapy: ensuring patient safety, radiation safety and regulatory issues in radiation oncology. *Health Phys.* 2008;95:658–665.

33. Ortiz LP, Cosset JM, Dunscombe O, et al. Preventing accidental exposures from new external beam radiation therapy technologies. *Ann ICRP.* 2009;39:1–86.

34. Petroski H. *To Engineer Is Human: The Role of Failure in Successful Design.* New York, NY: Vintage Books; 1992.

35. Haskins C, Forsberg K, Krueger M, et al. *Systems Engineering Handbook: A Guide for System Life Cycle Processes and Activities.* San Diego, CA: INCOSE; 2007.

36. Dhillon BS. *Medical Device Reliability and Associated Areas.* Boca Raton, FL: CRC Press; 2000.

37. Hughes TP. *Rescuing Prometheus.* New York, NY: Pantheon Books; 1998.

38. Chassin MR. Is health care ready for Six Sigma quality? *Milbank Q.* 1998;76:565–591.

39. Pande PS, Neuman RP, Cavanagh RR. *The Six Sigma Way: How GE, Motorola, and Other Top Companies Are Honing Their Performance.* 1st ed. New York, NY: McGraw-Hill Professional; 2001.

40. Hammer M. Process management and the future of Six Sigma. *MIT Sloan Manag Rev.* 2002:26–32.

41. Pyzdek T, Keller PA. *The Six Sigma Handbook.* Vol. 486. New York, NY: McGraw-Hill; 2003.

42. Harry MJ, Schroeder RR. Six Sigma: the breakthrough management strategy revolutionizing the world's top corporations. *Broadway Business.* 2005;1(1):43–50.

43. Guinane CS, Davis NH. The science of Six Sigma in hospitals. *Am Heart Hosp J.* 2004;2:42–48.

44. Trusko BE, Pexton C, Harrington J, et al. *Improving Healthcare Quality and Cost With Six Sigma.* 1st ed. Upper Saddle River, NJ: FT Press; 2007.

45. Corn JB. Six Sigma in health care. *Radiol Technol.* 2009;81:92–95.

46. Gamal AM. Six Sigma quality: a structured review and implications for future research. *Int J Qual Reliab Manag.* 2010;27(3):268–317.

47. DelliFraine JL, Langabeer JR II, Nembhard IM. Assessing the evidence of Six Sigma and Lean in the health care industry. *Qual Manag Health Care.* 2010;19:211–225.

48. Glasgow JM, Scott-Caziewell JR, Kaboli PJ. Guiding inpatient quality improvement: a systematic review of Lean and Six Sigma. *Jt Comm J Qual Patient Saf.* 2010;36:533–540.

49. Pawlicki T, Mundt AJ. Quality in radiation oncology. *Med Phys.* 2007;34:1529–1534.

50. Rath F. Tools for developing a quality management program: proactive tools (process mapping, value stream mapping, fault tree analysis and failure modes and effects analysis). *Int J Radiat Oncol Biol Phys.* 2008;71(Suppl 1):S187–S190.

51. Hendee WR, Herman MG. Improving patient safety in radiation oncology. *Med Phys.* 2011;38:78–82.

52. Marks LB, Jackson M, Xie L, et al. The challenge of maximizing safety in radiation oncology. *Pract Radiat Oncol.* 2011;1:2–14.

53. Kapur A, Potters L. Six Sigma tools for a patient safety-oriented, quality-checklist driven radiation medicine department. *Pract Radiat Oncol.* 2012;2:86–96.

54. Pawlicki T, Chera B, Ning T, et al. The systematic application of quality measures and process control in clinical radiation oncology. *Semin Radiat Oncol.* 2012;22(1):70–76.

55. Lohr KN, ed. *Medicare: A Strategy for Quality Assurance.* Washington, DC: National Academy Press; 1990.

56. Institute of Medicine. *Crossing the Quality Chasm: A New Health System for the 21st Century.* Washington, DC: National Academy Press; 2001.

57. Blumenthal D. Quality of care—what it is? *N Engl J Med.* 2006;335:891–894.

58. Ford EC, Santos LF, Pawlicki T, et al. Consensus recommendations for incident learning database structures in radiation oncology. *Med Phys.* 2012;39:7272–7290.

59. Institute of Medicine. *Performance Measurement: Accelerating Improvement.* Washington, DC: National Academy Press; 2005.

60. Brook RH, McGlynn EA, Cleary PD. Quality of health care, part 2: measuring quality of care. *N Engl J Med.* 1996;335:966–970.

61. Rubin HR, Pronovost P, Diette GB. From a process of care to a measure: the development and testing of a quality indicator. *Int J Qual Health Care.* 2001;13:489–496.

62. Hayman JA. Measuring the quality of care in radiation oncology. *Semin Radiat Oncol.* 2008;18:201–206.

63. Albert JM, Das P. Quality assessment in oncology. *Int J Radiat Oncol Biol Phys.* 2012;83:773–781.

64. Donabedian A. Evaluating the quality of medical care [reprinted from the *Milbank Memorial Fund Q* 1966;44(3):166–203]. *Milbank Memorial Fund Q.* 1996;44:166–206.

65. Donabedian A. *Explorations in Quality Assessment and Monitoring.* Vols. I–III. Ann Arbor, MI: Health Administration Press; 1985.

66. Donabedian A. The quality of care: how can it be assessed? *JAMA.* 1988;260:1743–1748.

67. Donaldson H, Cao J, French J, et al. Quality standards in radiation medicine. *Pract Radiat Oncol.* 2014;4(4):208–214.

68. Ohri N, Shen X, Dicker AP, et al. Radiotherapy protocol deviations and clinical outcomes: a meta-analysis of cooperative group clinical trials. *J Natl Cancer Inst.* 2013;105:387–393.

69. Earle CC, Emanuel EJ. Patterns of care studies: creating "an environment of watchful concern." *J Clin Oncol.* 2003;21(24):4479–4480.

70. Palta JR, Efstathiou JA, Bekelman JE, et al. Developing a national radiation oncology registry: from acorns to oaks. *Practical Radiat Oncol.* 2012;2(1):10–17.

71. Leape LL. Reporting of adverse events. *N Engl J Med.* 2002;347(20):1633–1638.

72. American Society for Radiation Oncology. *RO-ILS: Radiation Oncology Incident Learning System.* Reston, VA: American Society for Radiation Oncology; 2014.

73. Hoopes DJ, Dicker AP, Eads NL, et al. RO-ILS: Radiation Oncology Incident Learning System: a report from the first year of experience. *Pract Radiat Oncol.* 2015;5(5):312–318.

74. Tamuz M, Harrison MI. Improving patient safety in hospitals: contributions of high-reliability theory and normal accident theory. *Health Serv Res.* 2006;41(4, Pt 2):1654–1676.

75. Mallon B. *Ernest Amory Codman: The End Result of a Life in Medicine.* Philadelphia, PA: WB Saunders; 2000.

76. Codman EA. *A Study in Hospital Efficiency.* Oakbrook Terrace, IL: Joint Commission on Accreditation of Healthcare Organizations Press; 1996.

77. Walton M. *The Deming Management Method.* New York, NY: Prentice Hall; 1972.

78. Deming WE. *Out of the Crisis, Massachusetts Institute of Technology.* Cambridge, MA: Center for Advanced Engineering Study; 1986:510.

79. Deming WE. *The New Economics for Industry, Government, Education.* 2nd ed. Cambridge, MA: MIT Press; 2000.

80. Shewhart WA, Deming WE. In memoriam: Walter A. Shewhart, 1891–1967. *Am Stat.* 1967;21(2):39–40.

81. Bacon F. *The New Organon.* In: Anderson F, ed. The library of the liberal arts Indianapolis & New York: Bobbs-Merrill, 1960.

82. Landrigan CP, Parry GJ, Bones CB, et al. Temporal trends in rates of patient harm resulting from medical care. *N Engl J Med.* 2010;363:2124–2134.

83. Classen DC, Resar R, Griffin F, et al. "Global trigger tool" shows that adverse events in hospitals may be ten times greater than previously measured. *Health Aff (Millwood).* 2011;30:581–589.

84. Shojania KG, Thomas EJ. Trends in adverse events over time: why are we not improving? *BMJ Qual Safety*. 2013;22(4):273–277.

85. Akao Y. Development history of quality function deployment. In: Mizuno S, Akao Y, eds. *QFD, the Customer-Driven Approach to Quality Planning and Deployment*. 1st ed. Tokyo, Japan: Asian Productivity Organization; 1994:339–351.

86. Gremyr I, Raharjo H. Quality function deployment in healthcare: a literature review and case study. *Int J Health Care Qual Assur*. 2013;26(2):135–146.

87. Moores BM. Radiation safety management in health care—the application of quality function deployment. *Radiography*. 2006;12(4):291–304.

88. Bonilla C, Pawlicki T, Perry L, et al. Radiation oncology Lean Six Sigma project selection based on patient and staff input into a modified quality function deployment. *Int J Six Sigma and Competitive Advantage*. 2008;4(3):196–208.

89. Senders JW. FMEA and RCA: the mantras of modern risk management. *Qual Saf Health Care*. 2004;13:249–250.

90. Kapur A, Goode G, Riehl C, et al. Incident learning and failure-mode-and-effects-analysis guided safety initiatives in radiation medicine. *Front Oncol*. 2013;3:305.

91. Ishikawa K, Ishikawa K. *Guide to Quality Control*. Vol. 2. Tokyo, Japan: Asian Productivity Organization; 1982.

92. Ford EC, Gaudette R, Myers L, et al. Evaluation of safety in a radiation oncology setting using failure mode and effects analysis. *Int J Radiat Oncol Biol Phys*. 2009;74:852–858.

93. Huq MS, Fraass BA, Dunscombe PB, et al. A method for evaluating quality assurance needs in radiation therapy. *Int J Radiat Oncol Biol Phys*. 2008;71(suppl 1):S170–S173.

94. George ML. Lean Six Sigma: combining Six Sigma quality with Lean production speed. New York, NY: McGraw-Hill Education; 2002.

95. Kim CS, Hayman JA, Billi JE, et al. The application of Lean thinking to the care of patients with bone and brain metastasis with radiation therapy. *J Oncol Pract*. 2007;3(4):189–193.

96. Kapur A, Riebling N, Galli BJ, et al. Streamlining the head and neck treatment process in radiation medicine using a kaizen approach. *Int J Radiat Onc Biol Phys*. 2012;84(3, Suppl):S151.

5 | Error Prevention and Risk Management

Suzanne B. Evans and Derek Brown

INTRODUCTION

This chapter discusses the nature of error, the classification of error, concepts in quality management, types of error mitigation, hierarchy of interventions, and the role of culture in error prevention.

PSYCHOLOGY OF ERROR: UNDERSTANDING OUR INHERENT BIASES

An exploration of the psychology of error is useful, as it provides context and insight that can help us understand the causes of error and develop functional error mitigation strategies.

The way we look at the world is often not rational. Our impressions are largely guided by heuristics, or "rules of thumb," as to how the world usually works. Psychologists have proposed a dual system processing theory for thought (1,2). There are many different modifications and permutations of this theory, but they all center on a similar basic concept: the belief that there is one mode of thinking in which a person is carefully considering the information in front of him or her, and making a rational judgment based on the information at hand. In the other mode of thinking, one is not thinking deliberately, and mental shortcuts are used to make snap judgments about a situation. These modes have been called systems 1 and 2 (2), central and peripheral (1), or slow and fast thinking (3), respectively. Clearly, the process of "fast thinking" leaves the individual much more prone to error; however, it is argued that this is the predominant mode of how we process interactions in our daily lives.

While we cannot remove ourselves from the tendencies and biases that we are subject to, it is helpful for all members in the department of radiation therapy to understand that these sorts of cognitive processes are not aberrant, but rather a natural part of human interactions. Therefore, the strategies for error mitigation include awareness of biases we are subject to, as well as avoiding error mitigation strategies that include the elimination of these biases, as this is impossible. An appreciation for the ubiquity of bias in medicine will aid in the understanding of how errors can occur. Consider, if you will, the following biases, along with examples of how they might be evident in radiation oncology.

Confirmation bias

This is the tendency to believe, seek out, and interpret information that supports one's own preconceptions (4). This is similar to myside bias (5). For instance, a clinical example of this is a patient who arrives with a diagnosis of metastatic breast cancer and known bony metastases. She reports early satiety, intermittent fever, weight loss, and night sweats. Imaging reveals a large amount of axillary, supraclavicular, inguinal, and also periportal adenopathy. Her endocrine therapy is adjusted, and for 2 months there is progression. A biopsy is performed, and later diffuse large B-cell lymphoma is diagnosed. Another example is a physicist trying to troubleshoot a pretreatment quality assurance (QA) of an intensity-modulated radiation therapy (IMRT) plan that is off by more than 5%. The physicist may attribute this discrepancy to poor QA equipment setup, incorrect normalization of the verification plan, or poor choice of measurement location, when, in fact, there is a mechanical problem with the linac and the plan is not being delivered correctly.

Availability bias

This is the tendency to overestimate the occurrence of events that are known to the individual. Events may be more "available" depending on how unusual or emotionally charged they are (6). An example of this in radiation oncology is a treatment team that traumatically lost a patient to aortic dissection on the treatment table after the patient complained of chest pain and was hypotensive. The next patient who comes in with chest pain and hypotension is sent to the emergency department for a workup rather than treated for his radiation esophagitis and dehydration. Additionally, one can witness admitting inpatient teams "running specials" on a given disease process, as they are admitting multiple people with the same "available" diagnosis.

Ambiguity effect

The tendency to avoid choices for which information is missing makes the probability of a given effect seem "unknown" (7). For instance, a radiation oncology team is faced with a choice of two boards for prone positioning. After a detailed physics evaluation showing the two to be equivalent, the team decides to go with the more expensive, better-known company rather than the cost-effective start-up, whose service record is "unknown."

Sunk cost fallacy (also known as irrational escalation)

This occurs when individuals continue with a poor decision, based on a perceived prior amount of work already invested in that decision (8). A clinical example might be a radiation oncologist and dosimetrist who have spent many hours planning a treatment for IMRT to the head and neck, whose plan has already undergone quality assurance by the physicist. At chart rounds, peer review suggests that an additional lymph node basin should be included. The radiation oncologist decides not to include this nodal basin based on sunk cost fallacy.

Inattentional blindness

This is the phenomenon of items in plain sight remaining invisible to the viewers because they are not looking for these items or expecting to find them (9). An example of this is a very large thyroid mass being overlooked on a CT simulation for breast cancer, as the radiation oncologist is focused on definition of the lumpectomy cavity, the field design, and the heart and lung contours. Another example of this is a physicist checking a treatment plan, paying very close attention to doses to organs at risk and planning target volume coverage, but missing a 150% hotspot in unsegmented normal tissue.

Outcome bias

This is the tendency to judge a decision or action by its eventual outcome, rather than the quality of the decision at the time it was made (10). An example in radiation oncology might be regretting a decision to install an orthovoltage machine in a clinic seeing a tremendous amount of skin cancer, once reimbursement for orthovoltage treatments plummets.

Intervention bias

This describes the tendency of the treatment team (and sometimes the patient or family) to prefer intervention, whether it is with drugs, diagnostic tests, noninvasive procedures, or surgeries, when supportive care would be a reasonable alternative (11). A common example in radiation therapy is the preference of the medical team (and often the patient) to perform palliative radiation treatment on a patient with a massive burden of disease when it is unlikely to be of benefit, and the patient is clearly at the end of life. An additional example is an incident of minor severity and low occurrence frequency prompting institution of a lengthy therapy checklist to prevent its reoccurrence, out of an intrinsic preference for action.

Counterfactual thinking

This is the tendency of individuals to create alternative, imaginative outcomes after the actual outcome is known but has an undesirable result (12,13). An example in radiation oncology is a decision to treat an apical lung tumor at the high end or low end of acceptable doses. Out of concern for the brachial plexus and lung doses, the radiation oncologist elects to treat at the lower end of the acceptable dose. The patient subsequently suffers a local recurrence. The radiation oncologist spends significant time imagining a choice for a higher dose, imagining cure rather than serious radiation pneumonitis or brachial plexopathy.

Cognitive dissonance

This refers to the mental anxiety experienced by an individual who holds several contradictory beliefs or values at the same time, or is faced with new information that contradicts existing beliefs or values (14,15). An example in radiation oncology might be the treatment team who consider themselves exceptionally careful, yet make a catastrophic error in treatment. It is this sort of affront to one's positive self-concept that makes errors so challenging to recognize and admit.

Situational awareness

This refers to the ability of individuals to process what is happening around them in order to inform decision making (16). Loss of situational awareness may also be colloquially termed "losing the forest for the trees." Consider the tragic situation of Elaine Bromiley, a 37-year-old mother of two, who was admitted for an elective endoscopic sinus surgery and septoplasty (17). She suffered hypoxic brain damage, ultimately fatal, during the induction of general anesthesia, largely because of loss of situational awareness by the physician team. They were unable to intubate or ventilate her—a situation that calls for emergency tracheostomy—but they were caught up in the tasks of repeated attempts to intubate or ventilate her, ignoring the passage of time with profound hypoxia.

As evidenced by the preceding examples of bias, it is clear that the process of information processing and cognitive reasoning is quite complex, and subject to many biases even under the best conditions. But, as the later sections explore, the best conditions are not always present, and error can result.

CLASSIFICATIONS OF ERROR: HUMAN FACTORS ANALYSIS AND CLASSIFICATION SYSTEM

The accurate and timely classification of error forms the backbone of retrospective quality and safety improvement efforts and is the basis for prospective error mitigation strategies. Error classification also enables aggregate trending over time and comparisons across departments and institutions—both valuable tools in the effort to improve quality and safety.

Historically, when an incident occurs in the health care environment, teams of experts use root cause analysis (RCA) to classify the incident and to determine the underlying, root causes. More recently, a classification system based on Reason's error categorization, Human Factors Analysis

and Classification System (HFACS), has been demonstrated to improve standardization of error classification, increase the specificity of error classification, and facilitate the development of actionable corrective plans (18).

Before we discuss HFACS in more detail, it is useful to describe several other error categorization schemes that can be used in addition to those presented in HFACS. Errors can be classified as *sporadic*, where the same incident is unlikely to occur again in the same process step or under the same conditions; or *systematic*, where, given the same conditions, the same error is likely to occur again. Errors can also be classified as "active" and "latent" (19). Active errors occur at the point of contact between a human and some aspect of a larger system. Latent errors are less apparent failures of organization or design that contributed to the occurrence of errors. As we examine HFACS, we will attempt to identify error categories as either systematic/sporadic or active/latent.

The HFACS methodology, originally designed for use within the U.S. Navy and Marine Corps to identify common root causes among aviation-related accidents, looks at an incident from the perspective of Reason's four

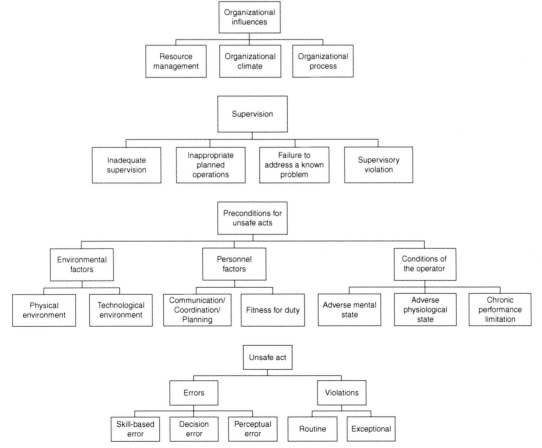

FIGURE 5.1 Human Factors Analysis and Classification System (HFACS) framework. (*Source*: From Ref. (18). Diller T, Helmrich G, Dunning S, et al. The Human Factors Analysis Classification System (HFACS) applied to health care. *Am J Med Qual.* 2014;29(3):181–190, with permission.)

levels of error causation: (a) Unsafe Act, (b) Preconditions for Unsafe Acts, (c) supervision, and (d) organizational influences (20,21). Each level contains several causal categories that act as bins for "nanocodes," which are similar to the root causes used in a RCA. Figure 5.1 shows the HFACS framework.

Because errors and violations are associated with human performance, it is worthwhile considering the performance categories that individuals are working in when the error occurs. Rasmussen defined three human performance categories: (a) skill-based, (b) rule-based, and (c) knowledge-based (22). Skill-based activities are typically straightforward routine tasks that have been performed for some time. Rule-based activities are more complex or critical tasks that may be only occasionally performed, and error results from improper application of a rule or a plan. Knowledge-based activities deal with unfamiliar and/or unprepared-for tasks, and the intended outcome may not be achieved because of a knowledge deficit. Unsafe acts are therefore categorized into errors (skill-based, perceptual, decision) and violations. Errors represent normal accepted behavior that fails to meet the desired outcome, whereas violations are the result of intentional departures from accepted practice. A decision error occurs when information, knowledge, or experience is lacking, whereas skill-based errors occur because of inattention or memory failure. A perceptual error occurs when sensory input is somehow unintelligible or unusual. Because unsafe acts occur while the individual is performing the task, these are typically seen as active errors, and depending on whether the error is skill-based, decision, or perception, unsafe acts can be categorized as either sporadic or systematic.

Preconditions for Unsafe Acts refer to causal factors, such as the work environment and conditions that existed at the time of the incident. These include environmental factors, personnel factors, and the conditions of the operator. Environmental factors include both the physical environment and the technological environment. Personnel factors relate to how people work together and communicate with one another. The *conditions of the operator* describe situations in which the person performing the task is either distracted or incapable of performing the task. Preconditions for Unsafe Acts may be either active or latent, depending on whether the causal factor related to the condition of the operator or environmental factors, and are more likely to be categorized as systematic when similar conditions would likely result in the same error.

The supervision category outlines factors that relate to leadership and administration and how these may have played a role in the incident. There are four subtypes in this category: leadership (provision of inadequate training, guidance, or oversight), operational planning (scheduling and the assignment of work), failure to correct known problems, and supervisory ethics (permitting individuals to perform work outside of their scope). Supervisory

factors are latent errors because these factors are typically "once removed" from the incident, and are likely to be systematic because similar conditions would likely result in the same error.

Organizational influences describe factors such as resource management and organizational culture that can directly affect supervisors and also contribute to incidents. The three subtypes in this category are resource management (allocation of human resources and equipment budgets), organizational climate (culture), and operational processes (high-level policies and procedures). Organizational influences, like supervision factors, are considered latent, systematic errors.

For further consideration, in an alternative but similar methodology, the Health Care Performance Initiative has further classified failure modes into individual or system failures. It divides individual failure modes into five categories: those related to competency, consciousness, communication, critical thinking, or compliance (23). Table 5.1 lists these in further detail. It divides system failure modes into five categories as well: those related to structure, culture, process, policy and protocol, or technology and environment (23). Table 5.2 lists these in further detail.

CONCEPTS IN QUALITY MANAGEMENT

Much like Socrates, to whom is attributed the quote that "The unexamined life is not worth living," one might say that failure to examine one's department for quality measures decreases the possibility that a quality department might exist. Without understanding one's event rates, one cannot understand whether small improvements or major overhauls are required. Several theories about the ideal strategy for this analysis, which will be explored now.

Dr. W. Edwards Deming (24) initially spoke about this process in regard to the Shewhart cycle (25): design the product, make the product, test the product through market research, and then redesign the product. From this came the Deming cycle, which espouses the principles "plan, do, study, act" (PDSA). The planning phase encompasses identification of areas for improvement, and identification of changes required. The "do" phase is for implementation. The study phase is for measurement of the success of the process or the outcome measure. The "act" phase refers to the need to make further changes based on those results. The intent with this system is that it is viewed as a cycle that is never completed, leading to continuous quality improvement, or continuous process improvement. This principle is applied to the optimization of medical processes for the purposes of increasing quality of care and increasing patient safety. It is important to note that the "check" or "study" piece of this process means that routine audits will have to be performed in order to measure progress or identify interventions that were less effective than hoped.

Table 5.1 Taxonomy of Individual Failure Modes

Competency (Knowl-edge and Skills)	Consciousness (Attention)	Communication (and Information Processing)	Critical Thinking (Cognition)	Compliance (Motivation)
Unformed skills/ habits (inability to do something well; while possessing knowledge, lacks performance reli-ability gained through experience)	Inattention (preoc-cupied; rushing or hurrying; not paying attention)	Incorrect assump-tion (assuming a thing to be true or correct that was in fact wrong)	Situational awareness (unawareness or lack-ing knowledge of what is going on; failure to perceive that acts or conditions deviated from desired path)	Indifference (in-adequate care or attention to people or things of respon-sibility; careless-ness, informality, or casual attitude, yet with no deliberate intention to cause harm)
Normalized deviance (conforming to an individual's standard, type, or custom, where behavior is sharply different from the generally accepted standard)	Distraction (divided or diverted attention)	Misinterpretation (forming an un-derstanding that is not correct from something that is said or done)	Failure to validate/ verify (failure to find or test the truth of something; failure in the cognitive process of establishing a valid proof)	Shortcut (deliber-ate, conscious act to take a quicker or more direct route—a route that deviates from the designated or opti-mal path)
Inadequate knowledge (lacks fundamental knowledge-in-the-head of operating proce-dures or principles, or knowledge of available protocols)	Habit intrusion or reflex (act performed without conscious thought; a settled or regular tendency or practice)	Information overload (overbur-dened with too much sensory or cognitive input or information)	Mindset (primed or biased by pattern or preconceived notion; a fixed mental attitude or disposition that pre-determines a person's response to interpreta-tions or situations)	Overconfident (ex-cessively confident or presumptuous; failure to stop when questions arise; proceeding in the face of uncertainty)
	Spatial disorientation (feeling lost or con-fused, especially with respect to direction or position; confused because of mislead-ing information)		Tunnel vision (the tendency to focus exclusively on a single or limited objective or view; overly focused on details of task; failure to see the big picture)	Reckless (acting without thought or care for the conse-quences of one's acts; acting overtly with full knowledge that an act could cause harm)
	Bored, fatigued, or unfit for duty (feeling weary; extreme tired-ness because one is unoccupied; has no interest because of physical or mental activity or external influence)			
	Lapse (a momentary fault or failure in behavior; inadequate mental tracking; in-advertently forgot to complete something)			

Source: Adapted from Ref. (23). Tjia I, Rampersad S, Varughese A, et al. Wake up safe and root cause analysis: quality improvement in pediatric anesthesia. *Anesth Analg*. 2014;119(1):122–136. Adapted with permission from HPI.

Table 5.2 Taxonomy of System Failure Modes

Structure	Culture	Process	Policy and Protocol	Technology and Environment
Structure model (wrong model, incompatible missions)	Inadequate vision or mission (lacking or poorly executed mission)	Omitted actions (key activity is missing or incomplete)	Lacking or informal (no policy or protocol)	Input/output (visual display, alarms, control configuration)
Inadequate structure (span of control, levels of leadership, leveraging positions and experience)	Noncollaboration (disruptive competition, defensiveness, poor teamwork, low morale)	Excessive actions (contains low-value activities)	Usability (poor presentation or information depiction, low credibility, poor access)	Human capability (symbols, codes, anthropometry, devices, human control, physical work)
Inadequate job function (overlap or gaps in roles, responsibilities, or expectations)	Operational leadership (lacking or inadequate command, prioritization, or assignment in response to emergent or emerging issues)	Poorly sequenced (poor flow, excessive branching of work process activities)	Understandability (difficult to comprehend because guidance detail is lacking or inadequate for the knowledge and skill level of the user)	Arrangement (physical arrangement of work space, department, facility, or campus negatively impacting performance)
Resource allocation (insufficient infrastructure, people, budget, equipment, or other resources)	High-reliability environment (setting does not incorporate error prevention expectations and focus including competency, consciousness, critical thinking, communication, compliance)	Inadequate interface (lack of or poorly designed handoffs of information, resources, or products)	Knowledge in environment (inadequate or underutilized job aids, forcing functions)	Environment (lighting, noise, climate, motion negatively impacting performance)
Collaboration mechanisms (wrong or inadequate collaboration mechanisms)		Inadequate checks (lack of or poorly designed checks, inspections, or reviews)		

Source: Adapted from Ref. (23). Tjia I, Rampersad S, Varughese A, et al. Wake up safe and root cause analysis: quality improvement in pediatric anesthesia. *Anesth Analg*. 2014;119(1):122–136. Adapted with permission from HPI.

As part of this attitude toward continuous improvement, the department is encouraged to adopt the practice of systems thinking (26). This refers to an analytic focus on the systems and complex interplays involved in the delivery of health care, rather than on individual error. This thinking paradigm seeks the systems approach solution to what is nearly always a multifactorial problem. This can be quite challenging, as there has always been an emphasis in health care on individual training and individual responsibility. However, the practice of blame and shame is counter to patient safety, as it inhibits future incident reporting and damages safety culture.

When looking at a quality management system, it is also useful to consider the International Organization for Standardization (ISO) 9000 and Six Sigma approaches. The concept of sigma is a metric that indicates how well a given process is performing (27,28). If the value of sigma

is high, then the performance quality of the process is also high. Essentially, sigma measures the ability of a process to result in defect-free work, with patient dissatisfaction considered a defect. "Six Sigma" refers to the concept that product defects (or error) would occur at a rate of six standard deviations away from being a matter of chance (29). Part of this process is the cycle "design, measure, analyze, improve, control" (DMAIC), which is similar to PDSA; however, it contains the additional step of control. *Control* refers to sustaining gains made through quality improvement. Part of the Six Sigma process is the generation of fishbone diagrams, in which the causes of a certain event are identified for later remediation. ISO 9000 is another quality management approach that is based on the principles of customer focus, leadership, involvement of people, process approach, systems approach to management, continual improvement, factual approach to decision making, and mutually beneficial supplier relationships (30). Criticisms of both ISO 9000 and Six Sigma (31) include the large time and financial investments required for their implementation.

The final approach mentioned here for quality management is the practice of peer review. There is no question that the practice within radiation oncology of reviewing cases on a routine basis with one's peers is somewhat exceptional in medicine. This is partially because of the tangible work product in radiation oncology—the treatment plan, which lends itself to review, unlike the surgical technique or diagnostic acumen, which is much more challenging to review for each and every patient treated, and certainly is less easy to adjust midstream. Peer review is an integral part of QA (32,33), and has been shown to result in changes in management in a nontrivial percentage of patients (34,35). Readers are directed to the guidance from the American Society for Radiation Oncology (ASTRO) on this subject for a detailed treatise on the components of peer review (36).

TYPES OF ERROR MITIGATION— PROACTIVE MITIGATION STRATEGIES AND RETROSPECTIVE CORRECTIVE ACTIONS

Whether in response to an incident or as part of a quality improvement project, the development of effective error mitigation strategies is unquestionably important. This is where the "rubber meets the road." You have done your prospective analysis, your RCA, or, better yet, your HFACS. You have figured out where the problems are and all the different pathways and factors that contributed, or could have contributed, to an incident. Now it is time to design, or redesign, a process, modifying or including new steps that will reduce the likelihood that an incident will occur.

Where do you turn for ideas? How would you know whether the newly implemented strategy will be effective? What about communicating the plan to everybody in your department? These are important questions, and if they are not adequately addressed, your error mitigation strategy is more likely to fail. In what follows we offer a brief, prescriptive approach to the development and implementation of error mitigation strategies.

Once you know where the problems are, the *first step* is to brainstorm potentially useful error mitigation strategies. The Hierarchy of Interventions can be useful in providing guidance on what broad type of error mitigation strategy might be appropriate (37). Another option is to see what others have done and then adapt this to your specific clinical situation. Sutlief (38) has performed an extensive review of 11 sources that describe more than 1,000 incidents and corrective actions . The relative distribution of corrective actions is shown in Figure 5.2. The safety barrier category includes corrective actions such as additional QA steps and checklists/time-outs.

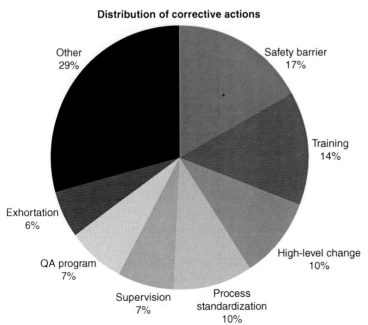

Distribution of corrective actions

- Other 29%
- Safety barrier 17%
- Training 14%
- High-level change 10%
- Process standardization 10%
- Supervision 7%
- QA program 7%
- Exhortation 6%

FIGURE 5.2 Relative frequency of corrective actions used—analysis of more than 1,000 reported incidents and corrective actions. (*Source*: Adapted from Ref. (38). Sutlief S, Brown D. Taxonomy of corrective actions in radiotherapy. *Med Phys*. 2014;41(6):433.) With permission.

Once you have decided on your error mitigation strategy, the *second step* is to implement it safely and effectively. Safe implementation involves: (a) making sure that the error mitigation strategy will actually address the problems you have identified and (b) ensuring that you do not make things worse by creating negative downstream effects. One way to do this is to redo the analysis that found the problems with the new error mitigation strategy in place. Another is to test the error mitigation strategy in a mock setting. This is a great way to see whether it actually works and will help significantly in elucidating any potential negative downstream effects.

Effective implementation involves: (a) generating buy-in from colleagues who are directly impacted and (b) understanding corrective actions as behavior changes. Generating buy-in is incredibly important, and is largely dependent on good communication. Some strategies for generating buy-in include involving as many stakeholders in the process as possible, communicating to individuals and groups through conversations and presentations, and valuing and acting on feedback from your colleagues. Some strategies for promoting behavior change are practice rehearsal (discussed earlier), the use of clinical guidelines and care maps, and the inclusion of reminders—checklists or time-outs—that improve compliance with new processes (39).

The *third step* is to realize that the error mitigation strategy that you have developed will very likely have to be modified once it is implemented system-wide. You should continually seek feedback and be open to adjusting the error mitigation strategy as necessary.

HIERARCHY OF INTERVENTIONS

The Hierarchy of Interventions provides a structured evaluation of the effectiveness of different broad types of error mitigation strategies. Vaida, working at the Institute for Safe Medication Practices, first developed the hierarchy in 1999, and Woods et al presented a modified version in 2008 (37,40). In the order of most effective to least effective, the Hierarchy of Interventions is presented as follows: (a) forcing functions; (b) automation, computerization, and technology; (c) standardization and protocols; (d) staffing organization; (e) policies, rules, and expectations; (f) checklists and double-checks; (h) risk assessment and communication error; (i) education and information; and (j) personal initiative—vigilance. This hierarchy is often represented as a pyramid, as in Figure 5.3.

It is potentially illustrative to categorize the most commonly cited corrective actions, presented in section IV based on the Hierarchy of Interventions. Table 5.3 presents this categorization.

Interestingly, none of the most commonly cited corrective actions fall into either of the two most effective intervention categories: "Forcing functions" and "Automation,

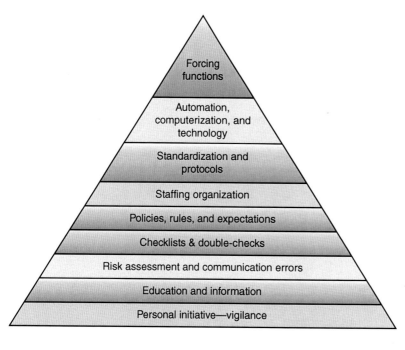

FIGURE 5.3 Hierarchy of interventions. (*Source:* Adapted from Ref. (40). Woods DM, Holl JL, Angst D, et al. Improving clinical communication and patient safety: clinician-recommended solutions. In: Henriksen K, Battles JB, Keyes MA, et al, eds. *Advances in Patient Safety: New Directions and Alternative Approaches.* Rockville, MD: Agency for Healthcare Research and Quality (US); 2008. *Performance and Tools; vol 3.*) With permission.

Table 5.3 Categorization of Most Commonly Cited Corrective Actions Based on the Hierarchy of Interventions

Hierarchy of Interventions	Corrective Actions
1. Forcing functions	
2. Automation, computerization, and technology	
3. Standardization and protocols	Process standardization
4. Staffing organization	High-level change
5. Policies, rules, and expectations	Supervision
6. Checklists & double-checks	QA program/safety barrier
7. Risk assessment and communication errors	
8. Education and information	Training
9. Personal initiative—vigilance	Exhortation

computerization, and technology." This omission is likely because technology in radiation oncology clinical practice is largely controlled by vendors, making clinic-specific implementation of forcing functions and automation extremely difficult. Also interesting is the observation that the two most commonly cited corrective actions—"safety barriers" and "training"—fall near the bottom of the hierarchy. Although training is categorized as not being very effective, it is possible that training should be split into two groups: (a) retraining staff who are already competent but who nonetheless made an error—likely not very effective; and (b) providing baseline clinical training to staff who never received it, were not competent, and made an error—potentially extremely effective.

THE ROLE OF CULTURE IN ERROR PREVENTION

A strong safety culture is essential to patient safety. Nebulous and difficult to change, safety culture can play a significant role in the instigation and resulting investigation of errors. Dekker (41) defined *safety culture* as "a culture that allows the boss to hear bad news." The Nuclear Regulatory Commission defines three levels of safety culture: (a) leadership, (b) management, and (c) individual (42). Leadership should show commitment to safety in their decisions and behaviors. Management should implement processes with an eye to safety, be open to identifying and finding resolutions to problems, and promote an environment that allows employees to raise concerns. Individuals should take personal accountability for maintaining professionalism by using safe practices, creating a respectful learning environment, and demonstrating a commitment to continuous learning.

At a more practical level, an unfortunate reality is that team members experience burnout, with subsequent erosion of their professionalism (43,44). The term in medicine is the *disruptive individual:* the team member who exhibits derogatory, hypercritical, aggressive, or angry responses in the workplace. This disruptive behavior impacts patient safety in a negative fashion (45). While some individuals display inappropriate behavior as a response to fatigue, stress, or burnout, it is nonetheless essential that the institution or clinic does not tolerate this behavior. There is an emerging realization that there has to be a dedicated effort to promote professionalism by the institution (46). The Brigham model (46) approaches this from the frame that support is needed for the clinician, and a tiered approach to interventions is followed to help individuals correct their negative behavior pattern. This starts with an awareness of how actions were perceived, with an emphasis on helping these persons understand the *impact* of their intentions, while recognizing that their *intent* was sometimes radically different. Although many of the efforts are best developed at the physician level, these principles should be followed for the whole team. Physicians are called upon to lead by example (47), and while a formalized professionalism initiative may be outside the reach of many clinics, at the very least, leadership should exhibit exemplary professionalism.

SUMMARY

An effective quality management program depends on a robust understanding of error, appropriate classification of error, the application of a systems approach to problem solving, the careful choice and implementation of error mitigation strategies, and a commitment to continuous improvement. With a lot of hard work and ingenuity, clinics can be made safer.

REFERENCES

1. Petty R, Cacioppo J. The elaboration likelihood model of persuasion. *Adv Exp Soc Psychol.* 1986;19:123–181.

2. Stanovich KE, West RF. Individual difference in reasoning: implications for the rationality debate? *Behav Brain Sci.* 2000;23:645–726.

3. Stanovich KE, West RF, Toplak ME. Myside bias, rational thinking, and intelligence. *Curr Dir Psychol Sci.* 2013;22:259–264.

4. Kahneman D. *Thinking, Fast and Slow.* 1st ed. New York, NY: Farrar, Straus & Giroux; 2011.

5. Oswald ME, Grosjean S. Confirmation bias. In: Pohl RF, ed. *Cognitive Illusions: A Handbook on Fallacies and Biases in Thinking, Judgement and Memory.* Hove, UK: Psychology Press; 2004:79–96.

6. Schwarz N, Bless H, Strack F, et al. Ease of retrieval as information: another look at the availability heuristic. *J Pers Soc Psychol.* 1991;61(2):195–202.

7. Baron J. *Thinking and Deciding.* 2nd ed. Cambridge, UK: Cambridge University Press; 1994.

8. Arkes R, Ayton P. The sunk cost and Concorde effects: are humans less rational than lower animals? *Psychol Bull.* 1999;125:591–600.

9. Mack A, Rock I. *Inattentional Blindness.* Cambridge, MA: MIT Press; 1998.

10. Petrocelli J. Pitfalls of counterfactual thinking in medical practice: preventing errors by using more functional reference points. *J Public Health Res.* 2013;2(3):e24.

11. Foy AJ, Filippone EJ. The case for intervention bias in the practice of medicine. *Yale J Biol Med.* 2013;86(2):271–280.

12. Kahneman D, Tversky A. The simulation heuristic. In: Kahneman D, Slovic P, Tversky A, eds. *Judgment Under Uncertainty: Heuristics and Biases.* New York, NY: Cambridge University Press; 1982:201–208.

13. Roese NJ, Olson JM. Counterfactual thinking: a critical overview. In: Roese NJ, Olson JM, eds. *What Might Have Been: The Social Psychology of Counterfactual Thinking.* Hillsdale, MI: Lawrence Erlbaum Associates; 1995:1–55.

14. Festinger L. *A Theory of Cognitive Dissonance.* Redwood City, CA: Stanford University Press; 1957.

15. Festinger L. Cognitive dissonance. *Sci Am.* 1962;207(4):93–107.

16. Endsley MR. Toward a theory of situation awareness in dynamic systems. *Hum Factors.* 1995;37(1):32–64.

17. Kamensky J. The power of Elaine's story: a personal reflection. *J Perioper Pract.* 2014;24(3):50–55.

18. Diller T, Helmrich G, Dunning S, et al. The Human Factors Analysis Classification System (HFACS) applied to health care. *Am J Med Qual.* 2014;29(3):181–190.

19. Reason J. Human error: models and management. *BMJ.* 2000;320(7237):768–770.

20. Wiegmann DA, Shappell SA. Human error analysis of commercial aviation accidents: application of the Human Factors Analysis and Classification System (HFACS). *Aviat Space Environ Med.* 2001;72(11):1006–1016.

21. Reason JT. *Human Error.* New York, NY: Cambridge University Press; 1990.

22. Rasmussen J. Skills, rules, and knowledge: signals, signs, and symbols, and other distinctions in human performance models. *IEEE Trans Syst Man Cybern.* 1983;13(3):257–266.

23. Tjia I, Rampersad S, Varughese A, et al. Wake up safe and root cause analysis: quality improvement in pediatric anesthesia. *Anesth Analg.* 2014;119(1):122–136.

24. Berwick DM. Controlling variation in health care: a consultation from Walter Shewhart. *Med Care.* 1991;29(12):1212–1225.

25. Best M, Neuhauser D. W Edwards Deming: father of quality management, patient and composer. *Qual Saf Health Care.* 2005;14(4):310–312.

26. Henriksen K, Battles JB, Marks ES, et al., eds. *Advances in Patient Safety: From Research to Implementation.* Rockville, MD: Agency for Healthcare Research and Quality (US); 2005. *Prologue: Systems Thinking and Patient Safety*; vol 2 (Concepts and Methodology).

27. Guinane CS, Davis NH. The science of Six Sigma in hospitals. *Am Heart Hosp J.* 2004;2(1):42–48.

28. Kapur A, Potters L. Six Sigma tools for a patient safety-oriented, quality-checklist driven radiation medicine department. *Pract Radiat Oncol.* 2012;2(2):86–96.

29. Gawande A. *Complications: A Surgeon's Notes on an Imperfect Science.* New York, NY: Metropolitan Books; 2002.

30. Sroufe R, Sime C. An examination of ISO 9000:2000 and supply chain quality assurance. *J Oper Manag.* 2008;26(4):503–520.

31. Benedetto AR. Six Sigma: not for the faint of heart. *Radiol Manage.* 2003;25(2):40–53.

32. Fogarty GB, Hornby C, Ferguson HM, et al. Quality assurance in a radiation oncology unit:

the Chart Round experience. *Australas Radiol.* 2001;45:189–194.

33. Boxer M, Forstner D, Kneebone A, et al. Impact of a real-time peer review audit on patient management in a radiation oncology department. *J Med Imaging Radiat Oncol.* 2009;53:405–411.

34. Johnstone PA, Rohde DC, May BC, et al. Peer review and performance improvement in a radiation oncology clinic. *Qual Manag Health Care.* 1999;8:22–28.

35. Brundage MD, Dixon PF, Mackillop WJ, et al. A real-time audit of radiation therapy in a regional cancer center. *Int J Radiat Oncol Biol Phys.* 1999;43:115–124.

36. Marks LB, Adams RD, Pawlicki T, et al. Enhancing the role of case-oriented peer review to improve quality and safety in radiation oncology: executive summary. *Pract Radiat Oncol.* 2013;3(3):149–156.

37. Medication Error Prevention Toolbox. 1999. www.ismp.org/newsletters/acutecare/articles/19990602.asp.

38. Sutlief S, Brown D. Taxonomy of corrective actions in radiotherapy. *Med Phys.* 2014;41(6):433.

39. Woodward CA, Department of Organization of Health Services Delivery, World Health Organization. *Strategies for Assisting Health Workers to Modify and Improve skills: Developing Quality Health Care: A Process of Change.* Geneva, Switzerland: World Health Organization; 2000.

40. Woods DM, Holl JL, Angst D, et al. Improving clinical communication and patient safety: clinician-recommended solutions. In: Henriksen K, Battles JB, Keyes MA, et al, eds. *Advances in Patient Safety: New Directions and Alternative Approaches.* Rockville, MD: Agency for Healthcare Research and Quality (US); 2008. *Performance and Tools*; vol 3.

41. Dekker SWA. *Patient Safety: A Human Factors Approach.* Boca Raton, FL: CRC Press; 2011.

42. Keefe M, Frahm R, Martin K, et al. Safety Culture Common Language (NUREG-2165). 2014. www.nrc.gov/reading-rm/doc-collections/nuregs/staff/sr2165.

43. West CP, Shanafelt TD. Physician well-being and professionalism. *Minn Med.* 2007;90(8):44–46.

44. Dyrbye LN, Massie FS Jr, Eacker A, et al. Relationship between burnout and professional conduct and attitudes among US medical students. *JAMA.* 2010;304(11):1173–1180.

45. Dang D, Bae SH, Karlowicz KA, et al. Do clinician disruptive behaviors make an unsafe environment for patients? *J Nurs Care Qual.* 2016;31:115–123.

46. Shapiro J, Whittemore A, Tsen LC. Instituting a culture of professionalism: the establishment of a center for professionalism and peer support. *Jt Comm J Qual Patient Saf.* 2014;40(4):168–177.

47. Marks LB, Rose CM, Hayman JA, et al. The need for physician leadership in creating a culture of safety. *Int J Radiat Oncol Biol Phys.* 2011;79(5):1287–1289.

6 | Quality, Value, and the Assessment of New Technology

Ronald C. Chen, James R. Broughman, and Jeff M. Michalski

INTRODUCTION

Radiation oncology is a field with rapidly advancing technologies that continue to improve treatment accuracy and/or reduce doses to bystander organs and tissues. Newer technologies are often associated with increased cost, which can be justified if they result in significant improvements in patient outcomes such as improved cancer control and/or reduced side effects.

Assessment of the quality and value of new technologies is a very important issue in the current health care environment, where policymakers must decide how to prioritize spending with limited health care resources. In recent years, there has been increasing awareness of the importance of "comparative effectiveness research," which aims to directly compare different available treatment options to inform decisions by patients, clinicians, and policymakers (1). Comparative effectiveness research can have direct implications regarding insurance coverage of newer treatments and technologies. For example, the Agency for Healthcare Research and Quality (AHRQ) Technology Assessment Program summarizes research data to inform national coverage decisions for Medicare and Medicaid. Much of comparative effectiveness research has focused on comparing older and newer technologies, which is directly relevant to radiation oncology. This chapter describes several types of studies that can be used to assess new technologies in radiation oncology.

RANDOMIZED CLINICAL TRIALS TO ASSESS NEW TECHNOLOGY

Randomized clinical trials are often considered the "gold standard" for comparing the efficacy of different treatments. Indeed, several randomized trials have compared radiotherapy technologies including intensity-modulated

radiation therapy (IMRT), proton therapy, stereotactic radiotherapy, and brachytherapy in a variety of cancers (Table 6.1).

In prostate cancer, a trial by Shipley et al (3) randomized 202 patients with stage T3–T4 prostate cancer to 50.4 Gy by four-field photons followed by either a 25.2 cobalt gray equivalent proton boost or a 16.8 Gy photon boost. This trial found that 5-year local control was significantly improved in the proton arm, which also delivered a higher total dose (64% for photons alone vs. 94% for photons + protons; $P = .001$) for patients with poorly differentiated cancers; but there were also higher rates of rectal bleeding (12% for photons alone vs. 32% for photons plus protons; $P = .002$) and urethral strictures (8% vs. 19%; $P = .07$). Two randomized trials compared conventional radiotherapy with 3D conformal radiotherapy (3DCRT). In one trial by Koper et al (4), 266 patients with stage T1–T4N0M0 prostate cancer were randomized to 66 Gy delivered by conventional radiotherapy versus 3DCRT. A second trial by Dearnaley et al (6) included 225 men with stage T1–T4N0 prostate cancer and had a similar comparison. Both trials showed that 3DCRT decreased toxicity compared with conventional radiotherapy, including acute gastrointestinal toxicity and radiation-induced proctitis. In the Dearnaley trial, 5-year local control was reported and not different in the two arms (78% for 3DCRT vs. 83% for conventional; $P = .4$). A smaller trial of 78 patients showed that IMRT compared with 3DCRT was associated with lower rates of acute grade 2 or greater gastrointestinal toxicity (20% vs. 61%, $P = .001$), but no difference in urinary toxicity or disease control (11).

In head and neck cancers, two randomized studies have compared 3DCRT with IMRT. In a trial by Pow et al (8), 51 patients with T2N0–1M0 nasopharyngeal carcinoma were randomized to either conventional radiotherapy (68 Gy total dose) or IMRT (68–72 Gy total dose). At 1

Table 6.1 Randomized Trials Comparing Radiation Technologies

Study	Type of Cancer	Number of Patients (N)	Treatments Compared	Overall Survival	Cancer-Specific Survival	Other Outcomes
Randomized Trials Comparing Charged Particle RT Versus Photon RT						
Lindstadt et al (2)	Pancreatic	49	5-FU + helium RT (60–70 Gy)	7.8 mo (median)	N/A	N/A
			5-FU + photon RT (60 Gy)	6.5 mo (P = .29)	N/A	N/A
Shipley et al (3)	Prostate	202	Photon RT (50.4 Gy) + proton boost (25.2 cGE)	75%	86%	Rectal bleeding: 32% Urethral stricture: 19%
			Photon RT (50.4 Gy) + photon boost (16.8 Gy)	80% (NS)	83% (NS)	Rectal bleeding: 12% (P = .002) Urethral stricture: 8% (P = .07)
Randomized Trials Comparing 3D Conformal RT Versus Conventional RT						
Koper et al (4,5)	Prostate	266	Conventional RT (66 Gy)	N/A	N/A	Grade 2 GI toxicity: 32%
			3D Conformal RT (66 Gy)	N/A	N/A	Grade 2 GI toxicity: 19% (P = .02)
Dearnaley et al (6)	Prostate	225	Conventional RT (64 Gy)	N/A	N/A	Grade 2 + proctitis: 15% 5-Y local control: 83%
			3D Conformal RT (64 Gy)	N/A	N/A	Grade 2+ proctitis: 5% (P = .01) 5-Y local control: 78% (P = .4)
Randomized Trials Comparing Intensity-Modulated RT (IMRT) Versus Conventional or 3D Conformal RT						
Kam et al (7)	Nasopharyngeal carcinoma	60	Conventional RT (66 Gy)	N/A	N/A	Severe xerostomia: 82%
			IMRT (66 Gy)	N/A	N/A	Severe xerostomia: 39% (P = .001)
Pow et al (8)	Nasopharyngeal carcinoma	51	Conventional RT (68 Gy to nasopharynx; 66 Gy to neck)	N/A	N/A	SWS recovery: 5% SPS recovery: 10%
			IMRT (GTV 68–72 Gy; PTV 66–68 Gy)	N/A	N/A	SWS recovery: 50% (P < .05) SPS recovery: 83% (P < .05)
Pignol et al (9)	Breast	358	Conventional RT (50 Gy) + optional electron boost (16 Gy)	N/A	N/A	Moist desquamation: 48%
			IMRT (50 Gy) + optional electron boost (16 Gy)	N/A	N/A	Moist desquamation: 31% (P = .002)

Table 6.1 Randomized Trials Comparing Radiation Technologies (Continued)

Randomized Trials Comparing Intensity-Modulated RT (IMRT) Versus Conventional or 3D Conformal RT						
Donovan et al (10)	Breast	306	Conventional RT (50 Gy) + electron boost (11.1 Gy)	N/A	N/A	Palpable induration: 32%
			IMRT (50 Gy) + electron boost (11.1 Gy)	N/A	N/A	Palpable induration: 21% (P = .02)
Al-Mamgani et al (11)	Prostate	78	3D conformal (78 Gy)	N/A	N/A	GI toxicity: 61% GU toxicity: 69%
			IMRT (78 Gy)	N/A	N/A	GI toxicity: 20% (P = .001) GU toxicity: 53% (P = .3)
Randomized Trials Comparing Stereotactic Radiosurgery (SRS) Alone Versus SRS Plus WBRT						
Aoyama et al (12)	Brain metastases	132	SRS alone (18–25 Gy, based on tumor size)	8.0 mo (median)	N/A	1-y brain tumor recurrence: 76.4%
			SRS + WBRT (30 Gy)	7.5 mo (P = .42)	N/A	1-y brain tumor recurrence: 46.8% (P < .001)
Chang et al (13)	Brain metastases	58	SRS alone (dose based on tumor size)	15.2 mo (median)	N/A	4-mo decline in learning and memory: 24%
			SRS + WBRT (30 Gy)	5.7 mo (P = .003)	N/A	4-mo decline in learning and memory: 52% (P < .05)
Randomized Trials Comparing Brachytherapy (BT) Versus External Beam RT (EBRT)						
Weigensberg et al (14)	Endometrial	105	BT (6,000–6,500 mg/hr)	N/A	N/A	10-y DFS: 67% Toxicity: 46%
			EBRT (40 Gy)	N/A	N/A	10-y DFS: 59% (P = .02) Toxicity: 24% (P < .02)
Randomized Trials Comparing Neutron RT Versus Photon RT						
Laramore et al (15)	Salivary gland	32	Neutrons (17–22 nGy)	25%	LRC: 56%	N/A
			Photons/electrons (55 Gy or 70 Gy)	15% (NS)	LRC: 17% (P = .009)	N/A
Maor et al (16)	Squamous cell carcinoma	169	Neutrons (20.4 nGy)	27%	LRF: 63%	Complete response: 70%
			Photons (70 Gy)	27% (NS)	68% (NS)	Complete response: 52% (P = .006)

BT, brachytherapy; DFS, disease-free survival; EBRT, external-beam radiotherapy; GI, gastrointestinal; GTV, gross tumor volume; GU, genitourinary; IMRT, intensity-modulated radiotherapy; LRC, local regional control; LRF, local regional failure; N/A, not available; NS, not significant; PTV, planning target volume; SPS, stimulated parotid saliva; SRS, stereotactic radiosurgery; SWS, stimulated whole saliva; WBRT, whole brain radiotherapy.

year posttreatment, significantly more patients in the IMRT arm had recovered at least 25% of their baseline stimulated whole saliva flow (5% conventional patients vs. 50% IMRT patients; P <.05) and stimulated parotid flow (10% vs. 83%; P <.05). A second trial by Kam et al (7) randomized 60 patients with T1-2bN0-1 nasopharyngeal carcinoma to 66 Gy delivered by conventional radiotherapy versus IMRT followed by an intracavitary boost. At 1 year posttreatment, patients in the IMRT arm had lower rates of observer-rated severe xerostomia (82% for conventional vs. 39% for IMRT; P = .001) as well as higher fractional stimulated parotid flow rates (0.05 vs. 0.9; P < .0001) and stimulated whole saliva flow rates (0.2 vs. 0.4; P = .001). There was, however, no significant difference in patient-reported xerostomia (P = .32).

Two randomized trials compared 3DCRT with IMRT in breast cancer. In a trial by Donovan et al (10), 306 women with early-stage breast cancer were randomized to 50 Gy delivered by conventional radiotherapy versus IMRT followed by an 11.1 Gy electron boost. After 5 years of follow-up, significantly fewer women in the IMRT arm developed palpable induration of the breast (32% for conventional vs. 21% for IMRT; P = .02). Further, patients receiving conventional radiotherapy were 1.7 times more likely to have a change in breast appearance compared with those receiving IMRT (P = .008). A later trial by Pignol et al (9) randomized 358 patients with early-stage breast cancer to 50 Gy delivered by conventional radiotherapy versus IMRT plus an optional 16 Gy electron boost. The frequency of moist desquamation during the 6 weeks following radiation treatment was significantly decreased among women in the IMRT arm (48% for conventional vs. 31% for IMRT; P = .002).

Trials have also assessed whole-brain radiotherapy (WBRT) and stereotactic radiosurgery (SRS) for the treatment of brain metastases. A first trial by Aoyama et al (12) compared SRS alone with SRS plus WBRT, and showed that adding WBRT significantly improved the control of intracranial disease at 1 year, but there was no difference in overall survival in the two arms. A smaller trial similarly showed that adding WBRT improved freedom from intracranial recurrence (27% for SRS alone vs. 73% for SRS with WBRT, P = .0003), but WBRT was associated with a detriment in learning and memory function and worse overall survival (13).

Results from these randomized trials have helped define the potential patient benefits from newer radiation technologies, and therefore led to adoptions in use of IMRT for head and neck cancers, 3DCRT and subsequently IMRT for prostate cancer, and SRS for brain metastases. However, it is not practical to evaluate every new technology with randomized trials, because of the long time required to complete each trial (while patients wait to receive the potentially beneficial new treatment), and common patient and physician reluctance regarding randomization. Therefore, other types of studies—such

as retrospective institutional studies, population-based data analyses, and prospective single-arm trials—are also needed to assess new technologies in radiation oncology.

NONRANDOMIZED STUDIES TO ASSESS NEW TECHNOLOGY

A common type of study design to compare patient outcomes of older versus newer treatments is analysis of population-based data such as the Surveillance, Epidemiology, and End Results (SEER). SEER is a National Cancer Institute–sponsored collection of population-based cancer registries across the United States, and provides information related to patients' sociodemographics, cancer diagnosis, and survival. SEER data can be linked with Medicare data, which provide claims and additional diagnostic information for patients who are 65 years and older (17). SEER-Medicare is a powerful data resource because it contains large numbers of patients for analysis, and provides results that are more generalizable than randomized trials (which often enroll younger and healthier patients who may not be representative of the overall patient population). Select nonrandomized studies that have compared different radiation technologies are summarized in Table 6.2.

An analysis of SEER-Medicare data by Sheets et al (18) compared the long-term morbidity in prostate cancer patients treated with older conformal, IMRT, or proton therapy. This study reported that IMRT compared with older conformal radiotherapy was associated with less gastrointestinal morbidity, fewer hip fractures, and less receipt of future cancer treatments (implying reduced cancer recurrence). In the same study that also compared IMRT with proton therapy, there was no difference in long-term outcomes except that IMRT was associated with a lower rate of gastrointestinal morbidity. In a complementary study by Yu et al (19) that analyzed Medicare data and focused on short-term outcomes, proton radiotherapy was associated with lower urinary morbidity at 6 months compared with IMRT (5.9% for proton vs. 9.5% for IMRT; P = .03), but at 12 months, there was no difference in urinary or gastrointestinal morbidity between the two treatments. Of note, an ongoing randomized trial of proton therapy versus IMRT for low- and intermediate-risk prostate cancer (NCT01617161) will add further information to this comparison. The primary endpoint of this trial is bowel quality of life at 2 years.

Another newer technology in prostate cancer treatment is stereotactic body radiotherapy (SBRT). As is common in the assessment of new treatments, SBRT early evaluations in prostate cancer involved prospective, single-arm trials to examine its cancer control efficacy and safety (toxicity). A study published by King et al (21) was a combined analysis of single-arm trials from multiple institutions, and included a total of 1,100 patients.

Table 6.2 Select Nonrandomized Studies Comparing Radiation Technologies

Study	Design	Number of Patients (N)	Treatments Compared	Overall Survival	Cancer-Specific Survival	Other Outcomes
Prostate Cancer Studies						
Sheets et al (18)	Retrospective, SEER-Medicare	12,976	IMRT vs. proton vs. conformal RT	N/A	N/A	(IMRT vs. conformal) GI morbidity: RR 0.91 ($P < .001$) Hip fracture: RR 0.8 ($P = .006$) (IMRT vs. proton) GI morbidity RR = 0.66 ($P < .05$)
Yu et al (19)	Retrospective, Medicare	27,647	IMRT vs. proton	N/A	N/A	(Urinary toxicity) 6-mo: 9.5% IMRT vs. 5.9% proton ($P = .03$) 12-mo: 17.5% IMRT vs. 18.8% proton ($P = .6$)
Yu et al (20)	Retrospective, Medicare	4,005	SBRT vs. IMRT	N/A	N/A	(Urinary toxicity) 6-mo: 15.6% SBRT vs. 12.6% IMRT ($P = .009$) 24-mo: 43.9% SBRT vs. 36.3% IMRT ($P = .001$)
King et al (21)	Prospective, multi-institution	1,100	SBRT	N/A	N/A	(5-y biochemical RFS) Low risk 95%, intermediate risk 83%, high risk 78%
SBRT Vs. Conventional RT for Metastases						
Hunter et al (22)	Retrospective, single-institution	110	SBRT vs. conventional RT	N/A	N/A	Complete pain relief: 12% conventional vs. 33% SBRT ($P = .01$)
Amini et al (23)	Retrospective, single-institution	46	SBRT vs. conventional RT	N/A	N/A	Symptom control at 10 mo: 75% SBRT vs. 44% conventional ($P = .02$)

(Continued)

Table 6.2 Select Nonrandomized Studies Comparing Radiation Technologies (Continued)

Study	Design	Number of Patients (N)	Treatments Compared	Overall Survival	Cancer-Specific Survival	Other Outcomes
Lung Cancer Studies						
Yom et al (24)	Retrospective, single-institution	290	3DCRT vs. IMRT	N/A	N/A	Grade $\geq$3 pneumonitis: 32% 3DCRT vs. 8% IMRT (P = .002)
Liao et al (25)	Retrospective, single-institution	409	3DCRT vs. IMRT	HR = 0.64 favoring IMRT (P = .04)	N/A	Grade $\geq$3 pneumonitis: HR = 0.33 favoring IMRT (P = 0.02)
Grills et al (26)	Retrospective, single-institution	124	SBRT vs. surgery	(30-mo) Surgery: 87% SBRT: 72% (P = .01)	(30-mo) Surgery: 93% SBRT: 94% (P = .5)	Local recurrence at 30 mo: 20% surgery vs. 4% SBRT (P = .07)
Crabtree et al (27)	Retrospective, single-institution	538	SBRT vs. surgery	(3-y) Surgery: 54% SBRT: 38% (P = .27)	(3-y) Surgery: 77% SBRT: 86% (P = .7)	Local control at 3-y: 88% surgery vs. 90% SBRT (P = .9)

3DCRT, three-dimensional conformal radiotherapy; GI, gastrointestinal; HR, hazard ratio; IMRT, intensity-modulated radiotherapy; N/A, not available; RFS, recurrence-free survival; SBRT, stereotactic body radiotherapy.

This study reported promising results, with 5-year relapse-free survival of 95% for low-risk and 84% for intermediate-risk patients. In a separate publication that included 864 patients with available quality-of-life data, the same group of authors reported favorable long-term patient-reported gastrointestinal and urinary function (28). However, in a comparative study using Medicare data, Yu et al (20) reported that SBRT was associated with higher rates of urinary morbidity than IMRT at both 6 months (16% for SBRT vs. 13% IMRT; $P = .009$) and 24 months (44% vs. 36%; $P = .001$).

There are emerging retrospective institutional studies evaluating the use of SBRT (with hypofractionation) to treat tumors traditionally considered to be radioresistant. A study by Hunter et al (22) compared conventional radiotherapy with SBRT among 110 patients with painful spinal metastases from renal cell carcinoma. SBRT was associated with a higher rate of complete pain response (12% for conventional vs. 33% SBRT; $P = .01$). A second study, by Amini et al (23), included 46 patients with bone metastases also from renal cell carcinoma. After a median follow-up of 10 months, symptom control rates were significantly better after SBRT (44% for conventional vs. 75% for SBRT; $P = .02$).

In lung cancer, studies have evaluated 3DCRT, IMRT, and SBRT. Two retrospective institutional studies compared patient outcomes of 3DCRT versus IMRT. In Yom et al (24), 290 patients with non–small cell lung cancer were analyzed. After a median follow-up of 8 to 9 months, IMRT was associated with lower rates of grade ≥ 3 pneumonitis (32% for 3DCRT vs. 8% IMRT; $P = .002$). Another study, by Liao et al (25), with 409 patients, similarly showed lower rates of pneumonitis from IMRT compared with 3DCRT, and also better overall survival with IMRT. An emerging treatment for early-stage lung cancer is SBRT, but, unfortunately, attempts at randomized trials to compare SBRT with surgical resection have failed owing to poor accrual. However, retrospective studies suggest that SBRT provides similar or potentially better cancer-specific survival and local control rates compared with surgical resection.

An important limitation of all nonrandomized studies is the potential for uncontrolled confounding, which can bias study results (29). While sophisticated analytic methodologies can be used to minimize confounding with big data analyses, residual confounding can remain, which may affect the results from these studies. Another significant limitation of nonrandomized trials is that big data registries such as SEER and the National Cancer Data Base (NCDB) lack detailed clinical information. For example, cancer recurrence data are not available in SEER or NCDB, and few big data sources have patient-reported quality of life. In addition, big data resources that are available for research are at least 2 to 3 years behind current practice because of the time needed for data processing and quality assurance. After factoring in the additional time needed for data analysis and publication,

the reported quality assessment results are typically at least 5 years old—and thus no longer reflective of "current" practice or quality gaps.

COST-EFFECTIVENESS ANALYSES FOR NEW TECHNOLOGY

A formal way to assess the value of a new technology is with cost-effectiveness analysis. Briefly, these analyses can be used to compare a new technology with an older/standard technology, and the result is usually reported as a ratio (called the incremental cost-effectiveness ratio, ICER) with the cost difference as the numerator and effectiveness difference as the denominator (30). Commonly, the effectiveness measure is the quality-adjusted life-year (QALY)—a composite measure that encompasses survival and quality of life. The magnitudes of difference between newer versus older technologies in terms of cost (numerator) and effectiveness (denominator) are the key to this evaluation; an ICER of $50,000 per QALY is commonly considered to be cost-effective (30).

Table 6.3 summarizes select examples of cost-effectiveness analyses of radiation technologies. A recent study by Savitz et al (31) examined the cost-effectiveness of multiple newer radiation technologies for brain metastases, including the currently investigational hippocampal-avoidance WBRT. Hippocampal-avoidance WBRT is more costly than conventional WBRT, but can also be more effective by reducing neurocognitive sequelae. This analysis showed that for patients with life expectancy of 1 year or longer, hippocampal-avoidance WBRT can be cost-effective ($42,872/QALY for patients with 1-year life expectancy, and $24,701/QALY for patients with 2-year life expectancy), likely because the benefit of hippocampal-avoidance compared with conventional WBRT is more commonly realized in patients who live longer. Additional studies have also evaluated the cost-effectiveness of IMRT in breast cancer (32) and IMRT for head and neck cancers (33).

A study by Konski et al (34) assessed the cost-effectiveness of proton therapy compared with IMRT for prostate cancer. This analysis assumed that proton therapy (91.8 cobalt gray equivalent) improved cancer control compared with IMRT (81 Gy) (5-year freedom from biochemical failure 83% IMRT to 93% proton); with this assumption, the ICER was $55,725/QALY.

When using cost-effectiveness analyses to assess the value of a new technology, it is important to realize that both cost and effectiveness data evolve over time. As the cost of a new technology decreases, it will reduce the ICER, making a technology cost-effective on the basis of the $50,000/QALY threshold. Further, accumulation of mature research data on a technology can better inform the "effectiveness" part of the cost-effectiveness analyses; it is possible that early cost-effectiveness studies of a new technology could have incorporated unrealistic expectations

Table 6.3 Select Cost-Effectiveness Studies of Radiation Technologies

Study	Cancer Type	Treatments Compared	Mean Cost	QALY	ICER
Konski et al (34)	Prostate	Proton vs. IMRT	(60 y/o man) Proton: $64,989 IMRT: $39,355 (70 y/o man) Proton: $63,511 IMRT: $36,808	(60 y/o man) Proton: 9.9 IMRT: 9.5 (70 y/o man) Proton: 8.5 IMRT: 8.1	Proton: (60 y/o man) $55,726/QALY (70 y/o man) $63,578/QALY
Sen et al (32)	Breast	No RT vs. conventional RT vs. IMRT	(70–74 y/o women) No RT: $20,077 Conventional: $29,500 IMRT: $37,710	(70–74 y/o women) No RT: 5.2 Conventional: 5.4 IMRT: 5.5	EBRT (vs. no RT): $44,600/QALY IMRT (vs. EBRT): $89,300/QALY
Kohler et al (33)	Head and neck	3DCRT vs. IMRT	(65 y/o patient) 3DCRT: $11,336 IMRT: $20,606	(2-y posttreatment) 3DCRT: 1.8 IMRT: 1.9	IMRT (2-y posttreatment): $101,100/QALY IMRT (15-y posttreatment): $34,523/QALY
Savitz et al (31)	Brain metastases	SRS vs. WBRT vs. HA-WBRT vs. SRS + WBRT vs. SRS + HA-WBRT	(24-mo) WBRT: $21,276 HA-WBRT: $24,668	(24-mo) WBRT: 1.66 HA-WBRT: 1.80	HA-WBRT (vs. WBRT, 24-mo): $24,701/QALY

3DCRT, three-dimensional conformal radiotherapy; EBRT, external beam radiotherapy; HA-WBRT, hippocampal-avoidance whole brain radiotherapy; ICER, incremental cost-effectiveness ratio, IMRT; intensity-modulated radiotherapy; QALY, quality-adjusted life-years; SRS, stereotactic radiosurgery; WBRT, whole-brain radiotherapy; y/o, year old.

of effectiveness, which would have to be revised as primary research data accumulate.

ADOPTION OF NEW TECHNOLOGY BASED ON EMERGING EVIDENCE: COVERAGE WITH EVIDENCE DEVELOPMENT

Assessments of new radiation technologies must focus on patient outcomes such as survival, cancer control, toxicity, and quality of life, as demonstrated by the studies discussed previously and summarized in the tables. Demonstration of improvements in patient outcomes, by randomized clinical trials and/or other nonrandomized studies, is necessary to facilitate the broad adoption of a new technology as the standard of care.

However, assessment of a new technology takes many years; while formal evaluations are occurring through clinical trials and other studies, patients often have no easy access to promising new treatments and other technologies. A compromise solution that allows patients early access to new technologies is "coverage with evidence development," where reimbursement is provided for new technologies with a requirement for formal assessment and data collection (35). The first example of this policy was for positron emission tomography (PET) scans, where Medicare reimbursed these scans if and only if a patient participated in the National Oncology PET Registry with prospective data collection (36). More recently, this policy has also been used for Medicare reimbursement of SBRT for early prostate cancer. The idea of coverage with evidence development is to allow patients access to promising new technologies while simultaneously mandating formal evaluation. After a defined period of time, collected data are analyzed, and if the new technology is found to be ineffective, reimbursement stops.

Coverage with evidence development has the potential to be a win–win for both patients and policymakers; however, it has some potential disadvantages. Importantly, reimbursement of a new technology can encourage its broad and rapid dissemination, and therefore discourage patient and physician participation in randomized clinical trials. For example, since the start of coverage with evidence development for PET scans in 2005, this technology has become widely available, but no randomized trial has been published comparing the efficacy of posttreatment follow-up PET with more traditional (CT or MRI) scans on patient outcomes. Given these considerations, the use of this policy should be selective, and reserved only for the most promising technologies for which accessibility to patients cannot wait until after research is completed.

In conclusion, radiation oncology is a rapidly advancing field in which newer technologies are continually developed. Although newer technologies are often more costly, this may be justified if they lead to improved patient outcomes. Randomized trials, nonrandomized studies, and cost-effectiveness analyses are all important ways of assessing the value and effectiveness of new technologies. Coverage with evidence development is a policy that can grant patients access to promising new technologies while formal research is being conducted, although this strategy must be used selectively.

REFERENCES

1. Chen RC. Comparative effectiveness research in oncology: the promise, challenges, and opportunities. *Semin Radiat Oncol.* 2014;24(1):1–4.

2. Linstadt D, Quivey JM, Castro JR, et al. Comparison of helium-ion radiation therapy and split-course megavoltage irradiation for unresectable adenocarcinoma of the pancreas: final report of a Northern California Oncology Group randomized prospective clinical trial. *Radiology.* 1988;168(1):261–264.

3. Shipley WU, Verhey LJ, Munzenrider JE, et al. Advanced prostate cancer: the results of a randomized comparative trial of high dose irradiation boosting with conformal protons compared with conventional dose irradiation using photons alone. *Int J Radiat Oncol Biol Phys.* 1995;32(1):3–12.

4. Koper PC, Stroom JC, van Putten WL, et al. Acute morbidity reduction using 3DCRT for prostate carcinoma: a randomized study. *Int J Radiat Oncol Biol Phys.* 1999;43(4):727–734.

5. Koper PC, Jansen P, van Putten W, et al. Gastrointestinal and genito-urinary morbidity after 3D conformal radiotherapy of prostate cancer: observations of a randomized trial. *Radiother Oncol.* 2004;73(1):1–9.

6. Dearnaley DP, Khoo VS, Norman AR, et al. Comparison of radiation side-effects of conformal and conventional radiotherapy in prostate cancer: a randomised trial. *Lancet.* 1999;353(9149):267–272.

7. Kam MK, Leung S-F, Zee B, et al. Prospective randomized study of intensity-modulated radiotherapy on salivary gland function in early-stage nasopharyngeal carcinoma patients. *J Clin Oncol.* 2007;25(31):4873–4879.

8. Pow EH, Kwong DL, McMillan AS, et al. Xerostomia and quality of life after intensity-modulated radiotherapy vs. conventional radiotherapy for early-stage nasopharyngeal carcinoma: initial report on a randomized controlled clinical trial. *Int J Radiat Oncol Biol Phys.* 2006;66(4):981–991.

9. Pignol J-P, Olivotto I, Rakovitch E, et al. A multicenter randomized trial of breast intensity-modulated radiation therapy to reduce acute radiation dermatitis. *J Clin Oncol.* 2008;26(13):2085–2092.

10. Donovan E, Bleakley N, Denholm E, et al. Randomised trial of standard 2D radiotherapy (RT) versus intensity modulated radiotherapy (IMRT) in patients prescribed breast radiotherapy. *Radiother Oncol.* 2007;82(3):254–264.

11. Al-Mamgani A, Heemsbergen WD, Peeters ST, et al. Role of intensity-modulated radiotherapy in reducing toxicity in dose escalation for localized prostate cancer. *Int J Radiat Oncol Biol Phys.* 2009;73(3):685–691.

12. Aoyama H, Shirato H, Tago M, et al. Stereotactic radiosurgery plus whole-brain radiation therapy vs stereotactic radiosurgery alone for treatment of brain metastases: a randomized controlled trial. *JAMA.* 2006;295(21):2483–2491.

13. Chang EL, Wefel JS, Hess KR, et al. Neurocognition in patients with brain metastases treated with radiosurgery or radiosurgery plus whole-brain irradiation: a randomised controlled trial. *Lancet Oncol.* 2009;10(11):1037–1044.

14. Weigensberg IJ. Preoperative radiation therapy in stage I: endometrial adenocarcinoma II: final report of a clinical trial. *Cancer.* 1984;53(2):242–247.

15. Laramore G, Krall JM, Griffin TW, et al. Neutron versus photon irradiation for unresectable salivary gland tumors: final report of an RTOG-MRC randomized clinical trial. *Int J Radiat Oncol Biol Phys.* 1993;27(2):235–240.

16. Maor MH, Errington RD, Caplan RJ, et al. Fast-neutron therapy in advanced head and neck cancer: a collaborative international randomized trial. *Int J Radiat Oncol Biol Phys.* 1995;32(3):599–604.

17. Virnig BA, Warren JL, Cooper GS, et al. Studying radiation therapy using SEER-Medicare-linked data. *Med Care.* 2002;40(8):IV-49–IV-54.

18. Sheets NC, Goldin GH, Meyer A-M, et al. Intensity-modulated radiation therapy, proton therapy, or conformal radiation therapy and morbidity and disease control in localized prostate cancer. *JAMA.* 2012;307(15):1611–1620.

19. Yu JB, Soulos PR, Herrin J, et al. Proton versus intensity-modulated radiotherapy for prostate cancer: patterns of care and early toxicity. *J Natl Cancer Inst.* 2013;105(1):25–32.

20. Yu JB, Cramer LD, Herrin J, et al. Stereotactic body radiation therapy versus intensity-modulated radiation therapy for prostate cancer: comparison of toxicity. *J Clin Oncol.* 2014;32(12):1195–1201.

21. King CR, Freeman D, Kaplan I, et al. Stereotactic body radiotherapy for localized prostate cancer: pooled analysis from a multi-institutional consortium of prospective phase II trials. *Radiother Oncol.* 2013;109(2):217–221.

22. Hunter GK, Balagamwala EH, Koyfman SA, et al. The efficacy of external beam radiotherapy and stereotactic body radiotherapy for painful spinal metastases from renal cell carcinoma. *Pract Radiat Oncol.* 2012;2(4):e95–e100.

23. Amini A, Altoos B, Bourlon MT, et al. Local control rates of metastatic renal cell carcinoma (RCC) to the bone using stereotactic body radiation therapy: is RCC truly radioresistant? *Pract Radiat Oncol.* 2015;5(6):e589–e596.

24. Yom SS, Liao Z, Liu HH, et al. Initial evaluation of treatment-related pneumonitis in advanced-stage non-small-cell lung cancer patients treated with concurrent chemotherapy and intensity-modulated radiotherapy. *Int J Radiat Oncol Biol Phys.* 2007;68(1):94–102.

25. Liao ZX, Komaki RR, Thames HD Jr, et al. Influence of technologic advances on outcomes in patients with unresectable, locally advanced non-small-cell lung cancer receiving concomitant chemoradiotherapy. *Int J Radiat Oncol Biol Phys.* 2010;76(3):775–781.

26. Grills IS, Mangona VS, Welsh R, et al. Outcomes after stereotactic lung radiotherapy or wedge resection for stage I non-small-cell lung cancer. *J Clin Oncol.* 2010;28(6):928–935.

27. Crabtree TD, Denlinger CE, Meyers BF, et al. Stereotactic body radiation therapy versus surgical resection for stage I non-small cell lung cancer. *J Thorac Cardiovasc Surg.* 2010;140(2):377–386.

28. King CR, Collins S, Fuller D, et al. Health-related quality of life after stereotactic body radiation therapy for localized prostate cancer: results from a multi-institutional consortium of prospective trials. *Int J Radiat Oncol Biol Phys.* 2013;87(5):939–945.

29. Meyer AM, Wheeler SB, Weinberger M, et al. An overview of methods for comparative effectiveness research. *Semin Radiat Oncol.* 2014;24(1):5–13.

30. Sher DJ, Punglia RS. Decision analysis and cost-effectiveness analysis for comparative effectiveness research—a primer. *Semin Radiat Oncol.* 2014;24(1):14–24.

31. Savitz ST, Chen RC, Sher DJ. Cost effectiveness analysis of neurocognitive sparing treatments for brain metastases. *Cancer.* 2015;121(23):4231–4239.

32. Sen S, Wang S-Y, Soulos PR, et al. Examining the cost-effectiveness of radiation therapy among older women with favorable-risk breast cancer. *J Natl Cancer Inst.* 2014;106(3):dju008.

33. Kohler RE, Sheets NC, Wheeler SB, et al. Two-year and lifetime cost-effectiveness of intensity modulated radiation therapy versus 3-dimensional conformal radiation therapy for head-and-neck cancer. *Int J Radiat Oncol Biol Phys.* 2013;87(4):683–689.

34. Konski A, Speier W, Hanlon A, et al. Is proton beam therapy cost effective in the treatment of adenocarcinoma of the prostate? *J Clin Oncol.* 2007;25(24):3603–3608.

35. Chen AB. Comparative effectiveness research in radiation oncology: assessing technology. *Semin Radiat Oncol.* 2014;24(1):25–34.

36. Tunis S, Whicher D. The National Oncologic PET Registry: lessons learned for coverage with evidence development. *J Am Coll Radiol.* 2009;6(5):360–365.

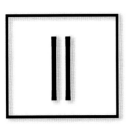

Quality in Radiation Physics

Eric C. Ford

7 Equipment and Software: Commissioning From the Quality and Safety Perspective

Indra J. Das and Aaron Andersen

INTRODUCTION

Radiation oncology is a technologically advanced field of medicine compared with other subspecialties. These advances have become even more complex in hardware and software, having progressed from a single cobalt-60 teletherapy machine to various advanced machines. In the course of its evolution, out of six vendors of linear accelerator (linac) providers, only three remain in the U.S.: Varian Medical System, Elekta, and Siemens. In fact, Siemens has been acquired by Varian, leaving only two manufacturers of standard linacs.

The evolution of machines from each vendor is directly linked to the advances made in treatment technology. For example, the Varian Clinac (clinical accelerator) series had Clinac-4, Clinac-6, and Clinac-18, where the number denoted the maximum photon energy. This was followed by the Clinac-C series (C stands for computerized), and then the CD (computerized and digital) series. Varian Trilogy had three features: very high dose rate, SRS feature (superior mechanical stability <1 mm), and imaging options, such as onboard imaging. During the same time, Varian IX machines were introduced, meant for imaging and treatment. Now the older models are being replaced with a new platform called Truebeam. Siemens had Mevatron machines designated with two-digit numbers, representing beam energy in terms of nominal depth dose at 10 cm. So Mevatron MD-67 stands for a magnetron-driven, digital machine that has a depth dose of 67%. For high energy, names like KD-77 stand for klystron, digital, and a depth dose of 77%. These were replaced with Primus, Oncor, and Artiste before the manufacturer closed its accelerator business. These were all mutileaf collimator (MLC)-based, but onboard imaging was the only standard feature beginning with Oncor. Similarly, Elekta started with the digital SL series, which stands for slalom magnet linear accelerator, in 1985. This was replaced with advanced features in each new platform like Synergy, Infinity, and Axesse. The latest digital machine, which is the sixth generation, is the Versa-HD, introduced in 2013.

Modern machines are all integrated for imaging and treatment, capable of delivering a very high dose rate and having the continuously fast-moving MLC that are required for volumetric modulated arc therapy (VMAT), a form of intensity-modulated radiation therapy (IMRT). This chapter discusses issues related to generic linac commissioning that are not specific to any vendor. However, familiarization with the device and differences in operation are beyond its scope and should be acquired from vendor-specific training on that type of machine.

This chapter provides the rationale for the need for commissioning and identifies its components. Software is another component that is directly interfaced with a machine to perform a certain task, and is vendor-specific. For example, record-and-verify systems that are integral to patient treatment should be validated for every component. This chapter deals with standard machine commissioning and does not cover advance data needed for specialized treatments such as SBRT, SRS, TBI, and TSEI, which are discussed further in Chapter 8.

ACCURACY AND PRECISION

The terms *accuracy* and *precision* are often used interchangeably. However, the distinction should be clearly understood. Figure 7.1 provides a schematic of these two concepts. In radiation oncology, both accuracy and precision should be maintained to achieve tumor control probability (TCP) and to reduce normal tissue complication

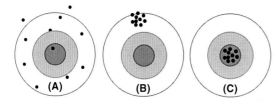

FIGURE 7.1 Three scenarios depicting the concept of accuracy and precision. (A) represents neither precision nor accuracy, (B) represents precision but not accuracy, and (C) both accuracy and precision. In radiation oncology, we need both accuracy and precision to irradiate the intended volume and achieve the goal of tumor control.

probability (NTCP). In Figure 7.1 (A), neither TCP nor NTCP can be achieved. In Figure 7.1 (B), the TCP will be minimal, and NTCP is expected to be very high, depending on the structure, whereas in Figure 7.1 (C), it is expected that TCP is high and NTCP is low, which is the goal of radiation oncology. To achieve accuracy and precision, radiation machines should have proper quality assurance and commissioning data, which is discussed in this chapter.

REQUEST FOR PROPOSAL/PURCHASE, ACCEPTANCE TESTING PROCESS, AND COMMISSIONING

The planning process to acquire, commission, and use a device may be very long and must be clearly understood. The accuracy and precision described in the previous section are part of the commissioning process, which is discussed in detail in a separate section.

Request for proposal/purchase

For any machine or device acquisition, a request for proposal (RFP) is needed. This is a process in which an institution indicates its desire to buy equipment. A written "wish list" should be included. However, most of the time RFPs are written on the basis of what a vendor can provide and are sometimes biased toward one particular vendor. Additionally, wish lists may not be met, and a modification is needed. When writing an RFP, it is important to clearly delineate the requirements, such as beam energy, dose rate, field size, type of MLC, stability, flatness, and symmetry. The RFP is a legal document and is binding between the institution and the vendor. It also includes costs associated with the acquisition and terms of delivery.

Acceptance testing process

After the RFP is issued, a vendor is selected, which delivers the product. Manufacturers have a set of testing criteria and tolerance limits for acceptance. Most parameters are

defined by the manufacturer and are documented in the acceptance testing protocol (ATP) manual. This manual is executed on site for operation and parameter verification and is strictly followed. One can argue for a national/international criterion for parameters, but at this stage the ATP is the guideline. For example, linear accelerator beam flatness can be stated as required by TG-45 (1) given in Eq. [1] or by a particular manufacturer in Eq. [2]. Please note that these two equations differ by a factor of 2. The relevant equations are:

$$\text{Flatness (\%)} = 100 \frac{(D_{max} - D_{min})}{(D_{max} + D_{min})} \qquad [1]$$

$$\text{Flatness (\%)} = 100 \frac{(D_{max} - D_{min})}{(D_{avg})}$$
$$= 100 \times 2 \frac{(D_{max} - D_{min})}{(D_{max} + D_{min})} \qquad [2]$$

where D_{max}, D_{min}, and D_{avg} are the maximum, minimum, and average dose respectively, in 80% field width (usually a field size of less than or equal to 20×20 cm^2). In spite of the factor of two, the ATP guideline in Eq. [2] will hold well based on vendor specification. Similarly, other parameters such as beam symmetry also differ in definition. Assigning beam energy could be controversial, and has been discussed in many references (2–6).

The user should not argue at the time of ATP, but follow strictly what is defined in the RFP. Usually, a machine manufacturer's document is taken as a reference at the time of ATP. At this time, many of the beam characteristics will be measured strictly in the vendor's terms by the machine engineer to verify that the machine meets the criterion, which may not be optimal, but there may be little recourse for the user. For example, beam flatness, symmetry, and percent depth dose (PDD) can be measured to satisfy the ATP criterion based on a small portable water tank that may differ from the actual data collection in a large scanning water tank with full scatter conditions. These differences could be as high as 2%, but should match the RFP and ATP. At the end of the ATP process, the vendor representative and the facility physicist should sign the ATP, which becomes a legal document. The ATP process is usually very intense and lasts several days (2–3 days). The vendor then files paperwork to process payments in terms of the agreement as defined in the RFP.

COMMISSIONING

The word *commissioning* is defined as "a process of bringing a newly designed or produced product into working condition." This holds good for treatment machines. Once the equipment has been accepted (i.e., meeting the manufacturer's working criteria), commissioning can start. TG-45 (1) provided a code of practice for linear accelerators. This publication served well for older generations of linear accelerators, but is not appropriate for modern machines. It also did not include beam data commissioning. A conceptual description of machine commissioning from the United Kingdom was provided in a monograph (7). Critical components and a "how-to" guide have also been published by the AAPM TG-106 (8). It is important to keep in mind that machine commissioning takes several weeks (8) because of the need for data collection for each beam energy in photon and electron beams. This, compared with ATP of only a few days. These data cannot be rushed, so the proper amount of time should be allocated.

Linear accelerator technology has matured enough that intermachine variability is shrinking rapidly. Although some advocate accepting golden data provided by the manufacturer, it is not prudent to do so, as discussed in the references (9,10). Additional analysis for the criterion of beam matching shown by Hrbacek et al (11) indicates that it is easy to match central axis data, but very hard to match the full set of data, and hence beam commissioning should be performed as discussed in TG-106 (8).

In the context of commissioning, it is interesting to consider the pathways for error. Error detection in radiation therapy is difficult and usually is managed by continuous checks and quality assurance. Examples include chart checks by an independent person, through which most errors can be detected. Bojecho et al (12) provided some error detection using electronic portal imaging;

however, such methods cannot trace all factors. The World Health Organization (WHO) published radiation incident data for the period 1976 to 2007, in which 3,125 adverse events were analyzed (13). Figure 7.2 shows the data, indicating that almost 90% of errors are related to treatment planning (54%), commissioning (24%) and data transfer (10%). It also provided a large set of data for errors in commissioning. In view of such a large error rate, it is prudent to follow guidelines for commissioning (8). Readers are encouraged to review TG-106, which covers every aspect of commissioning beam data.

Data for reference

Commissioning a machine means collecting machine-specific data that are true to its values and that are used as a reference in the future throughout the life of the machine, usually 15 years. Quality assurance and machine calibrations are periodically performed according to various protocols (14–17). The annual calibration of a machine is concise, and its performance is verified with respect to commissioned data. Hence, during commissioning, reference data should be collected that are a true representation of the machine in every aspect, mechanically and dosimetrically. The reference data are tabulated and kept in the department for daily use in clinical operation and for future reference. These data sets are comprehensively scanned from very

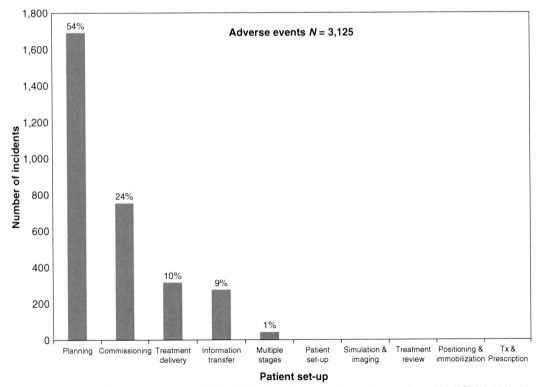

FIGURE 7.2 Source of adverse events compiled by WHO, drawn from actual data. (*Source*: From Ref. (13). World Health Organaization. *Radiotherapy Risk Profile, Technical Manual*. Geneva, Switzerland: World Health Organaization; 2008.)

small fields to large fields and represent every kind of data that are needed for patient treatment, such as PDD, tissue maximum ratio (TMR), output factor (OF), off-axis ratio (OAR), scatter factors (collimator, phantom, and total), MLC transmission, MLC gap, wedge factor, tray factor, field size factor for photon and depth dose, profile, bremsstrahlung, cone factor, virtual distance, and inverse square factors for electrons. The reference conditions also provide dosimetric parameter data for machine calibration as defined in TG-51 (14) or TRS-398 (16).

Data for treatment planning system

The treatment planning system (TPS) relies on actual measured data to account for planning. However, such planning does not account for tissue heterogeneity and does not provide the actual dose to the patient, but rather dose to water. For irregular fields, Clarkson integration (18) is still used on the assumption that the patient is composed of uniform water. The old generation TPSs that are factor-based have now been replaced with model-based wherein pencil beam, convolution/superposition, collapsed cone, Boltzmann transport, and, ultimately, Monte Carlo are increasingly used (19–25). However, most modern TPSs do not use a complete set of measured data but instead provide recommendations for commissioning and data collection. In general, a very limited data set (5×5, 10×10, 20×20, and 30×30 cm^2) is acquired for these TPSs. Most systems, however, require diagonal profile scans in the form of a star pattern. Absolute dose and various other factors are needed for a TPS. The details of can be found in the literature (26,27), but, more importantly, the data requirement of the TPS vendor should be followed. Monte Carlo–based derived parameters for TPSs have also been proposed (28–30). Unfortunately, widespread acceptance of such data is a long way away, and measured data are still preferred.

COMPONENTS OF DATA COLLECTION

The commissioning data of a machine can be divided into several components, namely, scanned and nonscanned (point) data, which are discussed in the following section. A detailed discussion can also be found in TG-106 (8).

Scanned data

A large water tank is essential and is now offered by most radiation therapy vendors. They come in many forms, including rectangular, square, and cylindrical, with many attractive features and sophisticated software for processing and analyzing the measured data. Akino et al (31) showed that beam data are not dependent on the scanning system and thus most of them can collect accurate data. Selection of a scanning system should involve considering the ease of software in acquisition and the processing and creation of tables for later analysis. The data are taken after the tank is properly set up to collect accurate data by an experienced physicist. Many techniques are available and common sense is needed to set up the tank, level it, and select the detector for a specific job. Tanks should be set such that the movement of the three axes is orthogonal to one other and the beam axis matches with the depth axis. TG-106 (8) has provided details of these procedures. Figure 7.3 shows an example of data if the arm of the tank and gantry are not set properly. Small changes in tank set-up may not be reflected in normal conditions, but will be visible in wedge data, especially for large angles.

When scanning a beam, a reference detector should be used to eliminate the fluctuation in beam output. Placement of such a detector should be selected so that it does not shadow the scanned axis and remains in the beam from small fields to large. Recently, some

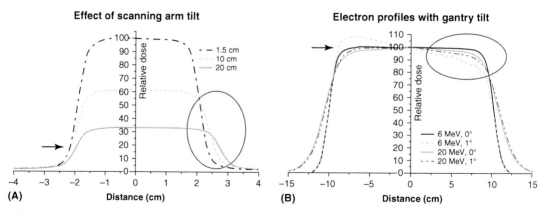

FIGURE 7.3 Effect of scanning arm is visible in profiles (see circle area) taken at different depths (A); also, if machine gantry is titled, electron profiles show skewed behavior (B). (*Source*: Adapted from Ref. (8). Das IJ, Cheng CW, Watts RJ, et al. Accelerator beam data commissioning equipment and procedures: report of the TG-106 of the Therapy Physics Committee of the AAPM. *Med Phys*. 2008;35:4186–4215.)

vendors have provided a transmission ion chamber for a reference detector that could be used if purchased. Another good option is to place the detector on the bottom of the tank, securely taped to the tank, so that it does not float. If none of these options are available, and the machine is unstable, a longer time for signal integration or use of a monitor ion chamber as reference can be explored.

Percent depth dose

Depth dose measurements are straightforward and the simplest of the measurements. Selection of the detector is critical, as variability in response due to energy dependence and extracameral effect should be avoided (32–34). In general, small volume (≈ 0.125 cm^3) ion chambers are best suited for standard data collection. Before data collection, the quality of the triaxial cable should be properly examined to eliminate error in data, especially when the signal is very low (small fields and penumbra or out-of-field measurements). It is good practice to collect null data or subtraction data without the beam in some systems before collecting any scanned data.

The direction of scanning (i.e., top to bottom or bottom to top) also affects the quality of data. Owing to the air–water interface and wake of water, it is strongly recommended that scanning be performed from bottom to top. Even in such situations, the buildup region or surface dose cannot be trusted with scanned beam.

TG-106 (8) has demonstrated the seriousness of beam data collection in the buildup region. If the buildup region is important, data should be acquired using a parallel plate ion chamber with proper corrections (35–38) after PDD data are collected. Another method based on curve fitting (39) can also be used. These methods, however, tend to be time consuming.

Tissue maximum ratio (TMR)

The TMR/TPR measurements are similar to the PDD, as discussed in the previous section, except that the detector is kept at the same distance and the water height is changed. Such measurements are very difficult unless a pressure sensing system is available to the scanning water tank. When performing TMR measurements, the same considerations must be taken into account while selecting the proper detector and direction of scanning and measurement in the buildup region, as mentioned in the previous section.

Most scanning systems provide software to convert PDD to TMR, which is shown mathematically in various references (5,8,40). The conversion from PDD to TMR requires extrapolation of field data, and hence very small field PDDs are needed that are difficult to measure (41, 42). Additionally, care should be taken not to blindly use converted data from software, as these have larger errors

in large fields and deeper depths (5,40,43). Spot checks of TMR are essential to make sure that calculated data are within at least 1% agreement. Although the assumption is made that TMR are source–surface distance independent, this ignores any scatter contribution arising from beam divergence at larger distances.

Profile/off-axis ratio

Profiles are needed for off-axis ratio (OAR) data that are required for isodose calculations as well as dose calculations to any point off-axis. Before setting up the water tank, care should be taken to ensure that the physical orientation of the tank and the direction of scanning correlate with the scanning software. If the tank is set up improperly, in-plane measurements can be incorrectly recorded as cross-plane and vice versa, thus creating confusion in selecting the correct profile for TPS or for future comparison. Scanning software can often be used to determine the radiation isocenter, which can minimize physical set-up errors using cross-hairs/lasers and result in more consistent data.

Selection of the detector (i.e., short axis or spherical chambers for high resolution) should be specified. It has been shown in many references that beam profiles are strongly dependent on the detector (8,44). Figure 7.4 shows actual data taken for the same machine and energy but with different detector orientations. Beam profiles should be taken in-plane and cross-plane. In general, there is very good agreement for a well-calibrated machine, but slight variations are expected, as X and Y jaw positions are nearly 8 cm apart, and thus the backscattering from jaw to ion chamber (45–47) and divergence of the beam make the profiles slightly ($\leq 0.5\%$) different.

Films (radiographic and radiochromic) can be used for profile measurements, provided proper precautions, as shown in references (48–50), are adopted. If radiochromic film is used for beam commissioning, flat-bed densitometer issues (spectrum, position, orientation, air gap, temperature, time, etc.) should be clearly understood (51) and benchmarking with respect to ion chamber readings should be performed. There are many other approaches, such as 3D detectors based on gel dosimetry; however, they are still limited to a few centers and are not in mainstream use.

NONSCANNED (POINT DOSE)

Once PDD, profiles, and diagonal scans are completed for photon (normal and wedge beams) and electron beams, point dose measurements are collected. Again, either a small water tank or a large tank with the option of point dose measurement in the software can be used. Many sets of data points are needed for TPS commissioning, as well as for monitor unit (MU) calculation, which is discussed later.

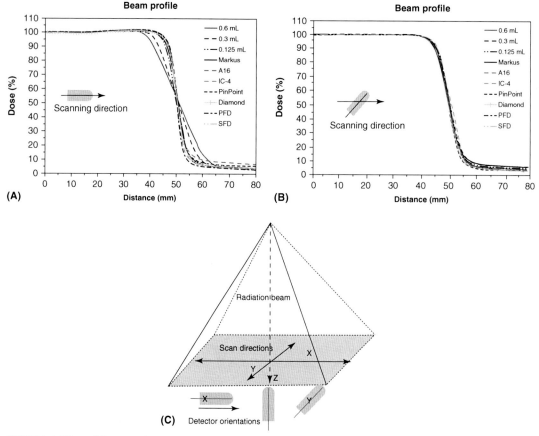

FIGURE 7.4 Effect of detector orientation on beam profile for a 6 MV beam. (A) Detector axis is the same as the scan direction, and (B) detector axis is perpendicular to the scan direction. For some detectors, beam and detector axis parallel can be explored if cable noise is minimal, as shown in (C). (*Source*: Adapted from Ref. (8). Das IJ, Cheng CW, Watts RJ, et al. Accelerator beam data commissioning equipment and procedures: report of the TG-106 of the therapy physics committee of the AAPM. *Med Phys*. 2008;35:4186–4215.)

Source: Adapted from Accelerator beam data commissioning equipment and procedures: Report of the TG-106 of the therapy physics committee of the aapm. Med Phys 2008;35:4186-4215.

Scatter factor

Scatter is a part of the radiation beam and should be quantified for each beam energy. In general, scatter is divided into collimator scatter (S_c), phantom scatter (S_p), and total scatter (S_{cp}). The names of these quantities have been changing over time, which is alluded to in TG-74 (52). According to the TG-74, S_c and S_{cp} should be called *in air output ratio* and *in water output ratio,* respectively. These factors are normalized to a reference field size, which is traditionally 10×10 cm^2 for standard radiation treatment.

Collimator scatter factor, Sc

There is a great deal of variation in the measurement of S_c. Traditionally, it has been measured with plastic buildup caps individualized for beam energy. However, as beam energy increases, the buildup caps become very large,

affecting the coverage of small fields at a standard 100 cm distance, and hence data lesser than 4×4 cm^2 are hard to achieve. Metallic buildup caps have been proposed, but these have the additional problem of interface effect and require corrections as shown (53,54). Zhu et al (55–57) provided a clear rationale for the mini-phantom approach to the S_c measurement, which is also advocated in TG-74 (58). Mini-phantoms tend to provide electronic equilibrium and remove electron contamination from the head (59–61). For irregular fields, Kim et al (62) provided a generalized method, but for commissioning, mainly square fields are used. For very small fields in SRS/SRT, metallic buildup caps have been suggested, but their use should be limited and proper corrections, as provided by Weber et al (54), should be used. In such situations, S_c can be measured at very long distances (3–5 m), either with a buildup cap or a mini-phantom advocated by TG-74. If long distances are used, the user should be aware that the air column does contribute to scatter and contaminate the condition.

Total scatter factor, S_{cp}

As described earlier, the scatter component associated with the collimator and phantom has many names, including total scatter factor, output factor, and now "in water output ratio," as defined by TG-74 (52). This is measured in a large water phantom under full electronic equilibrium. The definition of S_{cp} was originally meant for a dose at d_{max} normalized to a 10×10 cm^2 reference field (63). However, TG-74 recommended that S_{cp} be measured at greater depths where there is no contribution from electron contamination. It recommended that S_{cp} be measured at a reference depth (5 or 10 cm). These two definitions are noncongruent and have been discussed in detail by Cheng et al (64). If the output factor is measured at a variable distance, the dose normalized to the reference field is not unique, as shown in Figure 7.5. However, these two are related as in Eq. [3].

$$S_{cp}(A,d_{ref}) = \frac{PDD(A,\ d_{ref})}{PDD(A_{ref},\ d_{ref})} \times S_{cp}(A,d_{max})$$

where A is field size, d is depth, and ref stands for reference. If a correction is made to S_{cp}, the variation in Figure 7.5 converges to a single curve. Thus, it is important to specify and clarify the meaning of S_{cp} in terms of depth of measurement.

Phantom scatter, S_p

The S_p is not measured, but computed on the basis of $S_p = S_{cp}/S_c$. It is critical that the definition of S_{cp}, as discussed in the previous section, be compatible, so that the accuracy of S_c is maintained for accurate calculation of S_p, which is used in dose calculations in most TPS and MU calculation algorithms.

Wedge factor

Wedges are devices that modulate the dose profiles in a plane. Wedges are physical or electronic (called "soft wedge"). These soft wedges have unique names, depending on the vendor, and cannot be interchanged. Hence, enhanced dynamic wedge (EDW) (65–67), virtual wedge (68–72), and universal/omni wedge (73–75) are unique to Varian, Siemens, and Elekta machines, respectively. Physical wedges are falling out of favor in radiation oncology, because they change the beam characteristics, and the wedge factor is dependent on field size, depth, energy, and wedge angle (76–81). Additionally, Varian has two sets of physical wedges (upper and lower) that compound for extra work during commissioning. Cheng et al (82) showed that commissioning time can be reduced

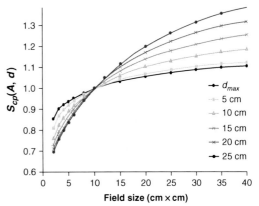

FIGURE 7.5 Total scatter factor as a function of depth of measurement. Note that S_{cp} was originally defined at d_{max} (63), whereas 5 to 10 cm is now advocated by TG-74 (52).

by spot checking, as lower and upper wedge factors are relatively similar.

Soft wedges evolved from the original concept proposed before computers came to be used more extensively in radiation therapy (83,84). However, implementation of modern soft wedges is credited to Petti et al (85), who suggested mixing a weighted 60° wedge profile with an open beam to create any possible wedge angle.

The wedge factor is a ratio of dose with wedge to the open beam for a field size, beam energy, and depth. Traditionally, the depth is chosen to be 10 cm in modern radiation treatment with a suitable ion chamber with adequate signal, since the large wedge angles attenuate the beam significantly and may give a poor signal.

Tray factor

Before the MLC era, most treatments were performed with cerrobend blocks that were mounted on a Lucite tray. Because trays attenuate the beam, the tray factor (TF) was measured. The TF is the ratio of dose with and without the tray. This is again measured at a 10 cm depth with the tray in place to open beam for a given field size and beam energy. One should be aware that it should not be measured at d_{max} because of significant electron contamination from the tray (86,87).

Cone factor

Apart from various commissioning scans for electron beams, the collection of cone factor data is essential. This is measured at the relevant d_{max} or d_{ref} for each electron energy. The cone factor is a ratio of dose in a given cone to the reference cone, usually 15×15 cm^2, as defined in various references (14,88,89).

NONSTANDARD TREATMENT

Apart from standard radiation treatment, special procedures for large fields such as total body irradiation (90) and total skin electron irradiation (91) require additional beam data that must be commissioned on the basis of the technique and institutional preference. In contrast, small fields require additional data for cranial irradiation (stereotactic radiosurgery [SRS]), stereotactic body radiotherapy (SBRT), Gamma Knife, Cyberknife, Tomotherapy, and linear accelerators. Small field dosimetry issues have been discussed in many references (92–96) and are beyond the scope of this chapter.

PEER REVIEW—TG-103

Peer review is an essential component for detection of possible errors in beam data commissioning and calibration. This is often accomplished by verifying the measured data published from similar machines from the Radiological Physics Center (RPC), now known as Imaging and Radiation Oncology Core (IROC) (97–99). Golden data can also be compared. However, when there is only one physicist at a center, there is no mechanism for a second set of checks of the beam parameters and calibration. TG-103 (100) was written in this context to have a friend or colleague thoroughly check every aspect of the beam and write a report after independently verifying it. The American College of Radiology (ACR) has adopted TG-103 for peer review for a solo practice.

EXTERNAL AUDITS VIA IMAGING AND RADIATION ONCOLOGY CORE OR THE EQUIVALENT

For centers that are part of collaborative clinical trials, radiological parameters are periodically checked by RPC/IROC. Ibbott et al (101) noted the challenges associated with credentialing the institutions by comparing the data. However, in a simpler version, only central axis reference condition data are checked annually by mail-order thermo-luminescent dosimeter (TLD) service. A set of TLDs are sent to an institution to expose in calibration conditions. These are returned for evaluation to IROC, which compares them with the known dose and writes a report. Several high-profile incidents have been discovered through such operation. IAEA/WHO and European countries have also adopted postal services for machine calibration validations (102–104).

SOFTWARE

Software error detection is a very difficult process. The industry is trying to eliminate software bugs, but it is expected that errors of nearly 0.2% are inherent in any code. These could create a major problem in health care. A software glitch associated with the Therac-25 killed many patients and forced this brand to be discontinued. Software errors can also be associated with device failures due to radiation or environmental conditions. Vendors usually test whether components meet strict guidelines, to provide a safe environment for their product (105). However, failures related to software are very hard to detect and exist even in a perfect system.

Major accidents

Although many accidents occur in every walk of life because of software errors, in radiation oncology, the most important and critical error was associated with Therac-25 linear accelerators that killed eight patients in Tyler and Yakima (106). A great deal has been written about this accident in the media and in journals. A recent accident involving an MLC control failure of a Varian machine was also highly publicized (107).

Error detection

Human–machine interface is the most common problem associated with major accidents. A culture of safety should be introduced at each workplace, emphasizing the critical nature of errors related to patient care. Recently, most societies have devoted considerable time to the culture of safety, as shown in reference (108). IAEA Safety Report 17 (109) provided a comprehensive analysis of error mitigation in radiation-related safety concerns including human–machine interface. Proper training in the use of equipment by the vendor and periodic training on critical components and upgrades is vital in reducing the chances of error. Interlock overrides, either in clinical, service, or research mode, should be viewed with extreme severity and should not be allowed. Any warning sign on screen cannot be ignored and should be fully investigated (107,109). A running log of the faults for each machine is vital in resolving issues with the maintenance engineer and also with the vendor. A periodic maintenance, also known as a preventive maintenance inspection (PMI), is critical for eliminating errors. During a PMI, engineers can repair and upgrade any software problem that has been detected by the vendor. The ACR accreditation process requires documentation of these services. There are various watchdog agencies that provide feedback on the safety aspect of the treatment machine that should be periodically evaluated. Patient-related data in the record-and-verify system should be periodically evaluated for overrides, and their consequences should be disseminated. Simple factors such as table coordinates can potentially provide a chance to detect possible error in treatment site.

SUMMARY

This chapter provides an overview of beam data commissioning, its components, and rationale. Some administrative approaches related to the beam data have also been added and terminology expanded. Detailed references, published since TG-106 (8), have also been listed. Differences in terminology that exist in the literature are pointed out. It is also emphasized that beam data for a machine should be collected with adequate allocation of time. Any similar set of data (golden) should be cross-referenced and should never be copied, even in an advanced machine. This chapter did not cover commissioning for small fields, which is an evolving subject and pending for the upcoming report TG-155 (93). Quality assurance and mechanical aspects of the machines are considered in other chapters in this book.

REFERENCES

1. Nath R, Biggs PJ, Bova FJ, et al. AAPM code of practice for radiotherapy accelerators: report of AAPM Radiation Therapy Task Group No. 45. *Med Phys.* 1994;21:1093–1121.

2. LaRiviere PD. The quality of high-energy x-ray beams. *Br J Radiol.* 1989;62:473–481.

3. Kalach NI, Rogers DWO. Which accelerator photon beams are "clinic-like" for reference dosimetry purposes? *Med Phys.* 2003;30:1546–1555.

4. Das IJ, Khan FM, Gerbi BJ. Interface dose perturbation as a measure of megavoltage photon beam energy. *Med Phys.* 1988;15:78–81.

5. Aird EGA, Burns JE, Day MJ, et al. Central axis depth dose data for use in radiotherapy: 1996, a survey of depth doses and related data measured in water or equivalent media. *Br J Radiol.* 1996;(Suppl 25).

6. Kosunen A, Rogers DW. Beam quality specification for photon beam dosimetry. *Med Phys.* 1993;20:1181–1188.

7. Institute of Physics and Engineering in Medicine. *Acceptance Testing and Commissioning of Linear Accelerators.* York, UK: Institute of Physics and Engineering in Medicine; 2007. IPEM Report 94.

8. Das IJ, Cheng CW, Watts RJ, et al. Accelerator beam data commissioning equipment and procedures: report of the TG-106 of the Therapy Physics Committee of the AAPM. *Med Phys.* 2008;35:4186–4215.

9. Das IJ, Njeh CF, Orton CG. Point/counterpoint: vendor provided machine data should never be used as a substitute for fully commissioning a linear accelerator. *Med Phys.* 2012;39:569–572.

10. Kapanen M, Sipila P, Bly R, et al. Accuracy of central axis dose calculations for photon external radiotherapy beams in Finland: the quality of local beam data and the use of averaged data. *Radiother Oncol.* 2008;86:264–271.

11. Hrbacek J, Depuydt T, Nulens A, et al. Quantitative evaluation of a beam-matching procedure using one-dimensional gamma analysis. *Med Phys.* 2007;34:2917–2927.

12. Bojechko C, Phillips M, Kalet A, et al. A quantification of the effectiveness of EPID dosimetry and software-based plan verification systems in detecting incidents in radiotherapy. *Med Phys.* 2015;42:5363–5369.

13. World Health Organization. *Radiotherapy Risk Profile, Technical Manual.* Geneva, Switzerland: World Health Organization; 2008.

14. Almond PR, Biggs PJ, Coursey BM, et al. AAPM's TG-51 protocol for clinical reference dosimetry of high-energy photon and electron beams. *Med Phys.* 1999;26:1847–1870.

15. Klein EE, Hanley J, Bayouth J, et al; Task Group AAPM. Task Group 142 report: quality assurance of medical accelerators. *Med Phys.* 2009;36:4197–4212.

16. International Atomic Energy Agency. *Absorbed Dose Determination in External Beam Radiotherapy: An International Code of Practice for Dosimetry Based on Standards of Absorbed Dose to Water.* Vienna, Austria: International Atomic Energy Agency; 2000. IAEA TRS 398.

17. World Health Organization. *Quality Assurance in Radiotherapy.* Geneva, Switzerland: World Health Organization; 1988.

18. Clarkson JR. A note on depth doses in fields of irregular shape. *Br J Radiol.* 1941;14:265–268.

19. Ahnesjö A, Aspradakis MM. Dose calculations for external photon beams in radiotherapy. *Phys Med Biol.* 1999;44:R99–R155.

20. Ahnesjö A, Saxner M, Trepp A. A pencil beam model for photon beam calculation. *Med Phys.* 1992;19:263–273.

21. Ahnesjö A. Collapsed cone convolution of radiant energy for photon dose calculation in heterogeneous media. *Med Phys.* 1989;16:577–592.

22. Fogliata A, Nicolini G, Clivio A, et al. Critical appraisal of Acuros XB and anisotropic analytic algorithm dose calculation in advanced non-small-cell lung cancer treatments. *Int J Radiat Oncol Biol Phys.* 2012;83:1587–1595.

23. Fogliata A, Nicolini G, Clivio A, et al. Accuracy of Acuros XB and AAA dose calculation for small fields with reference to RapidArc® stereotactic treatments. *Med Phys.* 2011;38:6228–6237.

24. Van Esch A, Tillikainen L, Pyykkonen J, et al. Testing of the analytical anisotropic

algorithm for photon dose calculation. *Med Phys.* 2006;33:4130–4148.

25. Knöös T, Ceberg C, Weber L, et al. The dosimetric verification of a pencil beam based treatment planning system. *Phys Med Biol.* 1994;39:1609–1628.

26. Fraass B, Doppke K, Hunt M, et al. American Association of Physicists in Medicine Radiation Therapy Committee Task Group 53: quality assurance for clinical radiotherapy treatment planning. *Med Phys.* 1998;25:1773–1829.

27. International Atomic Energy Agency. *Commissioning and Quality Assurance of Computerized Planning Sytems for Radiation Treatment of Cancer.* Vienna, Austria: International Atomic Energy Agency; 2004. IAEA TRS 430.

28. St. Aubin J, Steciw S, Kirkby C, et al. An integrated 6 MV linear accelerator model from electron gun to dose in a water tank. *Med Phys.* 2010;37:2279–2288.

29. Chetty IJ, Curran B, Cygler JE, et al. Report of the AAPM Task Group No. 105: issues associated with clinical implementations of Monte Carlo-based photon and electron external beam treatment planning. *Med Phys.* 2007;34:4818–4853.

30. Pena J, Franco L, Gomez F, et al. Commissioning of a medical accelerator photon beam: Monte Carlo simulation using wide-field profiles. *Phys Med Biol.* 2004;49:4929–4942.

31. Akino Y, Gibbon JP, Neck DW, et al. Intra- and inter-variability in beam data commissioning among water phantom scanning systems. *J Appl Clin Med Phys.* 2014;15(4):4850.

32. Fowler JF, Farmer FT. Insulators for radiological instruments. *Br J Radiol.* 1956;29:118–119.

33. Spokas JJ, Meeker RD. Investigation of cables for ionization chambers. *Med Phys.* 1980;7:135–140.

34. Gross B. The Compton current. *Zeit Phys.* 1959;155:479–487.

35. Gerbi BJ, Khan FM. Measurement of dose in the buildup region using fixed-separation plane-parallel ion chambers. *Med Phys.* 1990;17:17–26.

36. Gerbi BJ, Khan FM. Plane-parallel ionization chamber response in the buildup region of obliquely incident photon beams. *Med Phys.* 1997;24:873–878.

37. Mellenberg DE. Determination of buildup region over-response corrections for a Markus-type chamber. *Med Phys.* 1990;17:1041–1044.

38. Velkley DE, Manson DJ, Purdy JA, et al. Buildup region of megavoltage photon radiation sources. *Med Phys.* 1975;2:14–19.

39. Das IJ, Bushe HS, Copeland JF. Determination of exact point of measurement and surface dose in an electron beam with cylindrical ion chambers. *AMPI Med Phys Bull.* 1993;18:16–19.

40. Khan FM. *The Physics of Radiation Therapy.* 3rd ed. Philadelphia, PA: Lippincott Williams & Wilkins; 2003.

41. Francescon P, Beddar S, Satariano N, et al. Variation of k(fclin, fmsr, Qclin, Qmsr) for the small-field dosimetric parameters percentage depth dose, tissue-maximum ratio, and off-axis ratio. *Med Phys.* 2014;41:101708.

42. Cheng CW, Cho SH, Taylor M, et al. Determination of zero-field size percent depth doses and tissue maximum ratios for stereotactic radiosurgery and IMRT dosimetry: comparison between experimental measurements and Monte Carlo simulation. *Med Phys.* 2007;34:3149–3157.

43. Bjärngard BE, Zhu TC, Ceberg C. Tissue-phantom ratios from percentage depth doses. *Med Phys.* 1996;23:629–634.

44. Das IJ, Downes MB, Kassaee A, et al. Choice of radiation detector in dosimetry of stereotactic radiosurgery-radiotherapy. *J Radiosurgery.* 2000;3:177–185.

45. Hounsell AR. Monitor chamber backscatter for intensity modulated radiation therapy using multileaf collimators. *Phys Med Biol.* 1998;43:445–454.

46. Olofsson J, Georg D, Karlsson M. A widely tested model for head scatter influence on photon beam output. *Radiother Oncol.* 2003;67:225–238.

47. Huang PH, Chu J, Bjarngard BE. The effect of collimator backscatter radiation on photon output of linear accelerators. *Med Phys.* 1987;14:268–269.

48. Pai S, Das IJ, Dempsey JF, et al. TG-69: radiographic film for megavoltage beam dosimetry. *Med Phys.* 2007;34:2228–2258.

49. Niroomand-Rad A, Blackwell CR, Coursey BM, et al; American Association of Physicists in Medicine. Radiochromic film dosimetry: recommendations of AAPM Radiation Therapy Committee Task Group 55. *Med Phys.* 1998;25:2093–2115.

50. Devic S. Radiochromic film dosimetry: past, present, and future. *Phys Med.* 2011;27:122–134.

51. Rosen BS, Soares CG, Hammer CG, et al. A prototype, glassless densitometer traceable to primary optical standards for quantitative radiochromic film dosimetry. *Med Phys.* 2015;42:4055.

52. Zhu TC, Ahnesjo A, Lam KL, et al. Report of AAPM Therapy Physics Committee Task Group 74: in-air output ratio, S_c, for megavoltage photon beams. *Med Phys.* 2009;36:5261–5291.

53. Ciesielski B, Reinstein LE, Wielopolski L, et al. Dose enhancement in buildup region by lead,

aluminum, and lucite absorbers for 15 MVp photon beam. *Med Phys.* 1989;16:609–613.

54. Weber L, Nilsson P, Ahnesjö A. Build-up cap materials for measurement of photon head-scatter factors. *Phys Med Biol.* 1997;42:1875–1886.

55. Zhu TC, Bjarngard BE. The head-scatter factor for small field sizes. *Med Phys.* 1994;21:65–68.

56. Li J, Zhu TC. Measurement of in-air output ratios using different miniphantom materials. *Phys Med Biol.* 2006;51:3819–3834.

57. Li J, Zhu TC. Monte Carlo simulation of the effect of miniphantom on in-air output ratio. *Med Phys.* 2010;37:5228–5237.

58. Zhu TC, Ahnesjö A, Lam KL, et al. Report of AAPM Therapy Physics Committee Task Group 74: in-air output ratio, S_c, for megavoltage photon beams. *Med Phys.* 2009;36:5261–5291.

59. Hug B, Warrener K, Liu P, et al. On the measurement of dose in-air for small radiation fields: choice of mini-phantom material. *Phys Med Biol.* 2015;60:2391–2402.

60. van Gasteren JJ, Heukelom S, van Kleffens HJ, et al. The determination of phantom and collimator scatter components of the output of megavoltage photon beams: measurement of the collimator scatter part with a beam-coaxial narrow cylindrical phantom. *Radiother Oncol.* 1991;20:250–257.

61. Nilsson B, Brahme A. Electron contamination from photon beam collimators. *Radiother Oncol.* 1986;5:235–244.

62. Kim S, Palta JR, Zhu TC. A generalized solution for the calculation of in-air output factors in irregular fields. *Med Phys.* 1998;25:1692–1701.

63. Khan FM, Sewchand W, Lee J, et al. Revision of tissue-maximum ratio and scatter-maximum ratio concepts for cobalt 60 and higher energy x-ray beams. *Med Phys.* 1980;7:230–237.

64. Cheng CW, Tang WL, Das IJ. S_{cp} revisited. *J Med Phys.* 2016. (Under review).

65. Leavitt DD, Klein E. Dosimetry measurement tools for commissioning enhanced dynamic wedge. *Med Dosim.* 1997;22:171–176.

66. Moeller JH, Leavitt DD, Klein E. The quality assurance of enhanced dynamic wedges. *Med Dosim.* 1997;22:241–246.

67. Klein EE, Gerber R, Zhu XR, et al. Multiple machine implementation of enhanced dynamic wedge. *Int J Radiat Oncol Biol Phys.* 1998;40:977–985.

68. McGhee P, Chu T, Leszczynski K, et al. The Siemens virtual wedge. *Med Dosim.* 1997;22:39–41.

69. Desobry GE, Waldron TJ, Das IJ. Validation of new virtual wedge model. *Med Phys.* 1998;25:71–72.

70. van Santvoort J. Dosimetric evaluation of the Siemens virtual wedge. *Phys Med Biol.* 1998;43:2651–2663.

71. Rathee S, Kwok C, MacGillivray C, et al. Commissioning, clinical implementation and quality assurance of Siemen's virtual wedge. *Med Dosim.* 1999;24:145–153.

72. Verhaegen F, Das IJ. Monte Carlo modelling of a virtual wedge. *Phys Med Biol.* 1999;44:N251–N259.

73. Klein EE, Esthappan J, Li Z. Surface and buildup dose characteristics for 6, 10, and 18 MV photons from an Elekta Precise linear accelerator. *J Appl Clin Med Phys.* 2003;4:1–7.

74. Phillips MH, Parsaei H, Cho PS. Dynamic and omni wedge implementation on an Elekta SL linac. *Med Phys.* 2000;27:1623–1634.

75. Shackford H, Bjarngard BE, Vadash P. Dynamic universal wedge. *Med Phys.* 1995;22:1735–1741.

76. McCullough EC, Gortney J, Blackwell CR. A depth dependence determination of the wedge transmission factor for 4–10 MV photon beams. *Med Phys.* 1988;15:621–623.

77. Palta JR, Daftari I, Suntharlingam N. Field size dependence of wedge factors. *Med Phys.* 1988;15:624–626.

78. Knöös T, Wittgren L. Which depth dose data should be used for dose planning when wedge filters are used to modify the photon beam? *Phys Med Biol.* 1991;36:255–267.

79. Niroomand-Rad A, Haleem M, Rodgers J, et al. Wedge factor dependence on depth and field size for various beam energies using symmetric and half-collimated asymmetric jaw settings. *Med Phys.* 1992;19:1445–1450.

80. Heukelom S, Lanson JH, Mijnheer BJ. Wedge factor constituents of high energy photon beams: head and phantom scatter components. *Radiother Oncol.* 1994;32:73–83.

81. Thomas SJ. The effect on wedge factors of scattered radiation from the wedge. *Radiother Oncol.* 1994;32:271–273.

82. Cheng CW, Tang WL, Das IJ. Beam characteristics of upper and lower physical wedge systems of Varian accelerators. *Phys Med Biol.* 2003;48:3667–3683.

83. Cheng CW, Chin LM. A computer-aided treatment planning technique for universal wedge. *Int J Radiat Oncol Biol Phys.* 1987;13:1927–1935.

84. Kijewski PK, Chin LN, Bjärngard BE. Wedge-shaped dose distribution by computer controlled collimator motion. *Med Phys.* 1978;5:426–429.

85. Petti PL, Siddon RL. Effective wedge angles with universal wedge. *Phys Med Biol.* 1985;30:985–991.

86. Klein EE, Michalet-Lorenz M, Taylor ME. Use of a lucite beam spoiler for high-energy breast irradiation. *Med Dosim.* 1995;20:89–94.

87. Bova FJ, Hill LW. Surface doses for acrylic versus lead blocking trays for Co-60, 8 MV and 17 MV photons. *Med Phys.* 1983;10:254–256.

88. International Commission on Radiation Units and Measurements. *Radiation Dosimetry: Electron Beams with Energies Between 1 to 50 MeV.* Bethesda, MD: International Commission on Radiation Units and Measurements; 1984. ICRU Report 35.

89. Gerbi BJ, Antolak JA, Deibel FC, et al. Recommendations for clinical electron beam dosimetry: supplement to the recommendations of Task Group 25. *Med Phys.* 2009;36:3239–3279.

90. Van Dyk J, Galvin JM, Glasgow GP, et al. *The Physical Aspects of Total and Half Body Photon Irradiation.* New York, NY: American Association of Physicists in Medicine; 1986. AAPM Report No. 17.

91. Karzmark CJ. *Total Skin Electron Therapy: Technique and Dosimetry.* New York, NY: American Institute of Physics; 1988. AAPM Report No. 23.

92. Das IJ, Ding GX, Ahnesjö A. Small fields: non-equilibrium radiation dosimetry. *Med Phys.* 2008;35:206–215.

93. Das IJ, Francescon P, Ahnesjö A, et al. Small fields and non-equilibrium condition photon beam dosimetry: AAPM Task Group Report 155. *Med Phys.* (In review).

94. Alfonso P, Andreo P, Capote R, et al. A new formalism for reference dosimetry of small and non-standard fields. *Med Phys.* 2008;35:5179–5186.

95. Aspradakis MM, Bryne JP, Palmans H, et al. *Report No. 103: Small Field MV Dosimetry.* York, UK: Institute of Physics and Engineering in Medicine; 2010.

96. Yunice KM, Vinogradskiy Y, Miften M, et al. Small field dosimetry for stereotactic radiosurgery and radiotherapy. In: Benedict SH, Schlesinger DJ, Goetsch SJ, et al, eds. *Stereotactic Radiosurgery and Stereotactic Body Radiation Therapy.* Boca Raton, FL: CRC Press; 2014:265–286.

97. Tailor RC, Tello VM, Schroy CB, et al. A generic off-axis energy correction for linac photon beam dosimetry. *Med Phys.* 1998;25:662–667.

98. Tailor RC, Followill DS, Hanson WF. A first order approximation of field-size and depth dependence of wedge transmission. *Med Phys.* 1998;25:241–244.

99. Followill DS, Tailor RC, Tello VM, et al. An empirical relationship for determining photon beam quality in TG-21 from a ratio of percent depth doses. *Med Phys.* 1998;25:1202–1205.

100. Halvorsen PH, Das IJ, Fraser M, et al. AAPM Task Group 103 report on peer review in clinical radiation oncology physics. *J Appl Clin Med Phys.* 2005;6:50–64.

101. Ibbott GS, Followill DS, Molineu HA, et al. Challenges in credentialing institutions and participants in advanced technology multi-institutional clinical trials. *Int J Radiat Oncol Biol Phys.* 2008;71:S71–S75.

102. Espinosa Mdel M, Nunez L, Muniz JL, et al. Postal dosimetry audit test for small photon beams. *Radiother Oncol.* 2012;102:135–141.

103. Izewska J, Bera P, Vatnitsky S. IAEA/WHO TLD postal dose audit service and high precision measurements for radiotherapy level dosimetry. International Atomic Energy Agency. *Radiat Prot Dosimetry.* 2002;101:387–392.

104. Izewska J, Georg D, Bera P, et al. A methodology for TLD postal dosimetry audit of high-energy radiotherapy photon beams in non-reference conditions. *Radiother Oncol.* 2007;84:67–74.

105. Wilkinson JD, Bounds C, Brown T, et al. Cancer-radiotherapy equipment as a cause of soft errors in electronic equipment. *IEEE Device Maker Reliabil.* 2005;5:449–451.

106. Leveson NG, Turner CS. An investigation of the Therac-25 accidents. *IEEE Comput.* 1993;26:18–41.

107. Bogdanich W. Radiation offers new cures, and ways to do harm. *New York Times.* January 23, 2010.

108. Zietman AL, Palta JR, Steinberg ML. *Safety Is No Accident: A Framework for Quality Radiation Oncology and Care.* Fairfax, VA: American Society for Radiation Oncology; 2012.

109. International Atomic Energy Agency. *Lessons Learned from Accidental Exposures in Radiotherapy.* Vienna, Austria: International Atomic Energy Agency; 2000. IAEA Safety Reports Series No. 17.

8 | Equipment, Software, and Techniques for Quality Assurance

Baozhou Sun and Eric E. Klein

INTRODUCTION

Importance and concept of quality assurance in radiation safety

The radiation therapy (RT) process is very complex and involves understanding the principles of multiple disciplines, including medical physics, radiobiology, dosimetry, imaging, and radiation safety. In a typical radiation therapy clinic, the treatment process includes prescribing a treatment protocol, CT simulation, treatment planning, physics and physician plan review, pretreatment quality assurance (QA) and plan verification, treatment delivery, and follow-up evaluation and care. The International Commission on Radiation Units and Measurements (ICRU) recommends that the dose delivered to the patient should be within 5% of the prescribed dose (1). Taking into consideration the multiple steps involved in delivering dose to a target volume in a patient, each step in the integrated process in RT must be subject to quality control and QA to achieve this recommendation and to prevent errors. A series of articles in the *New York Times* in 2010 reported a number of serious and tragic accidents involving RT treatments (2–5). Some of the reported errors resulted from a failure to implement the QA program appropriately or insufficiency of the QA performed. A comprehensive QA program in radiation oncology must be implemented to ensure consistency of the medical prescription, and safe fulfillment of that prescription, with regard to the dose to the target volume with minimal dose to normal tissues, and minimal exposure to personnel. Several American Association of Physicists in Medicine (AAPM) Task Group reports (6,7) and American Society for Therapeutic Radiology and Oncology (ASTRO) reports (8) have been published to recommend QA in RT. A comprehensive QA program includes all aspects of patient care (e.g., physical, clinical, and medical aspects). In the physical aspect, one of the important elements of a QA program is equipment, software, and techniques.

Historical review

Every QA task is performed by human beings using certain hardware tools or automated with software tools. The hardware and software tools designed for quality assurance play a critical role in radiation therapy. Without dosimetric equipment, dosages delivered to patients cannot be verified. With the advent of image-guided RT (IGRT), the imaging quality is tested with imaging phantoms. The QA equipment is usually integrated with software to analyze results. Without proper tools, cannot be performed. If the QA equipment is not used appropriately, tragic errors and mistakes can occur. A faulty ionization chamber used in the commissioning of radiosurgery for small radiation beam resulted in an overdose of 76 patients in Missouri (5). A large portion of the market in RT consists of the tools used for quality assurance. Although several AAPM task groups publish details on various types of dosimeters (ionization chamber (9), diodes (10), and film dosimetry [11,12]), the hardware and software tools used for QA in RT cover a broad range of equipment, including phantom and imaging tools, commercial and in-house developed software, and techniques. A comprehensive review of this topic is not available in the literature.

New technologies in radiation therapy demand more comprehensive QA equipment, software, and techniques

New technologies have revolutionized RT over the past 10 to 15 years. These include intensity-modulated radiation therapy (IMRT), helical tomotherapy, volumetric modulated arc therapy (VMAT), stereotactic radiotherapy, IGRT including MRI-guided RT, adaptive radiotherapy, particle therapy, and 4D-motion management. The increased complexity of modern treatment modalities requires improved verification techniques. For example, with image-guided

RT, the imaging and treatment coordinate coincidence is critical to ensure a safe treatment. For stereotactic body radiation therapy (SBRT), the accuracy of isocenter is tighter than conventional therapy. For gating, a specific AAPM Task Group report (13) (TG 76) was published, and prescribes that the synchronization of the radiation beam with the patient's respiratory cycle has to be checked during the QA phase. The quantity of data created by an IMRT treatment plan that must be transferred to a linac, coupled with the complexity of the dose calculations, makes it impossible to "hand check" a treatment plan in the traditional sense. Modern adaptive RT creates more data. Data transfer QA and plan verification greatly rely on advanced QA techniques, equipment, and software tools. With the increased complexity of radiation treatment techniques, increased dependence on computers, and increased use of imaging modalities for treatment planning and delivery, a more comprehensive QA program is critical to ensure that patients are treated safely. A comprehensive program that includes more efficient, accurate, and effective QA demands advanced development of QA equipment, software tools, and techniques.

EQUIPMENT AND SOFTWARE USED FOR QUALITY ASSURANCE IN RADIATION THERAPY

Dosimetry instrumentation

Conventional dosimeters

Ionization chambers. Ionization chambers (ICs) are the basic instrumentation for QA in RT because of their excellent stability, linear response to absorbed dose, small directional dependence, beam-quality response independence, and traceability to a primary calibration standard. Most of the commercially manufactured ICs are not constructed with exactly known sensitive volume, and therefore require calibration, which is performed by an accredited dosimetry calibration laboratory (ADCL) or national laboratories that maintain standard IC and calibrated γ-ray beams. They are manufactured in various styles (cylindrical and parallel plate [PP]). Figure 8.1(A) and (B) show the two different types of chambers: cylinder type and plane-parallel ionization chamber. Cylindrical ICs can be traced directly to ADCL reference dosimetry, whereas PP ICs are cross-calibrated using cylindrical ICs. Well-guarded plane-parallel ICs are designed to minimize scattering perturbation effects and the replacement perturbation correction factor. An additional advantage of a PP IC is that the effective point of measurement is the same as the assigned location. In most cases, PP IC chambers are optimized for electron beam dosimetry, but they are also recommended for measurements for photons at shallow depths.

An IC can also be classified by its active volume. The first type is a standard chamber whose active volume for a standard Farmer-type cylindrical ionization chamber is on average 0.6 mL. The Farmer-type chamber is usually used for reference dosimetry of a standard megavoltage (MV) beam in a 10×10 cm^2 field size. The second type is a minichamber with an active volume of on average 0.05 mL. These ion chambers are usually used for beam scanning of percentage depth dose (PDD) or profile. The third type is microchambers whose active volume is approximately 0.007 mL; these are ideally suited for small field dosimetry such as radiosurgery, GammaKnife, CyberKnife, and IMRT. When selecting the size of the IC, one should consider that a larger IC will reduce the sensitivity of the measurements to positioning inaccuracies. However, there is a larger volume effect, and it may not be used for high-dose gradient areas. A small IC will be sensitive to positioning errors and give a noisier signal.

Another type of design is the well shape, which is usually used for low air kerma rate sources. This requires chambers of sufficient volume (~250 mL) for adequate sensitivity and is ideally suited for calibration and standardization of brachytherapy sources. Figure 8.1(C) shows a schematic diagram of a well-type chamber (HDR plus 1000). Well-type chambers should be designed to accommodate sources of the typical sizes and shapes that are in clinical use for brachytherapy. They are calibrated in terms of the reference air kerma rate for each source type calibrated. A pressurized well-type IC is also used as a dose calibrator to assay radiopharmaceuticals, but the instrument response is interpreted as activity in units of millicuries. Calibration of various isotopes is based on relative chamber response measured by intercomparison with the respective standards calibrated by the National Institute of Standards and Technology (NIST) directly in terms of activity (14).

Diodes. Semiconductor diode dosimeters are used widely for QA for both photon and electron beams. Figure 8.2(A) shows a typical diode used for dosimetry. Characteristics of diodes include quick response time (microseconds compared with milliseconds of an IC), excellent spatial resolution, absence of external bias, and high sensitivity (15). The relatively high atomic number of silicon in the diode detector leads to a greater sensitivity to low-energy photons. Therefore, diode detectors are usually used for small field dose distribution measurements, where there are relatively few low-energy photons. Certain diode dosimeters are particularly attractive for radiation dosimetry in an electron beam because of their energy independence of mass collision stopping power ratio (silicon and water for energy between 4 and 20 MeV). Diodes with a buildup encapsulation are also used in in vivo dosimetry on patients. Diodes show temperature, dose rate, energy, and angular dependence. AAPM TG 62 (10) provides a good reference of diode dosimetry. In addition, a diode detector may show long-term irreversible radiation damage that changes the sensitivity of the diode over time (16). Therefore, diodes are used for reference

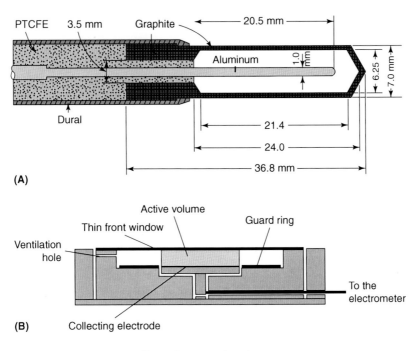

(A)

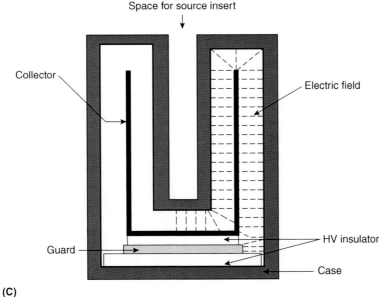

(B)

(C)

FIGURE 8.1 Schematic drawings of Farmer graphite/aluminum chamber (A). Nominal air volume, 0.6 mL. Parallel plate ion chamber (B) and well-type ion chamber (C).

dose measurements. Before using a diode detector, one should compare it with an IC measurement to confirm its correction operation and accuracy in measurement.

Thermoluminescent dosimeters and optically stimulated luminescent dosimeters. The most commonly used thermoluminescent dosimeters (TLDs) in RT are composed of LiF:Mg, Ti, LiF:Mg, Cu, P, and Li2B4O7:Mn, because of their tissue equivalence (Z = 8.1). Figure 8.2(B) shows the

typical TLDs and instruments for readout. TLDs are usually small in size and available in various forms (powder, chips, rods, and ribbons). TLDs show linear dose response over a wide range of doses used in RT, although it increases in the higher dose region and exhibits supralinear behavior. Before they are used, TLDs have to be annealed to erase the residual signal. Annealing cycles, including the heating and cooling rate, should be established and be reproducible. A TLD can also serve as a relative dosimeter. Calibration

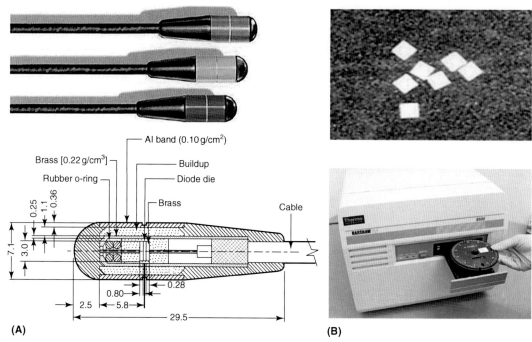

FIGURE 8.2 Typical diode dosimeter (A). Typical TLD chips and TLD reader from Thermo Scientific (B).

should be performed using the same beam energy, and a few correction factors should be applied, such as fading and dose response nonlinearity.

Optically stimulated luminescent dosimeters (OSLDs) are plastic disks infused with aluminum oxide doped with carbon (Al_2O_3:C). OSLDs are based on a principle similar to that of TLDs and have the same application possibilities as TLDs. The largest difference in the dosimetry process is the readout technique. Instead of heat, light from a laser is used to release the trapped energy in the form of luminescence.

Typical applications of TLDs and OSLDs in radiotherapy include in vivo dosimetry on patients as a routine quality assurance procedure or for dose monitoring in special cases (for example, complicated geometries, skin dose measurements, dose to critical organs, total body irradiation, and brachytherapy); verification of treatment techniques in phantoms; dosimetry audits (such as the RPC—Radiological Physics Center TLD dose audit program); and dose comparisons among hospitals.

Film. The most commonly used films in RT include radiographic and radiochromic film. Two AAPM task groups have been published for radiographic film (12) (AAPM TG 69) and radiochromic film (11) (AAPM TG 55). These are comprehensive and address many aspects of film dosimetry. Film is an excellent tool for 2D dose measurement because of its extremely high spatial resolution. Radiographic film is coated with a radiation emulsion of AgBr grains, which is a high-Z material. Silver halide–based radiographic film shows strong energy dependence. Unlike radiographic film, radiochromic film is nearly tissue-equivalent and does not require a processor for generating the optical density response to ionizing radiation. Radiochromic film exhibits less energy dependence. However, radiochromic films are generally less sensitive than radiographic films, requiring higher doses, although the dose response nonlinearity should be corrected in the upper dose region. Application of film dosimetry includes profile measurements, output factor measurement for small fields, and quality control of radiotherapy machine (e.g., congruence of light and radiation fields and the determination of the position of collimator axis). When film is used for IMRT quality assurance, a calibration curve of optical density versus dose should be established. Recommendations on the use of film for IMRT QA are summarized in reference (15).

2D array detectors. Use of 2D array detectors has become increasingly popular in view of their ease of use and immediate readout of the results. Two types of 2D detector arrays are commercially available for the primary purpose of providing patient-specific IMRT QA tools: the Mapcheck diode array, shown in Figure 8.3(A) (Sun Nuclear Corp., Melbourne, FL), and the ionization chamber array, shown in Figure 8.3(B) (ImRT MatriXX, IBA Dosimetry, Germany). Many other systems are available. The Mapcheck contains an array of 445 variably spaced diodes over an area of 22 × 22 cm2. The diode spacings are 7.07 and 14.14 mm in the central 10 × 10 cm^2 and outer regions, respectively. The diode

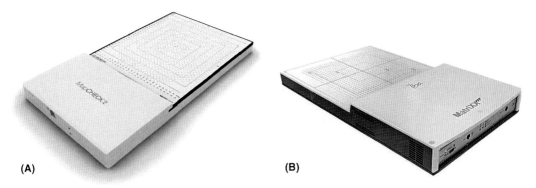

(A) **(B)**

FIGURE 8.3 MapCheck from SunNuclear (A) and matrix from IBA dosimetry (B).
Sources: (A) MapCHECK®from Sun Nuclear Corporation (diode array). Reprinted with permission from Sun Nuclear Corporation. (B) MatriXX from IBA dosimetry (ionization chamber array) Reprinted with permission from IBA Dosimetry GmbH

array detectors are small (<1 mm), and therefore ideal for measuring complex IMRT planar dose distributions with minimal volume averaging effect. However, diodes are known to suffer from radiation damage, and possess energy, field size, and dose-rate dependencies. The Mapcheck device is also used to verify the absolute and relative dose distribution on a beam-by-beam basis with beam irradiated at normal incidence to the devices. The Matrixx from IBA contains an ionization chamber array of 1,020 detectors with a spacing of 0.76 cm in a total area of 24.4×24.4 cm^2. The array exhibits long-term stability and no dose rate dependence. Typically, existing array detectors have low spatial resolution, generally >7 mm. Software interpolation of measured dose map provides a useful tool to evaluate 2D distribution during IMRT QA.

New developments

With more complicated and more efficient delivery systems, several new systems have been developed to perform machine QA and IMRT patient QA. The major development has been a shift to more robust, efficient, and reliable QA tools. One of the techniques recently published is electronic portal imaging devices (EPID)-base QA, which does not rely on third-party tools (17). With submillimeter spatial resolution and high-contrast resolution, EPID can be used as an ideal tool for linac QA. As both MV and kilovoltage (kV) detector panels are onboard, the set-up time for QA procedures can be greatly reduced. A phantom and a software tool have been developed to check linac performance, including output, flatness, symmetry, uniformity, tissue phantom ratio (TPR)$_{20/10}$, positional accuracy of the jaws and multileaf collimators (MLCs), wedge factor, and imaging quality (high- and low-contrast resolution of kV and MV imager). The dosimetry and mechanical and imaging performance are checked in one integrated system. Cloud-based EPID-based tools are under development, and will be expanded to multiple institutions (17).

EPID-based dosimetry has been implemented not only for pretreatment IMRT QA (18), but also for in vivo dosimetry measurement (19) using back-projection algorithms. Commercial software is available to analyze EPID-based

in vivo measurements and provide confirmation of dose delivered. The 3D dose can also be reconstructed on the basis of planning CT (20) and 3D gamma analysis, and dose volume histogram (DVH) comparisons are derived from in vivo EPID measurement.

A new 3D diode array (ArcCHECK, Sun Nuclear, Melbourne, FL) has been developed for routine QA of IMRT and VMAT (21,22). Figure 8.4 shows the ArcCHECK phantom and software. The ArcCHECK is a cylindrical water-equivalent phantom with a three-dimensional array of 1,386 diode detectors with 10 mm detector spacing. The device geometry is cylindrical, which ensures that detectors are always facing the delivery beam regardless of gantry angle and measure entry and exit dose for every angle. The detectors spiral down the cylinder with dimensions of 21 cm diameter and length in order to increase the spatial sampling rate and reduce detector overlap from the beam's eye view (BEV). The active detector size is 0.8×0.8 mm^2. There is a 15 cm diameter cavity in the phantom that can hold an insert with an ionization chamber for absolute dose measurement. The ArcCHECK measures in 50 ms intervals, saves all measurement data as a function of time, and makes both relative and absolute dose measurements. The system can assess the accuracy of MLC positions and the dose rate at each control point, as well as the gantry speed between control points at the same time (23). Many studies have been performed to commission and characterize the ArcCHECK device, and it has been shown that the short-term reproducibility, dose linearity, dose rate dependence, dose per pulse dependence, field size dependence, and out-of-field dependence of ArcCHECK are suitable for IMRT and VMAT QA (24). The ArcCHECK gives a higher confidence in terms of gamma comparison between measured and calculated dose distribution (25). This device is also MRI compatible and was used for IMRT QA in MRI-guided RT (26). Another 3D device that is available is the Delta4 (Scandidos AB, Uppsala, Sweden).

Another development of dosimeter is 3D gel dosimetry. Recently, new 3D dosimetry materials have been proposed with striking performance characteristics (27). The three main categories of 3D dosimeters are olyacrylamide gels,

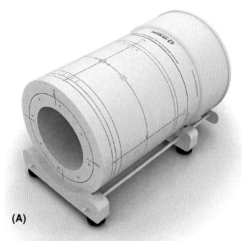

(A)

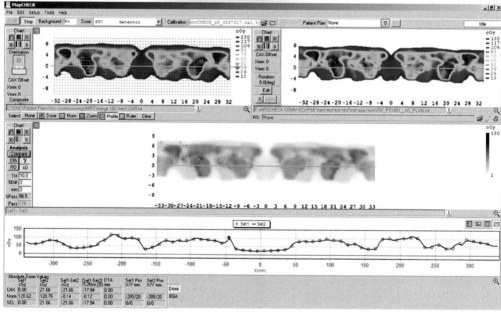

(B)

FIGURE 8.4 ArcCHECK and associated software.

Source: ArcCHECK® and associated software. Reprinted with permission from Sun Nuclear Corporation

Fricke gels, and radiochromic plastics, and the two main methods of dose readout are magnetic resonance (MR) imaging and optical computed tomography. Many of the 3D gel dosimeters are still at the development stage. The BANG gel system is commercially available from MGS Research. The BANG gel dosimeter is a 3D polymer dosimeter. In the presence of ionizing radiation, the active ingredient, methacrylic acid, undergoes free-radical polymerization. The concentration of polymer particles in the gel is directly related to the delivered dose. The particles are trapped in the gel, and they do not diffuse away; therefore, the resultant 3D image is permanent.

Imaging instrumentation

Various AAPM task group reports provide recommendations for QA of imaging systems integrated with medical accelerators, including MV planar imaging, kV planar imaging,

and MV or kV computer tomographic imaging (both serial and cone beam). These reports include AAPM TG-142 (7), TG-179, and the more recent TG-226 Medical Physics Practice Guideline; QA tests covered include geometric accuracy, image quality, and dosimetry measurements of the imager system. The suggested frequency of these tests varies between the reports.

Geometry test with a cube phantom

Positioning/repositioning accuracy is critical for the precise delivery of IGRT treatments. This can be tested using a cube phantom with a radiopaque marker (28,29). Figure 8.5(A) shows a picture of a cube phantom (Modus Medical Devices, Inc., London, Ontario, Canada), consisting of a tungsten sphere 8 mm in diameter embedded at the center of a 5 cm^3 plastic cube. The phantom is aligned with the cross-hair on the couch at the isocenter. Then, the phantom is shifted away from the isocenter by known displacements along three translational directions. With the orthogonal kV and MV imaging, the 2D/2D matching is performed, and the phantom is shifted back to the target position. The same phantom can be used to test imaging and treatment coordinate coincidence when the phantom is placed on the couch at the isocenter. Planar MV and KV images are then taken at four cardinal gantry angles (e.g., 0°, 90°, 180°, and 270°). The distances between the corresponding digital imaging centers and the target center are measured as the discrepancies of the coincidence.

Megavoltage imaging quality test with the Las Vegas phantom

The MV imaging quality can be tested by using the Las Vegas phantom, which is composed of holes of varying thickness and varying width embedded in aluminum; these holes represent spatial and contrast resolution benchmarks. Figure 8.5(B) shows the pattern of the holes of a Las Vegas phantom. Visualizing a certain hole implies a specific resolution for a given linear accelerator/EPID combination (30). During the testing, the Las Vegas phantom is placed on the top of the couch, and an MV detector is positioned at a standard clinical position (source to imager position at 150 cm). A planar MV image is acquired using 1 to 2 monitor units (MUs) at standard photon energy (e.g., 6 MV). As shown in Figure 8.5(B), the Las Vegas phantom has 28 circular holes in a matrix of 6 columns by 5 rows embedded in the block. The maximum row visible in the maximum columns determines contrast, and the maximum column visible in the maximum row determines resolution (31).

Kilovoltage imaging quality test with Leeds phantom

A Leeds phantom TOR 18FG (Leeds Test Objects Ltd, North Yorkshire, UK) can be used to quantify the spatial resolution and contrast of the planar kV imaging, as shown in Figure 8.5(C). The phantom has 18 disks of 8 mm diameter and 21 bar patterns. The spatial resolution and contrast can be specified by determining the lowest contrast disk and the smallest discernible group of bars visible in the image.

Beam quality test of 3D cone beam computer tomography with Catphan phantom

A Catphan 504 or Catphan 503 Phantom (The Phantom Laboratory, NY) is used for evaluation of the image quality of 3D CBCT, as shown in Figure 8.5(D). The phantom has various inserts, so it can be used to measure different aspects of the CBCT image quality, including geometric distortion, spatial resolution, low contrast, HU constancy, uniformity, and noise of CBCT (31).

Dosimetry measurement

Dosimetric characteristics of kV 2D imaging and 3D CBCT can be tested with the same equipment used for a diagnostic CT scanner. The Unfors Xi system (Unfors Instruments AB, Billdal, Sweden) tests multiple parameters of KV x-ray, including kVp, dose, dose rate, pulse, pulse rate, dose/frame, and time. Figure 8.5(E) shows the Unfors Xi system, including a base unit and R/F detector and CT detector. The detector is connected to the base unit, which displays the measured results. The two detectors are used to measure dosimetric characteristics of various modes, such as radioscopy/fluoroscopy (R/F) or computed tomography (CT). The R/F detector is a solid-state detector and has two sensors: R/F low for low dose-rate measurements, and R/F high for high dose-rate measurements. The CT detector is a long cylindrical ionization chamber designed to measure CT dose for applications such as dose length product (DLP) and computed tomography dose index (CTDI) (31).

Integrated systems to automate the image quality test

A few commercial products, including an imaging QA phantom and software, are available to review geometric accuracy and imaging quality of the kV and MV imager. One system is the EPID QC phantom and the associated software epidSoft marketed by PTW-Freiburg (Germany) (Figure 8.6). This system allows automatic image analysis of the QC phantom images, documentation of the QC results, and data storage and retrieval for long-term assessment of the performance of the EPID (32). A unique feature is the collection of imaging tools for EPID QA using a single phantom to evaluate several parameters, including: (a) geometric accuracy, including scaling and rotation tests; (b) linearity test through a pair of copper step wedges; (c) linearity; (d) signal-to-noise ratio (SNR); (e) low-contrast resolution through various holes in the aluminum slab; and (f) high-contrast spatial resolutions through modulation transfer function (MTF) determination in both the in-plane and cross-plane directions, because resolution depends on the focal spot, which varies in both directions (32).

Other equipment and software used for quality assurance in radiation therapy

Water tank

A 3D water tank larger than $40 \times 40 \times 40$ cm^3 is usually used to measure the beam data for commissioning and QA. TG-142 recommends that the beam symmetry, flatness, penumbra, field size, and energy be checked on an annual basis. The most accurate measurements are performed using a scanning ion chamber (micro ion chamber) and a scanning tank. Scanning systems should allow scanning in both cross- and in-planes (x and y directions) and depth dose (z direction). For the best results, it is desirable to have multiple scanning speeds so that the user can configure relatively slow speed in a high gradient area and higher speed in a plateau region. Figure 8.7 shows two commercial scanning systems: Blue Phantom by IBA (A) and 3D scanning tank by SunNuclear (B). The SunNuclear 3D tank provides a functionality of auto setup. It is time-consuming

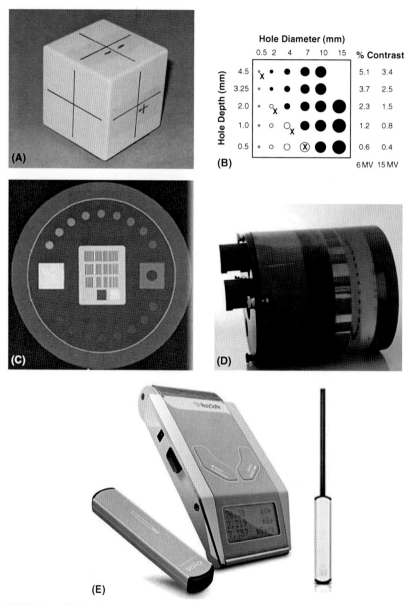

FIGURE 8.5 (A) A cube phantom used for IGRT tests. (B) Aluminum Las Vegas phantom for EPID image contrast and spatial resolution. (C) kV planar images of KV image of the Leeds phantom. (D) Catphan 504 phantom with different modules. (E) Unfors Xi system with R/F detector, base, and CT detector.

to set up a 3D tank for beam scanning because accurate alignment is critical to beam profile measurements. A 1D tank ($40 \times 40 \times 40$ cm^3) can be used for beam calibration per AAPM TG-51 protocol (33).

Plastic phantoms

Point dose measurements, particularly for relative dose measurements such as output factors, surface dose, leakage/transmission, wedge and tray factors, can be measured using a plastic phantom. The basic requirements in

phantom design are materials with mechanical strength and dosimetric properties closely matched to those of water (34). Several water-equivalent materials are on the market, manufactured to mimic the dosimetric behavior of water as closely as possible over a wide range of energies. Of the commercially available phantom materials, polymethyl methacrylate, polystyrene, and epoxy resin are most frequently used as dosimetric phantoms (35). For any plastic to be considered water equivalent, it should not introduce more than 1% uncertainty to the absorbed dose

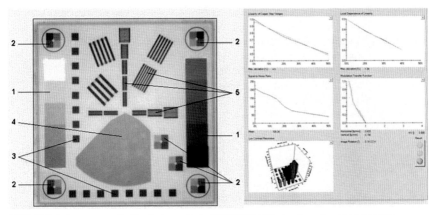

FIGURE 8.6 Arrangement of test elements in PTW EPID QC phantom: 1, signal linearity and signal-to-noise ratio; 2, isotropy of signal linearity; 3, geometric isotropy (distortion); 4, low-contrast resolution; 5, high-contrast resolution. Also shown are sample analyses in the epidSoft user interface.

Source: From Ref. (32). Das IJ, Cao M, Cheng C-W, et al. A quality assurance phantom for electronic portal imaging devices. J Appl Clin Med Phys. 2011;12(2):3350.

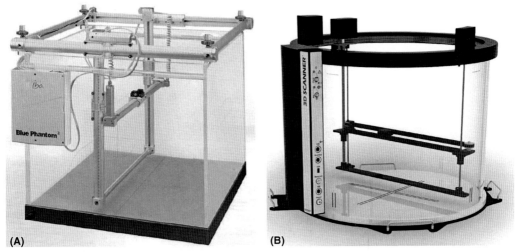

FIGURE 8.7 IBA Blue Phantom (A) and SunNuclear scanning tank (B).

Sources: (A) IBA Blue Phantom. Reprinted with permission from IBA Dosimetry GmbH (B) Right – 3D Scanner™ (Sun Nuclear Scanning Tank) Reprinted with permission from Sun Nuclear Corporation.

(36). If total uncertainties reach more than 1%, appropriate correction factors have to be applied (36). The quality of the phantom material should be checked with a CT scan for any artifacts and inhomogeneity in electron density via CT number. Note that these CT numbers may differ from water if the solid materials are designed to be water equivalent at megavoltage energies only.

Quality assurance software

There are many software tools used for quality assurance in RT. Most QA software is associated with a hardware tool or phantom and should be considered part of QA equipment. The main trend in software developments is to improve efficiency through automation with less human

interventions. Two QA software tools are discussed here as examples: RIT (a commercial software tool for film analysis) and dynaQA (an in-house developed software tool for data transfer and beam delivery accuracy).

RIT is a standalone software tool to analyze the QA images to automate the image QA for AAPM TG 142 (7). It can analyze images from EPID, 2D-array, film, and gel dosimeter. It also provides a tool to show the trend of particular QA parameters. RIT software includes the tools to analyze the film-based IMRT QA, MLC-QA (picket fence), CBCT analysis with the Catphan, Fluoro kV imaging from various phantoms, kV/MV imager coincidence from a cube phantom, star-shot film, etc.

The dynaQA software is an in-house software tool to perform an end-to-end data transfer integrity check and verify the beam delivery (37,38). Beam parameters such as monitor units (MU), gantry angle, couch angle, dose rate MLC positions, jaw positions, wedge angle, and beam energy can be extracted. The software reads the Varian linac log files, extracts the delivered parameters, and compares them against the original treatment planning data. It can check all the beam deliveries, including 3D conformal therapy, enhanced dynamic wedge delivery, IMRT, volumetric modulated RT, flattening filter-free mode, and electron therapy treatment. Log file–based dynaQA software is a valuable QA tool because it automatically checks all the beam parameters for each fraction and for each patient.

QUALITY ASSURANCE OF EQUIPMENT, SOFTWARE, AND TECHNIQUES

General consideration for implementation of new techniques requiring quality assurance

With the introduction of a new modality, such as IMRT including VMAT, TBI, intraoperative RT, stereotactic techniques (39), and dedicated special-purpose treatment units, a program must be in place to ensure the accuracy and precision of measurement equipment used for calibration and constancy checks of treatment machines and instruments used for patient dosimetry and imaging QA. Sufficient and efficient QA must be performed using proper QA equipment. Redundancy in dose calibration equipment is recommended to ensure that instruments are holding their calibration. It is recommended that both a local standard and a field dosimetry system be maintained and routinely compared. All the equipment and software used for QA must be tested before the first use and periodically.

Quality assurance of new equipment and software

A few examples, including dosimetry equipment and software tools, are discussed in the following sections, and each clinic should set its own procedures to perform QA or acceptance according to the clinic purpose and manufacturer recommendations.

Acceptance test of a new ion chamber

New ICs have to be tested for appropriate performance. These tests should be performed before calibration is obtained for the chamber. The following suggested tests are recommended (14,40):

1. Mechanical integrity should be checked using perpendicular radiographs and to ensure there are no cracks and that central electrodes are not tilted.

2. Leakage current should be measured with the electrometer to ensure that the system has a sufficiently low background and that any guard electrodes are performing properly. Leakage for a chamber is generally 1 to 10 fA.

3. The stem effect should be quantified by irradiating the ionization chamber at orientations that include and exclude the guarded portions of the chamber. If the guard electrodes are working properly, there should be a negligible difference in readings.

4. Microphonic currents generated by mechanically flexing the cables should be tested in the chamber, as well as in the cables and connectors that will be used with the ionization chamber.

5. Reproducibility of ion chamber readings should be tested. A properly working ionization chamber should provide reproducible measurements after at most two readings of approximately 200 cGy each.

6. Environmental correction (temperature and pressure correction) factor should be tested; check that the chamber obeys ideal gas-law scaling of sensitivity by mildly changing the temperature of the system.

7. Polarity factor should be measured for different energies. It is generally approximately 1% for a good ion chamber.

8. The recombination factors of the ionization chamber in the intended radiation fields should be measured at high voltage (-300 V) and low voltage (-150 V).

9. Orientation dependence must be determined and checked against specifications given by the manufacturer.

Verification and validation of scanner

Modern water scanning systems are extremely accurate and precise. However, some basic quality assurance, as suggested by Humphries and Purdy (40), should be adopted. A quality assurance procedure should be performed periodically or at least before use of the water tank (41). This includes the following:

1. The free movement of each arm, and the x, y, z, and diagonal motion, should be checked (34).

2. Accuracy and linearity should be checked over the long range of the scanning system. The vertical travel of the detector should be exactly vertical, without migration.

3. The physical condition of the tank, such as leaks, cracks, and mechanical stability, as well as the quality of connecting cables for leakage and reproducibility, should be checked.

4. Communication between the hardware and the software should be checked.

5. Annual preventive maintenance services offered by manufacturers should be performed.

6. The software features (e.g., normalization, smoothing, shifts, protocol to calculate symmetry and flatness, etc.) should be tested.

Quality assurance for quality assurance software

The software used for QA in RT should be tested and verified before use. All the functionality, including the analysis, display, and report, should be tested in real clinical situations. A preceding section discusses in-house developed dynaQA software. The approach to verify the QA software tool is to intentionally introduce errors (38); for example, to test whether the software tool accurately identifies differences between the intended plan from the treatment planning system and the delivered plan on the linac. As part of the testing, some field parameters were intentionally changed in the treatment management systems. The Y1 jaw position was displaced by 1 cm, and the gantry angle was changed by 90°. The MLC positions for beam 1A were changed by adding 2 mm to all leaves in the A bank and 2.5 mm to all leaves in the B bank. The plan was then delivered on the linac and analyzed using the software tool. The errors should be flagged when the software works properly.

Another example is the EPID-based QA tool previously described to detect the MLC positioning accuracy (17). To validate the positional accuracy of MLC leaves, known intentional errors were introduced in a number of leaf positions in the picket-fence (PF) pattern by applying displacements of 0.5, 1.0, and 1.5 mm to the gap width in opposite directions. The EPID images collected in conjunction with these known errors were analyzed using the daily QA software and compared with the introduced error to assess error detection accuracy. Figure 8.8 shows the verification results analyzed using an in-house–developed EPID daily QA tool.

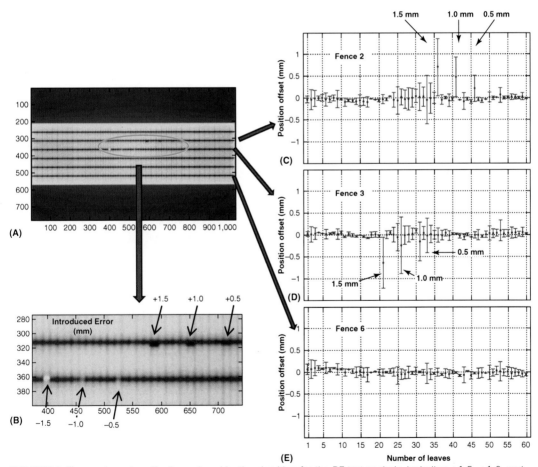

FIGURE 8.8 The graphs automatically produced by the algorithm for the PF test analysis, including ±1.5, ±1.0, and ±0.5 mm intentional errors. EPID image (A) enlarged portion for closer view of intentional errors (B). Peak positions of A bank and B bank leaves in fence 2, 3, and 6, respectively (C, D, and E). Upper boundary corresponds to the A bank leaf position, and lower boundary corresponds to the B bank leaf. The middle dot represents the central location of Gaussian fitting.

CONCLUSIONS

QA metrology, equipment, and software are very important components of RT. As treatment becomes more and more complicated, it is vital to implement more robust, accurate, and efficient QA techniques, including hardware and software tools, to ensure safe treatment. This is especially important because direct patient-related QA is less practical, making the need for phantom-based QA more vital. We hope this chapter aids the physicist in deciding what characteristics of devices fit the clinical needs of his or her facility.

REFERENCES

1. International Commission on Radiation Units and Measurements. *Determination of Absorbed Dose in a Patient Irradiated by Beams of X- or Gamma-Rays in Radiotherapy Procedures.* Bethesda, MD: International Commission on Radiation Units and Measurements; 1976. Report 24.

2. Bogdanich W. Radiation offers new cures, and ways to do harm. *New York Times.* January 23, 2010. www.nytimes.com/2010/01/24/health/24radiation.html.

3. Bogdanich W. As technology surges, radiation safeguards lag. *New York Times.* January 27, 2010. www.nytimes.com/2010/01/27/us/27radiation.html?pagewanted=all.

4. Bogdanich W. West Virginia hospital over irradiated brain scan patients, records show. *New York Times.* March 6, 2011. www.nytimes.com/2011/03/06/health/06radiation.html.

5. Bogdanich W. Radiation errors reported in Missouri. *New York Times.* February 24, 2010. www.nytimes.com/2010/02/25/us/25radiation.html?_r=0.

6. Kutcher GJ, Coia L, Gillin M, et al. Comprehensive QA for radiation oncology: report of AAPM Radiation Therapy Committee Task Group 40. *Med Phys.* 1994;21:581–618. http://scitation.aip.org/content/aapm/journal/medphys/21/4/10.1118/1.597316.

7. Klein EE, Hanley J, Bayouth J, et al. Task Group 142 report: quality assurance of medical accelerators. *Med Phys.* 2009;36:4197–4212. http://scitation.aip.org/content/aapm/journal/medphys/36/9/10.1118/1.3190392.

8. ASTRO. *Safety Is No Accident: A Framework for Quality Radiation Oncology and Care.* Arlington, VA: ASTRO; 2012. www.astro.org/Product-Catalog/Products/Publications/SafetyisNoAccident.

9. Almond PR, Attix FH, Humphries LJ, et al. The calibration and use of plane-parallel ionization chambers for dosimetry of electron beams: an extension of the 1983 AAPM protocol report of AAPM Radiation Therapy Committee Task Group No. 39. *Med Phys.* 1994;21:1251–1260. http://scitation.aip.org/content/aapm/journal/medphys/21/8/10.1118/1.597359.

10. Yorke E, Alecu R, Ding L, et al. *Diode In Vivo Dosimetry for Patients Receiving External Beam Radiation Therapy: Report of TG 62 of the Radiation Therapy Committee.* Madison, WI: Medical Physics Publishing; 2005. AAPM Report No. 87.

11. Niroomand-Rad A, Blackwell CR, Coursey BM, et al. Radiochromic film dosimetry: recommendations of AAPM Radiation Therapy Committee Task Group 55. *Med Phys.* 1998;25:2093–2115. http://scitation.aip.org/content/aapm/journal/medphys/25/11/10.1118/1.598407.

12. Pai S, Das IJ, Dempsey JF, et al. TG-69: radiographic film for megavoltage beam dosimetry. *Med Phys.* 2007;34:2228–2258. http://scitation.aip.org/content/aapm/journal/medphys/34/6/10.1118/1.2736779.

13. Keall PJ, Mageras GS, Balter JM, et al. The management of respiratory motion in radiation oncology report of AAPM Task Group 76. *Med Phys.* 2006;33:3874–3900. http://scitation.aip.org/content/aapm/journal/medphys/33/10/10.1118/1.2349696.

14. Gibbons JP, Khan FM. *Kahn's the Physics of Radiation Therapy.* Philadelphia, PA: Lippincott Williams & Wilkins; 2014.

15. Low DA, Moran JM, Dempsey JF, et al. Dosimetry tools and techniques for IMRT. *Med Phys.* 2011;38:1313–1338. http://scitation.aip.org/content/aapm/journal/medphys/38/3/10.1118/1.3514120.

16. Rikner G, Grusell E. General specifications for silicon semiconductors for use in radiation dosimetry. *Phys Med Biol.* 1987;32:1109. http://stacks.iop.org/0031-9155/32/i=9/a=004.

17. Sun B, Goddu SM, Yaddanapudi S, et al. Daily QA of linear accelerators using only EPID and OBI. *Med Phys.* 2015;42:5584–5594. http://scitation.aip.org/content/aapm/journal/medphys/42/10/10.1118/1.4929550.

18. Van Esch A, Depuydt T, Huyskens DP. The use of an aSi-based EPID for routine absolute dosimetric pre-treatment verification of dynamic IMRT fields. *Radiother Oncol.* 2004;71:223–234. www.sciencedirect.com/science/article/pii/S016781400400088X.

19. Ian MH, Vibeke NH, Igor O-R, et al. Clinical implementation and rapid commissioning of an EPID based *in-vivo* dosimetry system. *Phys Med Biol.* 2014;59:N171. http://stacks.iop.org/0031-9155/59/i=19/a=N171.

20. Mijnheer B, Olaciregui-Ruiz I, Rozendaal R, et al. 3D EPID-based in vivo dosimetry for IMRT and VMAT. *J Phys Conf Ser.* 2013;444:012011. http://stacks.iop.org/1742-6596/444/i=1/a=012011.

21. Yan G, Lu B, Kozelka J, et al. Calibration of a novel four-dimensional diode array. *Med Phys.* 2010;37:108–115. http://scitation.aip.org/content/aapm/journal/medphys/37/1/10.1118/1.3266769.

22. Petoukhova AL, Egmond JV, Eenink MGC, et al. The ArcCHECK diode array for dosimetric verification of HybridArc. *Phys Med Biol.* 2011;56:5411. http://stacks.iop.org/0031-9155/56/i=16/a=021.

23. Wang Q, Dai J, Zhang K. A novel method for routine quality assurance of volumetric-modulated arc therapy. *Med Phys.* 2013;40:101712. http://scitation.aip.org/content/aapm/journal/medphys/40/10/10.1118/1.4820439.

24. Li G, Zhang Y, Jiang X, et al. Evaluation of the ArcCHECK QA system for IMRT and VMAT verification. *Phys Med.* 2013;29:295–303. www.sciencedirect.com/science/article/pii/S1120179712000348.

25. Chaswal V, Weldon M, Gupta N, et al. Commissioning and comprehensive evaluation of the ArcCHECK cylindrical diode array for VMAT pretreatment delivery QA. *J Appl Clin Med Phys.* 2014;15(4):212–225.

26. Li HH, Rodriguez VL, Green OL, et al. Patient-specific quality assurance for the delivery of ^{60}Co intensity modulated radiation therapy subject to a 0.35-T lateral magnetic field. *Int J Radiat Oncol Biol Phys.* 2015;91:65–72. www.sciencedirect.com/science/article/pii/S0360301614040942.

27. Guo PY, Adamovics JA, Oldham M. Characterization of a new radiochromic three-dimensional dosimeter. *Med Phys.* 2006;33:1338–1345. www.ncbi.nlm.nih.gov/pmc/articles/PMC1616190.

28. Kry SF, Jones J, Childress NL. Implementation and evaluation of an end-to-end IGRT test. *J Appl Clin Med Phys.* 2012;13:46–53.

29. Yoo S, Kim G-Y, Hammoud R, et al. A quality assurance program for the On-Board Imager®. *Med Phys.* 2006;33:4431–4447. http://scitation.aip.org/content/aapm/journal/medphys/33/11/10.1118/1.2362872.

30. Herman MG, Balter JM, Jaffray DA, et al. Clinical use of electronic portal imaging: report of AAPM Radiation Therapy Committee Task Group 58. *Med Phys.* 2001;28:712–737.

31. Chang Z, Bowsher J, Cai J, et al. Imaging system QA of a medical accelerator, Novalis Tx, for IGRT per TG 142: our 1 year experience. *J Appl Clin Med Phys.* 2012;13(4):3754.

32. Das IJ, Cao M, Cheng C-W, et al. A quality assurance phantom for electronic portal imaging devices. *J Appl Clin Med Phys.* 2011;12(2):3350.

33. Almond PR, Biggs PJ, Coursey BM, et al. AAPM's TG-51 protocol for clinical reference dosimetry of high-energy photon and electron beams. *Med Phys.* 1999;26:1847–1870. http://scitation.aip.org/content/aapm/journal/medphys/26/9/10.1118/1.598691.

34. Das IJ, Cheng C-W, Watts RJ, et al. Accelerator beam data commissioning equipment and procedures: report of the TG-106 of the Therapy Physics Committee of the AAPM. *Med Phys.* 2008;35:4186–4215. http://scitation.aip.org/content/aapm/journal/medphys/35/9/10.1118/1.2969070.

35. Ramaseshan R, Kohli K, Cao F, et al. A dosimetric evaluation of Plastic Water-Diagnostic-Therapy (PWDT). *J Appl Clin Med Phys.* 2008;9:2761.

36. International Commission on Radiation Units and Measurements. *Tissue substitutes in radiation dosimetry and measurement.* Bethesda, MD: International Commission on Radiation Units and Measurements; 1989. ICRU Report 44.

37. Rangaraj D, Zhu M, Yang D, et al. Catching errors with patient-specific pretreatment machine log file analysis. *Pract Radiat Oncol.* 2013;3:80–90. www.sciencedirect.com/science/article/pii/S1879850012000677.

38. Sun B, Rangaraj D, Palaniswaamy G, et al. Initial experience with TrueBeam trajectory log files for radiation therapy delivery verification. *Pract Radiat Oncol.* 2013;3:e199–e208. www.sciencedirect.com/science/article/pii/S187985001200210X.

39. Benedict SH, Yenice KM, Followill D, et al. Stereotactic body radiation therapy: the report of AAPM Task Group 101. *Med Phys.* 2010;37:4078–4101. http://scitation.aip.org/content/aapm/journal/medphys/37/8/10.1118/1.3438081.

40. Humphries LJ, Purdy JA. *Advances in Radiation Oncology Physics Dosimetry, Treatment Planning, and Brachytherapy: AAPM Monograph.* Alexandria, VA: American Association of Physicists in Medicine;1992.

41. Mellenberg DE, Dahl RA, Blackwell CR. Acceptance testing of an automated scanning water phantom. *Med Phys.* 1990;17:311–314. http://scitation.aip.org/content/aapm/journal/medphys/17/2/10.1118/1.596510.

9 | Quality Considerations in External Beam Radiotherapy Simulation and Treatment Planning

Eric C. Ford

THE IMPACT OF PLAN QUALITY ON PATIENT OUTCOMES

Simulation and treatment planning have a key influence on the quality and safety of treatments in radiation oncology. Although this is obvious at an intuitive level, the evidence behind this statement is striking. Recent meta-studies have shown a strong link between plan quality and patient outcomes in cooperative group trials (1,2). Perhaps one of the most compelling data sets is from the RTOG 9704 trial on pancreatic cancer (3). In that study, the group of patients whose plans were "per protocol" had a median overall survival that was significantly longer than those whose plans did not conform to the protocol (1.74 vs. 1.46 years, $P < .008$). In addition, plan quality appeared to impact the trial endpoint. There was a significant difference in the RT + 5FU versus RT + gemcitibine arms of the trial, but only if the plans not per protocol were excluded. The specific issue of plan quality is discussed further in Chapter 13, which describes knowledge-based machine-learning tools to measure and improve the quality of plans.

Although plan quality is important, it must be noted that reports from cooperative group trials and other sources typically only include data from the treatment planning system itself. Other effects that can impact the quality of treatment are not included, for example, patient set-up and localization, accuracy of commissioning, and the performance and calibration of treatment machines. All of these effects appear to be important given the phantom dosimetry verification results from the Imaging and Radiation Oncology Core (IROC). The IROC head-and-neck phantom results showed that 30% of institutions did not meet the relatively lax criteria of 7%/4 mm agreement set forth by the agency (4). This is especially striking given that the clinics participating were

a highly selected group. The quality gap is likely larger in the community as a whole.

Taken as a whole, the data indicate that there are substantial gaps in the quality of care being delivered. These quality gaps significantly affect the outcomes of patients after treatment.

THE SOURCE OF QUALITY GAPS

There are many potential sources of error and unwanted variability, and these can occur at essentially any point in the radiotherapy workflow process. Studies of prospective risk assessment in radiation oncology dating back to 2009 have illustrated the many points where failures can occur (5). Errors in simulation and treatment planning are especially pernicious because they often affect the entire course of treatment.

An example of this is the effect of rectal filling in patients with prostate cancer and the effect on outcomes. The 2005 study from de Crevoisier et al (6) showed that patients who had a larger rectal filling at the time of simulation suffered from a reduced biochemical and local control rate. Since the effect was not appreciated at the time, it might not be called an "error" in the sense of an "act of omission leading to an undesirable outcome" (7). However, this example illustrates the problems that can occur in simulation and treatment planning and can propagate through the entire course of treatment.

Several studies in radiation oncology have suggested that treatment planning is a particularly risk-prone part of the radiotherapy workflow process. The studies of Clark et al (8,9) found that more than half of all incidents originated in the process of simulation or treatment planning, although most of these were caught before they reached the patient. Similarly, in Novak et al's study (10), 60% of reported near-miss events occurred in treatment planning or the workflow steps leading up to it, and, interestingly, the errors that occurred at the time of simulation were significantly more serious than other errors. The importance of treatment planning and simulation can be appreciated in the data in other studies as well (11–14).

COMMON QUALITY PROBLEMS AND THEIR UNDERLYING CAUSES

Numerous papers have appeared that describe the specific types of errors that can occur in radiation therapy (8,12,13,15). Although there is no common nomenclature or categorization schema to describe this, several patterns emerge. Table 9.1 summarizes the common types of error that are encountered in treatment planning and simulation, and gives specific examples.

The previous discussion describes *what* happened, but it is even more important to know *why* an error happened, that is, the contributing factors that led to the error. In identifying causal factors, it may be helpful to refer to the consensus study for an incident learning system from the American Association of Physicists in Medicine (AAPM), which includes a table of causal factors (16). The causal factors that occur frequently in practice (8) include communication, human behavior involving staff (e.g., slip), issues with policies and procedures (often inadequate or nonexistent policies), and equipment and design issues (including human factors engineering problems).

CASE STUDY: CALCULATION ERROR IN TREATMENT PLANNING

The tragic radiation overdose of Lisa Norris in Scotland in 2006 illustrates many of the quality problems outlined here and provides an opportunity to learn and close the quality gap so that future patients are not affected. The information

presented here is drawn from the very detailed and informative report from the Scottish Ministry of Health (17).

In essence, the error involved in this situation was a miscalculation in the process of treatment planning (as in the first row of Table 9.1). In September of 2005, Lisa Norris, then 15 years old, was referred for treatment of pineoblastoma. The intention was to treat her whole craniospinal axis with 175 cGy × 30 fractions followed by a 180 cGy × 11 fraction boost to the tumor bed. During the process of planning, however, a monitor unit (MU) factor of (MU/100 cGy) was input on the paper forms instead of (MU/175 cGy), as it should have been. The result was a calculated MU that was too high. This was due, in part, to an upgrade, 7 months before, of the Oncology Information System to Varis 7, which allowed a direct transfer of a prescription from RTChart into the Eclipse planning system. Under the workflow of the clinic, the user was supposed to click "no" to the option of importing the prescription, but in this case they selected "yes" to import. The error was further magnified when the radiographer (radiotherapy technician or RTT) followed the standard procedures of multiplying the output from planning (MU/100 cGy) by the prescription of the physician (175 cGy). The end result was a treatment with 159 MU instead of the correct setting of 94.5 MU—that is, a 68% overdose. The error was not identified by the plan checker. No in vivo dosimetry system was in use. The error was identified 19 fractions into treatment when the same planner made the same error in another plan and a different physicist caught it.

In the follow-up, gaps were identified in training and competency, staffing, and policies and procedures (i.e., the planner did not know of the existence of written procedures, and in any case, the documents dated back to 1998 and made no mention of normalization). Human factors design issues were also involved. It should be clear that these same contributing factors

Table 9.1 Common Types of Error in the Process of Simulation and/or Treatment Planning Along, With Example Error Scenarios

Error Type	Example of Specific Error
Calculation or normalization error in planning	An SBRT plan normalized to the 98% isodose line vs. intended 80% line.
Plan performed for incorrect dose or dose per fraction (mismatch to intended prescription)	Physician called for 200 cGy × 25 fractions, but plan performed for 250 cGy × 20 fractions.
Omission in the planning process or misplan	Plan performed with incorrect beam energy; or wrong treatment site planned.
Error in evaluating the treatment plan	Previous radiation therapy treatment not included in plan evaluation.
Problem with target or normal tissue delineation	Incorrect expansion from the clinical target volume (CTV) to the planning target volume (PTV) due to miscommunication.
Issue related to the isocenter location in treatment planning and communication	Incorrect shifts calculated from the simulation scan and/or miscommunication about these shifts.
Change to plan not executed or executed incorrectly	New plan completed by planner, but other staff not informed.

are involved in many errors in radiation therapy as discussed previously.

CLOSING THE QUALITY GAP

Although the issues outlined in this chapter are well appreciated and supported by a growing body of literature in radiation oncology, it is often unclear how they can be effectively managed. The topic of quality improvement ranges from design considerations (18) to risk management (19) to the understanding of what drives human error (20). This section focuses very narrowly on specific quality management measures that apply to external beam simulation and treatment planning. The tools described here can be considered essential features of a good quality management program.

Patient-specific safety barriers

The specific barriers listed in Table 9.2 are strongly advocated in the references listed there, many of them from national or international professional societies. The effectiveness of these various patient-specific barriers was addressed in a 2012 multi-institutional study of error (22). More recent studies of other databases have confirmed the trends noted in that study (14,58). A notable result of the 2012 study was that physics plan review appeared to be a particularly effective

safety barrier if performed with high fidelity. Other highly effective barriers were in vivo dosimetry measurements, a time-out by therapists before treatment, and a review of plans by a therapist before treatment. Pretreatment IMRT quality assurance (QA), surprisingly, could detect less than 2% of errors. However, it should be noted that IMRT QA has the capability to detect very serious errors that occur in the process of planning, and is also semiautomatic in nature and therefore likely more reliable. The topic of patient-specific QA is considered in more detail in Chapter 12.

Automatic error detection tools for plans

A handful of studies have appeared describing software-based tools designed to identify known errors in treatment plans or in the record-and-verify system (32–36,38–42). These are typically based on rules that describe parameters and matching that is allowed versus that which is not. At least one paper that has investigated the potential effectiveness of such tools concluded that roughly 55% of errors might be identified with such an approach (58). Recently, an alternative scheme has been proposed that uses probabilistic networks to search for anomalous patterns in the oncology information system (37). The sensitivity and specificity of this tool are promising (area under the curve [AUC] in excess of 0.8). To our knowledge, however, none of these tools are commercially available, even though these studies date back to 2007.

Table 9.2 Common Quality Management Tools

Quality Measure	References
Patient-specific safety barriers	
• Physics plan review	21–24
• RTT plan review	25–27
• Peer review	27 & Chapter 15
• Patient-specific QA	Chapter 12
• RTT time-out	24–26
• In vivo dosimetry check	28–31
Automatic error detection tools for plans	32–42
Plan quality tools	43–50 & Chapter 13
Validation tests	51,52 4,53
• End-to-end tests with phantom	
• IROC phantom tests	
Incident learning system	8,12,24,54,55
Prospective risk assessment	5,56
• Failure modes and effects analysis (FMEA)	
Safety profile assessment	57
• Online survey tool hosted by AAPM designed to assess compliance with established safety metrics	

Plan quality tools

Tools that automatically rate the quality of a treatment plan are in active development (43–50). The reader is referred to Chapter 13 for a thorough discussion.

Validation tests

Validation tests and end-to-end phantom studies are advocated by a number of professional societies, including the ASTRO White Papers from the American Society for Radiation Oncology (ASTRO) (51,59,60). External validation tests involve ordering a phantom test device from the IROC and then planning and irradiating it as if it were a patient. The embedded dosimetry devices are then measured and the accuracy of delivery assessed (53). End-to-end phantom tests are similar. The test phantom is treated as a patient, and the entire simulation, planning, and delivery process is tested for accuracy. At a more general level, validation of commissioning is also important. As the World Health Organization (WHO) *Radiotherapy Risk Profile* states, "Due to the pervasive impact of linear accelerator commissioning on subsequent usage, it is imperative to obtain independent review of commissioning documentation" (61). This is discussed further in AAPM TG-106 (62) and in Chapter 7.

Incident learning systems

Incident learning systems are a key component of enforcing process control and building a culture of safety. In the United States, the Radiation Oncology Incident Learning System, RO-ILS, launched by ASTRO and AAPM in June 2014, provides a framework for accomplishing this (63). Other international systems are available (64), and some clinics have developed their own solutions (54). Incident learning has been shown to reduce the rates of serious error (8,12) and to positively impact safety culture (14,65). Incident learning includes both misadministrations of treatment and (more commonly) near-misses that are identified before they reach the patient. The ASTRO Report *Safety Is No Accident* (24) strongly advocates engagement in incident learning, including near-misses.

Prospective risk assessment

Prospective risk assessment can take many forms, but the tool most commonly encountered in radiation oncology is failure mode and effects analysis (FMEA). This tool, first described in this context in 2009 (5), rates potential failures according to their severity and occurrence rate along with a score for how difficult it is to identify them. This allows a rational understanding and prioritization of risk for the purposes of quality improvement. Over the past 7 years, numerous reports have appeared, and a definitive work on the topic, AAPM Task Group 100, was published in 2016 (56).

Of all the various tools described in this chapter and listed in Table 9.2, it is unclear how widely each is used in clinical practice. Few of them are enforced by any regulations, except in the special case of brachytherapy. Most of the references in Table 9.2 are operational in nature, describing how the various tools are intended to work and not how they are actually used. The one exception is peer review, which has a body of related literature as discussed in Chapter 15.

An exception is a result drawn from the Safety Profile Assessment survey data of 114 clinics in the United States (66). These data showed excellent compliance with several safety indicators, including calibration of dosimetry equipment, performance of pretreatment IMRT QA, the review of plans and charts by a physicist, and the time-out for patient identification verification prior to treatment. However, there was relatively poor adoption of other tools, in particular physician peer review, review of near-miss safety events, an independent review of commissioning, a regular review of policies and procedures, and a review of staff competencies. Some of these tools appear in Table 9.2 and most are well established and advocated by national societies.

SUMMARY

Simulation and treatment planning are one of the highest risk points in the radiation oncology workflow. The errors that occur there have been shown to significantly impact patient outcomes. Although errors occur via many pathways, there are a few causal factors that are relatively common. There are well-established specific quality management tools that can help to avoid or mitigate these errors. These tools are known to be effective. However, their use does not appear to be as widespread as might be hoped. Increased adoption of these measures should improve the quality of care and the safety of patients.

REFERENCES

1. Ohri N, Shen XL, Dicker AP, et al. Radiotherapy protocol deviations and clinical outcomes: a meta-analysis of cooperative group clinical trials. *J Natl Cancer Inst.* 2013;105(6):387–393.

2. Fairchild A, Straube W, Laurie F, et al. Does quality of radiation therapy predict outcomes of multicenter cooperative group trials? a literature review. *Int J Radiat Oncol Biol Phys.* 2013;87(2):246–260.

3. Abrams RA, Winter KA, Regine WF, et al. Failure to adhere to protocol specified radiation therapy guidelines was associated with decreased survival in RTOG 9704—a phase III trial of adjuvant chemotherapy and chemoradiotherapy for patients with resected adenocarcinoma of the pancreas. *Int J Radiat Oncol Biol Phys.* 2012;82(2):809–816.

4. Ibbott GS, Followill DS, Molineu A, et al. Challenges in credentialing institutions and participants in advanced technology multi-institutional clinical trials. *Int J Radiat Oncol Biol Phys.* 2008;71(1):S71–S75.

5. Ford EC, Gaudette R, Myers L, et al. Evaluation of safety in a radiation oncology setting using failure mode and effects analysis. *Int J Radiat Oncol Biol Phys.* 2009;74(3):852–858.

6. de Crevoisier R, Tucker SL, Dong L, et al. Increased risk of biochemical and local failure in patients with distended rectum on the planning CT for prostate cancer radiotherapy. *Int J Radiat Oncol Biol Phys.* 2005;62(4):965–973.

7. *Concepts Underlying AHRQ's Common Formats.* Rockville, MD: Agency for Healthcare Research and Quality; 2011.

8. Clark BG, Brown RJ, Ploquin J, et al. Patient safety improvements in radiation treatment through 5 years of incident learning. *Pract Radiat Oncol.* 2013;3(3):157–163.

9. Clark BG, Brown RJ, Ploquin JL, et al. The management of radiation treatment error through incident learning. *Radiother Oncol.* 2010;95(3):344–349.

10. Novak A, Nyflot MJ, Ermoian R, et al. Targeting safety improvements through identification of incident origination and detection in a near-miss incident learning system. *Med Phys.* 2016;43:2053.

11. Shafiq J, Barton M, Noble D, et al. An international review of patient safety measures in radiotherapy practice. *Radiother Oncol.* 2009;92(1):15–21.

12. Arnold A, Delaney GP, Cassapi L, et al. The use of categorized time-trend reporting of radiation oncology incidents: a proactive analytical approach to improving quality and safety over time. *Int J Radiat Oncol Biol Phys.* 2010;78(5):1548–1554.

13. Hunt MA, Pastrana G, Amols HI, et al. The impact of new technologies on radiation oncology events and trends in the past decades: an institutional experience. *Int J Radiat Oncol Biol Phys.* 2012;84(4):925–931.

14. Mazur L, Chera B, Mosaly P, et al. The association between event learning and continuous quality improvement programs and culture of patient safety. *Pract Radiat Oncol.* 2015;5(5):286–294.

15. Bissonnette JP, Medlam G. Trend analysis of radiation therapy incidents over seven years. *Radiother Oncol.* 2010;96(1):139–144.

16. Ford EC, Fong de los Santos L, Pawlicki T, et al. Consensus recommendations for incident learning database structures in radiation oncology. *Med Phys.* 2012;39(12):7272–7290.

17. *Report into Unintended Overexposure of Lisa Norris at Beatson, Glasgow.* Scotland: Scottish Executive; 2006.

18. Grout JR. Mistake proofing: changing designs to reduce error. *Qual Saf Health Care.* 2006;15(Suppl 1):i44–i49.

19. Reasons JT. *Managing the Risks of Organizational Accidents.* Surrey, UK: Ashgate; 1997.

20. Dekker S, Dekker S. *The Field Guide to Understanding Human Error.* Burlington, VT: Ashgate; 2006.

21. ACR–ASTRO. *ACR–ASTRO Practice Parameter for Radiation Oncology.* Reston, VA: American College of Radiology; 2014.

22. Ford EC, Terezakis S, Souranis A, et al. Quality control quantification (QCQ): a tool to measure the value of quality control checks in radiation oncology. *Int J Radiat Oncol Biol Phys.* 2012;84(3):e263–e269.

23. Kutcher GJ, Coia L, Gillin M, et al. Comprehensive QA for radiation oncology: report of AAPM Radiation Therapy Committee Task Group 40. *Med Phys.* 1994;21(4):581–618.

24. Zeitman A, Palta J, Steinberg M. *Safety Is No Accident: A Framework for Quality Radiation Oncology and Care.* Arlington, VA: ASTRO; 2012.

25. *ASRT: The Practice Standards for Medical Imaging and Radiation Therapy.* Albuquerque, NM: American Society for Radiological Technologists; 2011.

26. Eatmon S. Error prevention in radiation therapy. *Radiat Ther.* 2012;21(1):59–74.

27. Marks LB, Adams RD, Pawlicki T, et al. Enhancing the role of case-oriented peer review to improve quality and safety in radiation oncology: executive summary. *Pract Radiat Oncol.* 2013;3(3):149–156.

28. International Atomic Energy Agency. *Development of Procedures for In Vivo Dosimetry in Radiotherapy.* Vol. 8. Vienna, Austria: International Atomic Energy Agency; 2013.

29. Mans A, Wendling M, McDermott LN, et al. Catching errors with in vivo EPID dosimetry. *Med Phys.* 2010;37(6):2638–2644.

30. Van Dam J, Marinello G. *Methods for In Vivo Dosimetry in External Radiotherapy.* Brussels, Belgium; 2006.

31. Yorke E, Alecu R, Ding L, et al. *Diode In-Vivo Dosimetry for Patients Receiving External Beam Radiation Therapy: Report of AAPM Task Group-62.* Madison, WI: Medical Physics; 1991:87.

32. Azmandian F, Kaeli D, Dy JG, et al. Towards the development of an error checker for radiotherapy treatment plans: a preliminary study. *Phys Med Biol.* 2007;52(21):6511–6524.

33. Dewhurst JM, Lowe M, Hardy MJ, et al. Auto-Lock: a semiautomated system for radiotherapy treatment plan quality control. *J Appl Clin Med Phys.* 2015;16(3):5396.

34. Ebert MA, Haworth A, Kearvell R, et al. Detailed review and analysis of complex radiotherapy clinical trial planning data: evaluation and initial experience with the SWAN software system. *Radiother Oncol.* 2008;86(2):200–210.

35. Furhang EE, Dolan J, Sillanpaa JK, et al. Automating the initial physics chart-checking process. *J Appl Clin Med Phys.* 2009;10(1):129–135.

36. Halabi T, Lu HM. Automating checks of plan check automation. *J Appl Clin Med Phys.* 2014;15(4):4889.

37. Kalet AM, Gennari JH, Ford EC, et al. Bayesian network models for error detection in radiotherapy plans. *Phys Med Biol.* 2015;60(7):2735–2749.

38. Li HH, Wu Y, Yang D, et al. Software tool for physics chart checks. *Pract Radiat Oncol.* 2014;4(6):e217–e225.

39. Nordstrom F, Ceberg C, Back SA. Ensuring the integrity of treatment parameters throughout the radiotherapy process. *Radiother Oncol.* 2012;103(3):299–304.

40. Siochi RA, Pennington EC, Waldron TJ, et al. Radiation therapy plan checks in a paperless clinic. *J Appl Clin Med Phys.* 2009;10(1):43–62.

41. Yang D, Moore KL. Automated radiotherapy treatment plan integrity verification. *Med Phys.* 2012;39(3):1542–1551.

42. Yang D, Wu Y, Brame RS, et al. Technical note: electronic chart checks in a paperless radiation therapy clinic. *Med Phys.* 2012;39(8):4726–4732.

43. Moore KL, Brame RS, Low D, et al. Quantitative metrics for assessing treatment plan quality. *Semin Radiat Oncol.* 2011;22:62–69.

44. Moore KL, Brame RS, Low DA, et al. Experience-based quality control of clinical intensity-modulated radiotherapy planning. *Int J Radiat Oncol Biol Phys.* 2011;81(2):545–551.

45. Olsen LA, Robinson CG, He GR, et al. Automated radiation therapy treatment plan workflow using a commercial application programming interface. *Pract Radiat Oncol.* 2014;4(6):358–367.

46. Tol JP, Delaney AR, Dahele M, et al. Evaluation of a knowledge-based planning solution for head and neck cancer. *Int J Radiat Oncol Biol Phys.* 2015;91(3):612–620.

47. Wu B, Ricchetti F, Sanguineti G, et al. Patient geometry-driven information retrieval for IMRT treatment plan quality control. *Med Phys.* 2009;36(12):5497–5505.

48. Wu BB, Ricchetti F, Sanguineti G, et al. Data-driven approach to generating achievable dose-volume histogram objectives in intensity-modulated radiotherapy planning. *Int J Radiat Oncol Biol Phys.* 2011;79(4):1241–1247.

49. Zhang X, Li X, Quan EM, et al. A methodology for automatic intensity-modulated radiation treatment planning for lung cancer. *Phys Med Biol.* 2011;56(13):3873–3893.

50. Zhu X, Ge Y, Li T, et al. A planning quality evaluation tool for prostate adaptive IMRT based on machine learning. *Med Phys.* 2011;38(2):719–726.

51. Moran JM, Dempsey M, Eisbruch A, et al. Safety considerations for IMRT: executive summary. *Pract Radiat Oncol.* 2011;1(3):190–195.

52. Donaldson L. *Towards Safer Radiotherapy.* London, UK: British Institute of Radiology, Institute of Physics and Engineering in Medicine, National Patient Safety Agency, Society and College of Radiographers, The Royal College of Radiologists; 2007.

53. Molineu A, Followill DS, Balter PA, et al. Design and implementation of an anthropomorphic quality assurance phantom for intensity-modulated radiation therapy for the radiation therapy oncology group. *Int J Radiat Oncol Biol Phys.* 2005;63(2):577–583.

54. Mutic S, Brame RS, Oddiraju S, et al. Event (error and near-miss) reporting and learning system for process improvement in radiation oncology. *Med Phys.* 2010;37(9):5027–5036.

55. Nyflot MJ, Zeng J, Kusano AS, et al. Metrics of success: measuring impact of a departmental near-miss incident learning system. *Pract Radiat Oncol.* 2015;5(5):e409–e416.

56. Huq MS, Fraass B, Dunscombe P, et al. Application of risk analysis methods to radiation therapy quality management: report of AAPM Task Group 100. *Med Phys.* 2016;43(7):4209-4262.

57. Dunscombe P, Brown D, Donaldson H, et al. Safety profile assessment: an online tool to gauge safety-critical performance in radiation oncology. *Pract Radiat Oncol.* 2015;5(2):127–134.

58. Bojechko C, Phillps M, Kalet A, et al. A quantification of the effectiveness of EPID dosimetry and software-based plan verification systems in detecting incidents in radiotherapy. *Med Phys.* 2015;42(9):5363.

59. Fraass BA, Marks LB, Pawlicki T. Safety considerations in contemporary radiation oncology: introduction to a series of ASTRO safety white papers. *Pract Radiat Oncol.* 2011;1(3):188–189.

60. Solberg T, Balter J, Benedict S, et al. Quality and safety considerations in stereotactic radiosurgery and stereotactic body radiotherapy: executive summary. *Pract Radiat Oncol.* 2012;2:2–9.

61. Donaldson L. *Radiotherapy Risk Profile: Technical Manual.* Geneva, Switzerland: World Health Organization; 2008.

62. Das IJ, Cheng CW, Watts RJ, et al. Accelerator beam data commissioning equipment and procedures: report of the TG-106 of the Therapy Physics Committee of the AAPM. *Med Phys.* 2008;35(9):4186–4215.

63. Hoopes DJ, Dicker AP, Eads NL, et al. RO-ILS: Radiation Oncology Incident Learning System: a report from the first year of experience. *Pract Radiat Oncol.* 2015;5(5):312–318.

64. Cunningham J, Coffey M, Knöös T, et al. Radiation Oncology Safety Information System (ROSIS)—profiles of participants and the first 1074 incident reports. *Radiother Oncol.* 2010;97(3):601–607.

65. Kusano AS, Nyflot MJ, Zeng J, et al. Measurable improvement in patient safety culture: a departmental experience with incident learning. *Pract Radiat Oncol.* 2015;5(3):e229–e237.

66. Ford EC, Brown D, Donaldson H, et al. Patterns of practice for safety-critical processes in radiation oncology in the United States from the AAPM safety profile assessment survey. *Pract Radiat Oncol.* 2015;5(5):e423–e429.

10 Quality Considerations in Brachytherapy

R. Adam B. Bayliss and Bruce R. Thomadsen

QUALITY IN BRACHYTHERAPY

Consideration of a quality management (QM) program begins with the setting of goals for quality assurance (QA). In brachytherapy, the key goals are the prevention of patient and staff injury and the minimization of downtime. While there is a strong temptation to expedite the process of starting treatments, a retrospective analysis of treatments as a means of establishing a QM program is prone to failure. A thoughtful design of policies, procedures, and responsibilities aimed at achieving the objectives of the treatments is critical. As will be made clear in subsequent paragraphs, proper delegation of responsibilities requires a commitment on the part of the facility to the hiring and training of sufficient personnel, and adequate execution of brachytherapy requires a large staff (1). Many of the concepts discussed in this chapter are considered in greater detail in Thomadsen (2).

GENERAL QUALITY MANAGEMENT PRACTICE

QM in brachytherapy does not differ tremendously from its use in other areas of radiation oncology. The key steps in the implementation of a QM program for brachytherapy are quality planning, QA, and quality audits (Figure 10.1). Upon deciding to provide a new treatment procedure, the Quality Management Committee consisting, in part, of medical physicists, radiation oncologists, radiation therapists, nurses, clerical staff, social workers and any other persons involved, creates a quality management plan. Within the plan is a listing of all the relevant equipment, staff, the accuracy goals required on a per-patient or procedure basis to meet the needs of an adequate accurate treatment. The stated treatment goals must be reconciled with the achievable accuracy of the treatment tools. Once the goals are identified and the procedure established, quality control procedures should be developed that ensure that a treatment satisfying the patient's need and an accurate delivery are possible. These QA parameters will include assurance of proper operation of planning systems and treatment equipment, plan quality, and proper execution of a plan. A systematic review of procedures, QA results, and individual cases should then be carried out with both independent and internal reviewers. These audits should determine whether the specified objective was attained and whether procedures were followed.

Several studies considered the failure modes that are possible within brachytherapy procedures using the failure modes and effects analysis (FMEA) risk-assessment methodologies of the American Association of Physicists in Medicine (AAPM) Task Group 100 (TG 100). These may be useful in designing a QM program. Mayadev et al (3) consider the gynecological treatments with high-dose rate (HDR) brachytherapy and list 50 specific error pathways and their causes. Most of these are covered by a QM program and are also included in the discussion here. Other brachytherapy risk-assessment studies include another study of HDR brachytherapy (4), a review of cervical cancer brachytherapy aimed at increasing efficiency (5), and HDR brachytherapy for skin cancer with special applicators (6).

The remainder of this chapter considers a potential QM program for brachytherapy. The program described would apply only to the facility for which it was developed. TG 100 of the AAPM discusses in detail how a facility can establish a quality program (7). The TG 100 approach uses a risk analysis for a particular facility, including process mapping, failure modes and effects analysis, and fault-tree analysis (see Section III, Chapter 25 in this book) (8). Because procedures differ markedly among facilities, the necessary quality procedures also vary, and one QA program cannot apply universally. That being understood, what follows constitutes common brachytherapy quality procedures. Before adopting any, a facility should perform its own analysis to assess which activities add value to its own quality program.

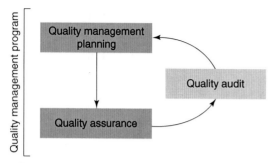

FIGURE 10.1 The quality management process.

QUALITY MANAGEMENT OF TREATMENT EQUIPMENT

Characterization of the sources, applicators, and measurement equipment is typically done first as part of acceptance tests and commissioning measurements. Acceptance tests verify that the characteristics of the equipment conform to expectations laid out in the agreement made to purchase the items. Commissioning typically builds on the acceptance testing by providing the necessary data for using the equipment in the clinic. After commissioning, periodic tests are made to confirm agreement with commissioning measurements and to verify continued functionality. Guidance for the frequency of such tests is given in the report of TG 100 (7).

Manual loading low-dose rate brachytherapy sources

Low-dose rate (LDR) brachytherapy sources can be divided into two groups: long-lived sources that are part of a permanent inventory, and shorter-lived sources that are ordered for administration during an individual patient's treatment. Although the maintenance of permanent inventories is increasingly rare in clinical practice, many of the tests inform management of custom sources.

Sources from a permanent inventory

Acceptance testing. The main requirements of acceptance testing for low-dose rate brachytherapy sources are the

verification of integrity, distribution of source activity, and source strength (Table 10.1).

Verifying integrity. Upon receipt of a source, the outer package should be checked for damage and any necessary contamination tests performed. Verification of source integrity is a visual inspection for mechanical damage such as cracks, dents, bends or weakness in the welds. Verification of lack of contamination is usually done through a wipe test.

A wipe test is optimally performed by rubbing the surface of the source with an alcohol-soaked glass fiber wipe, noting that several days may be required for contamination to build up again. In the United States, a reading of 185 Bq (0.005 µCi) or less identifies a source as contamination-free (9). When performing a leak test, consideration must be given to the statistical limitations of the measurement system. A comprehensive analysis was detailed by Altshuler and Pasternak and explained in Thomadsen (2,10). The process of analyzing a sample begins with determining the probability that for a given count rate, k_α, the system will incorrectly report activity when none is present (a false positive). The minimum significant count, C_S can be determined from the following equation:

$$C_S = k_\alpha \sigma_\beta \qquad [1]$$

where σ_β is the standard deviation in the measured background counts. The count rate is chosen on the basis of the desired level of uncertainty in the probability of determining a sample to have contamination when none is present. For example, choosing $k_\alpha = 2.576$ yields a probability of less than 0.5% of a false positive.

The alternative question is how low of a count rate would result in real activity in a sample being dismissed as background readings, that is, a false negative error. The process of determining this count rate is similar for counting systems and samples exhibiting Gaussian statistical behavior. A threshold probability for an acceptable likelihood of a false negative is set, defined as β. Then, based on integration over all possible count rates less than k_β, the detection limit, L_D, is

$$L_D = C_S + \sigma_S k_\beta \qquad [2]$$

where σ_S is the standard deviation in the count rate of the sample.

Table 10.1 Tests Typically Performed as Part of Acceptance-Testing a Source for a Permanent Source Inventory

Test	Goal
Integrity	No damage or contamination
Linear uniformity	Distribution of sources is as expected
Source strength	Activity meets stated values
Identification	Sources labeled or marked
Dose distribution	Measure penetration and dose distribution

Linear uniformity. It is verified by ensuring that the active radionuclide within the source casing is distributed consistently with manufacturer's specifications. Generally, this means the active source should produce a uniform radiation along its length at therapeutic distances. This test is most conveniently performed with GafChromic film, such as the RTQA2™ (Ashland Performance Materials, Ashland OH). The source activity distribution is verified through auto-exposure on the film, and orientation is captured with a kV exposure or careful marking of the physical boundaries of source on the film.

Identification of sources. This typically occurs while accepting a set of sources for addition to a permanent inventory. Photographic documentation of source identification supplied by the manufacturer and the markings on the sources should be performed.

Source strength. It is assayed using a calibrated well ionization chamber. All current standards from professional organizations recommend the use of air-kerma strength, S_k, that is, the air-kerma rate that would be produced by the source in vacuum at 1 m (11). For specification of source strength, to remove the dependence of the quantity on distance, the air-kerma rate at a meter is divided by the distance of specification (1 m), thus air-kerma strength carries the units $\mu Gy\ m^2\ h^{-1}$. The chamber should have at least secondary traceability to a National Institute of Standards and Technology (NIST) standard for each source model in the inventory. Additionally, a permanent inventory is optimally maintained by having at least one long-lived source that can be measured each time a well chamber is used, to verify the consistency of the well chamber calibration.

Penetration. Characterization of the ratio of response with and without attenuation within a stable measurement geometry, although not specifically recommended by the task groups of the AAPM, will provide a useful baseline over the life of the source to isolate contaminant isotopes should the source strength not follow expected decay.

Periodic testing. The recommended acceptance tests should be repeated at periodic intervals, based on the likelihood for change and the risk should a change not be detected.

Integrity. Most regulatory jurisdictions specify the frequency at which wipe testing of long-lived sources must occur.

Strength. The source strength should be checked after about 6 months from receipt, mostly to assess the possibility that the source material may have been contaminated with an isotope having a different half-life. If the source strength follows expectations on this check reading, intervals for subsequent checks can be extended. If the results are anomalous, the manufacturer should be contacted. A questionable reading should lead to reassessment in about 2 months and continue at frequent intervals until the issue is resolved.

Linear uniformity. When checking the source strength at the first six-month interval, imaging of the sources should be repeated to look for shifting in the source material. If the linear uniformity appears the same as when first assessed, the next check need not be for a couple of years, and thereafter at some longer interval. Most of the data in the literature for linear uniformity over time was for radium sources and is not relevant to more modern sources, so a period for such testing cannot be given here.

Source identification. Some forms of source identification—the markings that tell the strength of a source—wear off over time. At the time of periodic integrity testing, the condition of the identification marking should also be assessed and clarified as needed.

Penetration. Measurement of the penetration of the source radiation need not be repeated in the absence of changes in the measured source strength.

Sources for a particular patient

Sources ordered for a particular patient tend to be relatively short-lived (60 days or less). They usually are also implanted permanently in the patient shortly after receipt, so long-term measurements of consistency do not apply. All vendors of short-lived sources perform integrity checks on them before shipment. While opening a newly received package of sources, the packaging and the inside of the source container should be wipe-tested for contamination. Finding none, indicates that the source integrity has not been compromised. All such sources are quite small, so linear uniformity is also not an issue.

The remaining test, source strength, is important, but sometimes difficult to check. The recommendation from the AAPM is that in a batch of sources, 10% or 10, whichever is greater, should have the strength measured and compared with the vendor-specified average for the batch (12). If the calibration falls within 3%, nothing further need be done, but in case of a discrepancy of between 3% and 5%, the discrepancy should be investigated, possibly along with increasing the sample size. Discrepancies greater than 5% should be discussed with the vendor.

High-dose rate remote afterloaders

Much of the QA for a HDR remote-afterloading brachytherapy treatment unit is dictated by regulations. The regulations, found in 10 C.F.R. Subpart H for those facilities regulated by the U.S. Nuclear Regulatory Commission, have identical counterparts in the regulations of agreement states. Table 10.2 lists these activities, which must be followed. Other standard references for HDR brachytherapy include AAPM Task Group 59 (13), the ACR–ASTRO guidelines for the practice of HDR brachytherapy (14,15), the ASTRO Safety White Paper on HDR brachytherapy (16), and ESTRO Booklet Number 8 on safe practice in brachytherapy (17).

Table 10.2 Quality Assurance Steps Required for HDR Brachytherapy Treatment Units by Regulations of the U.S. Nuclear Regulatory Commission

Frequency	Required Check	Regulation Section
After each treatment	Exposure rate around patient (patient survey)	10 C.F.R. 35.604
Before first use after source installation	Calibration of source within 5% of vendor's value	10 C.F.R. 35.633(b)(1)
	Source positioning within 1 mm	10 C.F.R. 35.633(b)(2)
	Source retraction with backup battery	10 C.F.R. 35.633(b)(3)
	Length of transfer tubes	10 C.F.R. 35.633(b)(4)
	Timer accuracy and linearity over typical range of use	10 C.F.R. 35.633(b)(5)
	Length of applicators	10 C.F.R. 35.633(b)(6)
	Function of transfer tubes, applicators, and transfer-tube applicator interfaces	10 C.F.R. 35.633(b)(7)
Before first treatment of the day	Entrance interlocks	10 C.F.R. 35.643(d)(1)
	Source-exposed indicator lights	10 C.F.R. 35.643(d)(2)
	Video and intercom	10 C.F.R. 35.643(d)(3)
	Presence and operation of emergency equipment	10 C.F.R. 35.643(d)(4)
	Radiation detector potentially used to locate source	10 C.F.R. 35.643(d)(5)
	Timer accuracy	10 C.F.R. 35.643(d)(6)
	Time and date in unit's computer	10 C.F.R. 35.643(d)(7)
	Source activity in unit's computer compared with decay	10 C.F.R. 35.643(d)(8)

The tests listed after source installation apply anytime a source is installed in the unit, and also if the same source is removed and reinstalled.

For the most part, the required frequency for the tests satisfies the needs for quality and safety, with two exceptions. The first exception is the calibration of the source strength measured only at installation. Although it has been years since this problem occurred, there have been sources that were contaminated with a different radionuclide and exhibited anomalous decay. This would not be detected with a single measurement point. However, the likelihood of dosimetric problems from contaminated sources is slight. With 10% contamination, a very large proportion of a source strength, a contaminant with a 40-day half-life would just reach a 5% dosimetric error in 90 days, and would show as a 2% discrepancy from expected values with a reading 4 weeks after installation. For a contaminant with a longer half-life, a 10% contamination with a half-life of 140 days would yield a 5% dosimetric error at 90 days, just before source replacement, but would not give a 2% discrepancy from expected readings until 6 weeks after installation. Thus, contamination of a source with a different radionuclide is very unlikely to cause a problem over the life of the source, and would be difficult to distinguish from the normal uncertainty until 5 to 7 weeks after installation. Thus, it might be useful to check the source strength at about 6 weeks after installation, but that is unlikely to prevent a major error in dose to a patient.

The second parameter that may require checking more frequently than regulations recommend is the positioning accuracy of the source. The authors have seen the positioning accuracy suddenly change in the period between source changes. Many methods exist for verification of source positioning, and they have been discussed extensively in the literature; a detailed discussion can be found in Thomadsen (2). The following three methods are commonly used:

- Autoradiography, placing a catheter on a sheet of radiochromic film and marking two dwell positions as indicated by the unit's radiographic marker, separated by a distance such as 5 cm. Sending the source to the selected dwell positions will darken the film under the true dwell positions. This method was the standard for decades, but yields less precision than the other methods discussed next.

- Visualizing the position using the device's positioning rule and a television monitor, as illustrated in Figure 10.2. All of the units currently available come with rulers of this nature that can be used as part of a daily check if the room has a video monitor with a sufficiently high resolution and zoom.

- Measurements in a well chamber with a shielded insert (18). Figure 10.3(A) shows the insert. When the source falls behind the shielding, the reading falls to about a third of the reading outside the

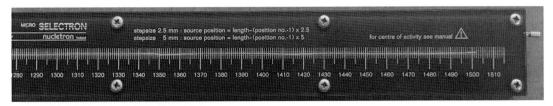

FIGURE 10.2 A picture of the HDR source in the vendor's ruler as seen on the in-room television monitor. The tip of the source should go to the programmed position for the center of the source plus 2 mm, accounting for half the length of the source capsule beyond the center.

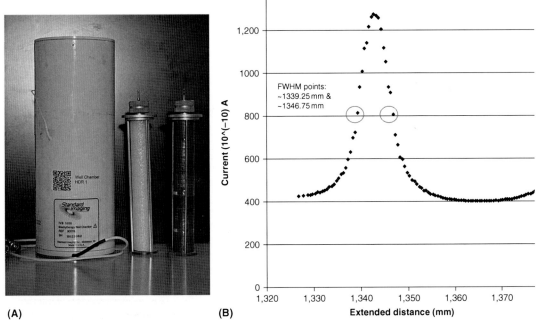

(A)   **(B)**

FIGURE 10.3 (A) A well chamber and its associated shielded insert. (B) Charge reading measured as the HDR source travels through the shielded insert. The readings with the source shielded are about a third of those appearing when the source is unshielded, and the gradient of the reading with source position is steep when the source is centered on the edge of the shield.

shielding. When the source is centered on the edge of the shielding, small variations in the actual position make large changes in the measured charge. Figure 10.3(B) shows a graph of the reading as the source moves along the chamber insert. Sending the source to the expected position of the edge of the shield and dividing the reading at that location by the reading at the maximum signal to eliminate decay gives a sensitive measure of the accuracy of source position. After the initial mapping of the relative intensity versus position in the chamber, this technique takes only a minute to set up and another to take the two readings.

Another potential problem that the required QA might not catch is more serious. Although the timer thus is unlikely to fail, the mechanism that drives the source indeed can. If the mechanism wears out, there can be a change in the time it takes the source to travel from the source safe to a dwell position in a catheter. Periodically measuring this time and comparing it with the time from an earlier determination can provide an alert that the mechanism should receive attention before the source movement fails. The measurement of the actual transit time is difficult, but a related quantity can serve as a surrogate. The surrogate can use two times—a short time, t_s, and a long time, t_l—for readings in the calibration well chamber. The readings can be R_s and R_1, respectively. From these, a quantity can be calculated that is related to the effect on the reading in the chamber due to the time the source takes to travel to the measurement position and then return to its safe. This quantity t_ϵ the equivalent time the source would be at the point of measurement to give the chamber reading equal to that during the time the source moves:

$$t_\epsilon = \frac{R_s}{\left(\dfrac{R_1 - R_s}{t_l - t_s}\right)} - t_s \qquad [3]$$

Sudden changes in the condition of the source movement are likely to trigger a friction interlock in the source drive. Thus, this effective time likely need only be calculated with source replacements.

Quality management of applicators and related treatment accessories

One of the most overlooked aspects of QA relates to the applicators and associated equipment used in the patient. The treatment appliances experience the most wear and hardest use of any parts used in brachytherapy. The vast variety of applicators used in brachytherapy, from gynecological tandems and rings through relatively simpler vaginal cylinders to simple implant catheters, makes covering the appropriate QM for each prohibitive. One of the references has a 30-page chapter covering just that (2). There are, however, some general principles that can guide the checking of applicators.

1. Pay attention to the expiration date of applicators and other equipment. Almost all applicators, and much of the equipment used in brachytherapy, have expiration dates. In some cases, no data exists supporting the dates, and they come from extremely safe estimates of how long operation can continue without parts failing. At other times, the dates come from experiences of equipment failures. A user does not know the basis for the dates. Particularly with applicators used in patients, the expiration date may factor in the effects of multiple sterilizations. The manufacturer cannot know the frequency of use an applicator would have in a given facility, so expiration dates often assume a frequency that is likely to be higher than the reality in most clinics. Regardless of the uncertainties involved, the use of outdated equipment puts a clinic at great legal risk should a patient suffer some untoward incident due to the treatment, regardless of whether the operation of the equipment was an issue or not.

2. All reusable applicators should be checked for operation (if applicable) and wear and tear of parts such as set screws when being cleaned *after* use preceding sterilization.

3. All applicators should be visually checked and, to the extent possible, checked for operation before insertion.

4. Damaged applicators, regardless of how slight the damage may be, should not be used. Several reported events resulted from use of applicators that were known to be damaged before insertion.

For HDR units, the regulations require testing of transfer tubes with each source change. There have not been many events involving damaged transfer tubes, although transfer tubes of the wrong length (that is, different from that expected in the plan) result in medical events every few years. The check of the transfer tube condition can be crafted to be quick and easy—slipping a cable of standard length down a tube, for example. A more valuable QM measure, which renders the true length of the transfer tube irrelevant, is performing localization imaging with radiographic markers that pass through the length of the transfer tube and all of the applicator, rather than short markers that only fill the applicator. In this way, the length to send the source is determined by the location of the marker after traveling the same path as the source eventually will. A problem that can develop with transfer tubes is that the mechanism that holds the applicator to the tube can fail, allowing the applicator to detach from the transfer tube during treatment. There is not much information about the failure pattern for the connectors, so the recommendation simply is to test the firmness of the hold by tugging gently on an attached applicator and visually inspecting the connector parts for wear.

ComfortCath™ (Elekta, Veenendaal, Netherlands) interstitial implant catheters have two parts: the catheters that reside in the patient for the duration of the treatment, and inserts that slide into the catheters and attach to transfer tubes to provide the source track. The inserts clip into the catheters with the distal tip touching the closed end of the catheter. In this way, the length of the catheter plays no part in the positioning of the source, but the length of the insert does. The catheter system assumes that the inserts all have a standard length. The length of the inserts should be checked, which can easily be performed in mass by holding a bunch of inserts together with their tips on a flat surface and comparing all the lengths with one for which the length had been measured (see Figure 10.4): Outliers become apparent. Another potential error is mistakenly using long inserts, used for catheters that pass through particularly thick body parts, instead of the standard-length inserts, resulting in a treatment shifted by several centimeters from the intended location. The likelihood of such an error only becomes significant when a mix of long and standard inserts are used in a patient.

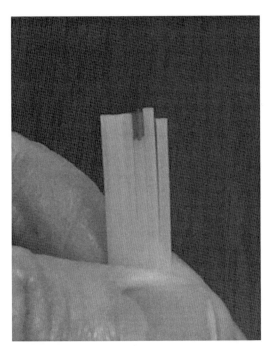

FIGURE 10.4 Checking the lengths of ComfortCath™ by comparison of a bunch with one that has been verified.

QUALITY MANAGEMENT FOR TREATMENT

Verification of applicator and patient set-up

Positioning of the applicator in the patient, regardless of the type, determines how well the treatment plan is mapped to the patient, and the ultimate success or failure of the treatment. In some cases, such as cervical brachytherapy using a tandem and ovoid, the positioning can be subject to movement while the patient is transferred to imaging devices and from patient movement. When considering the dose to neighboring organs, delays can degrade the accuracy of the calculated doses because of internal organ motion. Even interstitial treatments, where the needles may fix the geometry of the implant, can suffer dosimetric degradation should the patient's position change markedly from that during localization procedures. Together, these problems all center on the position of the applicator, that is, how well its position compares with that during imaging performed for dosimetry. To prevent problems, the position of the applicator should be checked before treatment begins. Usually, gynecological treatments can be checked visually, although the ability of the radiation oncologist to perceive changes in positions has not been quantified, and radiographs evaluated using skeletal landmarks may not be good benchmarks. Neither has the degree of conformance of the patient's position for interstitial

brachytherapy been assessed in the peer-reviewed literature. As a result, no recommendations for tolerances of applicator and patient set-up precision can be made, except that for treatment, both should be as close as possible to their positions when imaging for dosimetry was performed.

Verification of treatment parameters

High-dose rate treatments

Several key quality control procedures should be in place to prevent the errors that can happen during treatment (3). The first relates to verification of the program parameters in the treatment-unit computer. Most modern HDR treatments follow a program that has been sent to the treatment unit via intranet. Commissioning of the unit includes verification that treatment-program data sent from the treatment-planning computer is received reliably by the treatment-unit computer. Once confidence has been established, this check, per se, need not be repeated, assuming that some check of the program occurs with each patient. Only one event has been reported that resulted from a program changing when received by a treatment unit (and the software malfunction was corrected immediately by the vendor), so, although such a situation is possible, the probability is extremely low. There are more likely ways that the treatment-unit program may not be what is intended. Checking for the higher-probability errors also serves to verify the accuracy of the transfer of treatment information between computers.

The first check for the program in the treatment-unit computer verifies that it corresponds to the intended patient. Using the wrong patient's program results in a few medical events almost every year. Part of a time-out *just* before treating a patient should include verification of not only his or her identity and the procedure he or she will undergo, but also that the program in the treatment unit corresponds with the patient. This becomes more likely in a facility with several similar patients under treatment, particularly if the treatment room and unit have been set up for one patient some time ahead. A delay of the patient for whom the room was prepared, and bringing in a different patient, poses the danger that the unit operator may forget to reprogram the treatment unit.

Correct treatment requires correct programming of the dwell pattern: for each channel the proper length, step size or sizes, and right dwell time for each dwell position. The most common error in HDR treatments is the use of the wrong length, particularly, but not exclusively, when a length other than the default is intended (19). A check of the treatment program should always include a check of the length, even when the default value is planned. Likewise, the step size should be checked because, should that be different from the plan, the severity of the error could be extreme.

Assuming that the correct transfer of information to the treatment-unit computer has been validated, the only reason the dwell-time pattern should be wrong would be if the patient had more than one plan in the treatment-planning computer and the wrong one was forwarded to the treatment unit. Such an error could most likely be detected by checking the overall treatment time in the program compared with that on the treatment plan (corrected for decay as necessary, of course). There could be compensating changes in dwell times between plans, when time taken from one dwell position is added exactly to a different one. A general rule that will provide security in most cases is the following:

1. To check the overall treatment time compared with that in the treatment plan, corrected for decay, if the patient had only one plan in the treatment-planning computer.

2. To check the dwell times for each dwell position for the first fraction if the patient has more than one plan in the treatment-planning computer.

3. To check the overall treatment time for subsequent fractions after verifying the dwell pattern for the first fraction. For patients with multiple treatment programs in the treatment-unit computer, great care is needed to assure use of the correct program. In these cases, the check should be customized depending on the differences between the programs, possibly verifying the whole dwell pattern.

Low-dose rate treatments

QA for LDR treatments mostly consists of verifying that the source strength pattern matches that in the treatment plan and, for temporary implants, that the time for removal is known and there are procedures in the facility to make sure sources are removed on schedule. Checking the source strength for permanent implants is simply a matter of comparing the patient's plan with the assayed strength of the sources received from the vendor as part of the time-out before the procedure.

Verification of execution

High-dose rate treatments

During execution, the main concern is that the source progresses through the treatment pattern without getting stuck in any channel. After treatment, verification, as required by regulation, consists of checking that the treatment followed the program. Most treatment units simplify this task by printing side by side the treatment program and what was executed. There can be differences of 0.1 second between the programmed and executed times if a unit was programmed well before

the treatment, in which case the unit may increase the time for the treatment from that programmed to correct for source decay.

Low-dose rate treatments

For permanent implants using loaded needles, care must be taken during the procedure to assure that the correct needle is used in the correct template hole. One technique has the radiation oncologist call for a needle by template coordinate, and the physicist repeat the coordinates while picking up the needle and handing it to the radiation oncologist, who then restates the coordinates of the hole into which the needle is inserted. Implants using loose sources and devices such as the Mick applicator require increased diligence in accounting because, for each template hole, the depth to drop the sources must be communicated to the radiation oncologist. Each team should develop a method, perhaps using specially designed forms, to keep track of which sources have already been deposited. Final verification of the implant, regardless of the delivery method, comes with the CT used for dose calculation (20).

The source-strength pattern for temporary implants would be part of the source-strength assay check discussed earlier. At the time of insertion, procedures must assure that each ribbon is placed into the correct needle or catheter, and that the insertion places the ribbon in the correct location in the catheter, usually all the way to the end. The most usual method for keeping the source-strength patterns of the ribbons straight is having the vendor use ribbons of different colors for each loading pattern.

QUALITY MANAGEMENT OF TREATMENT PLANNING

One of the most common loci for errors in brachytherapy is in treatment planning, particularly in the gathering of data necessary to perform the treatment plan.

Localization and imaging

Because much of the treatment-planning information comes from imaging in modern brachytherapy, great attention must go toward QA of the imaging units. This section assumes that a facility has in place the routine QA for the imaging devices, both for the imaging proper and for the imaging used for external-beam treatments: for CT (21–24), for MRI (25,26), for ultrasound (27), and for radiography and fluoroscopy (28). The discussion here focuses on the particular QM needs of imaging instrumentation when used for brachytherapy applications. Applications in particular procedures will often inform the considerations.

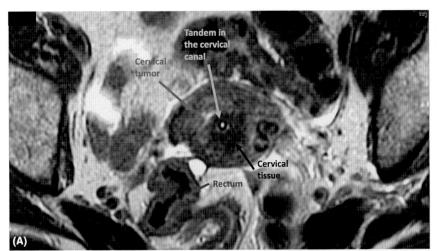

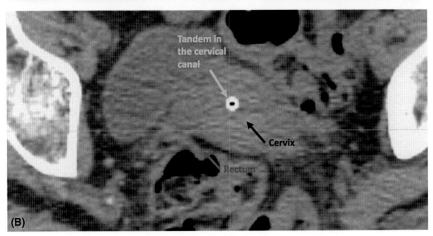

FIGURE 10.5 Images of a cervix with a tumor, as imaged by: (A) MRI, (B) CT.

Quality management for MRI guidance

MRI finds use in cervical brachytherapy because this imaging modality distinguishes between tumor, normal cervix, uterus, and pericervical tissues. Figure 10.5(A) shows an MRI of a cervix with the tumor highlighted. CT cannot make this differentiation, as shown in Figure 10.5(B). However, although MRI better shows different soft tissues, only CT can provide a measure of the radiation attenuation properties of tissue occupying a given voxel, a quantity necessary for dose calculations that account for tissue heterogeneity.

Brachytherapy differs from diagnostic applications of MRI by requiring not only the tissue-differential properties but also accurate geometric reconstruction. Usually, diagnoses require the ability to see anatomical changes from normal or measure physiological quantities such as flow. Often, the exact location of the features seen is not of paramount importance. Brachytherapy applications, in contrast, must determine the distances between source positions and points in the target or normal tissues at which dose is calculated.

Because of the inverse square relationship between distance and dose, the distances require high accuracy, and that, in turn, leads to several verifications needed during commissioning of the use of the imaging modality for brachytherapy and possibly on a per-patient basis.

- *Image isotropy (control of image distortion).* Modern MRI units have largely overcome the major image distortion problems prevalent with earlier units. Nevertheless, objects with permittivity very different from the surrounding tissue can create distortions in the magnetic field and thus the reconstructed image. Brachytherapy applicators can produce such distortions. Before using an applicator or needle types in patients, test images with the applicator in an appropriate phantom with known geometry are needed to assess the effects of the applicator on the image. Correction of such distortion is not possible at this time, so applicators that cause distortion sufficient to perturb the dose calculation more than desired should not be used.

- *Image reproduction.* Although image isotropy is a property of the imaging unit, bringing the images from the unit to the treatment planning system (TPS) also carries potential problems. The goal, of course, is to have the same image in the TPS as in the imaging system. Some potential problems include the following:

  - *Mismatch in the image spacing.* There have been events resulting from the TPS using a different interimage spacing. This failure produces 3D images that are either stretched out or compressed in the axial direction. Usually, errors of this nature can be found while describing an applicator (since it would not fit as expected), through QA of a treatment plan or simply comparing the images in the TPS with that in the imaging archive. Assuring that the TPS reads the image spacing correctly is part of the commission of the TPS.

  - *Failure of polarity or parity.* Another potential problem in importing images into the TPS is maintaining the correct polarity (i.e., the planar images stack correctly head to foot) and parity (right and left are indicated correctly). Failures of this nature can be systematic and again have to be addressed during commissioning. They can also occur in individual patients. Such failures can simply follow from a radiographer entering the wrong orientation in the scan information or from the patient being imaged in an unusual position without overriding the default settings in the header file. Because the images show greater soft-tissue detail, parity errors can be more easily noticed with MRI than CT, but if one focuses intently on a midline applicator, the clues may be missed. Polarity errors present as the patient appearing upside down from normal. If this occurs suddenly in a patient, it may be noticed. However, many departments have various planning systems, and some may routinely display the patient inverted, establishing the coordinate system looking down at the patient from the unit gantry. In such cases, seeing a patient inverted may seem quite normal. If an applicator description is being used from a library, the applicator would not match the patient's orientation, again giving a clue to the operator that something is amiss. However, entering the applicator from the images can result in incorrect dwell patterns or lengths, depending on how the planning system handles the data input.

  - *Grid resolution.* Combinations of modern TPS and MRI units should not have issues due to different grid sampling sizes, although these have caused problems in the past, and compatibility must be validated during commissioning.

Although the coarser sampling grid often used in a TPS should not cause geometric distortion, and the additional distance uncertainty should be small, the clarity of the soft-tissue differentiations can be reduced, or in some cases lost, in crucial locations. Usually in such cases, the image looks markedly degraded, which, again, give a clue to the operator to look at the original images before performing any contouring or dwell-position definition.

Locating the position of the first dwell in an applicator, or even the source channel, becomes a challenge in many cases under MRI guidance. This problem is so basic to the procedure that the GEC-ESTRO group that described the MRI-guided approach addressed this issue in one of its four founding articles on the technique (29). Some of the issues they note apply broadly across imaging modalities, such as dwell-position localization, as discussed later. Most relate specifically to MRI applicator reconstruction. Any facility starting a brachytherapy program using magnetic-resonance image guidance should study this document carefully.

One feature of MRI source or dwell reconstruction potentially affects any metallic applicators or needles. Such applicators cast axial shadows beyond the border of the applicator. Thus, the lumen of the applicator appears to extend past its physical end. This is the case not only for cervical applicators and needles but also for permanent sources in a prostate.

Quality management for CT guidance

Many of the potential problems discussed for MRI apply also to CT, such as the requirements for image isotropy and image reproduction. Detecting parity issues is simpler with CT than with MRI through the use of metallic markers on the image to indicate right and left.

Quality management for ultrasound guidance

Ultrasound finds application in brachytherapy mostly for prostate implants, gynecological tandem insertion guidance and target depth determination for skin cancers.

- *QA for transrectal ultrasound for prostate implants.* QA for transrectal ultrasound units is often forgotten. Poor image quality during prostate implants has contributed to several medical events in which the sources were implanted in totally wrong places. For this modality, it becomes useful to consider QA for the imaging proper simply because, generally, it is not covered in a hospital imaging QA program. The AAPM published a task group report describing a QA program for such units (30). Although still a very useful document, it came out just as more modern units with a different generation of display were entering the market. Tests, such as that of the grayscale, serve little purpose now. The first part of the report addresses imaging ability and accuracy. The first point, imaging ability, assesses how well, or even whether, the unit images either small high-contrast objects or moderate-sized objects with small differences in contrast. The second item, accuracy, addresses whether objects imaged appear in the correct location. Ultrasound units can have the image geometry altered accidentally—sometimes surprisingly easily. These tests require a phantom specifically made for testing transrectal units; at the time of writing, there were only two vendors of such phantoms. The second part of the report considers the congruence between the images and the patient and implantation system. On these units, the images show dots that correspond to where the ultrasound system estimates the needles should be based on the template. If the template is rotated with respect to the transducer or if the projected dots are out of calibration for distance, the needles, and thus the sources, will end up misplaced. The congruence between the indicator dots and the needles can be tested simply by placing the transducer, along with some needles in distant template holes, into a bucket of water and seeing whether the images of the needles are superimposed on their respective indicator dots, as shown in Figure 10.6. Because the speed of sound in room-temperature (20°C) water, 1,480 m s^{-1}, is slower than that in soft tissue at body temperature, 1,540 m s^{-1}, the ultrasound unit will indicate echoes from needles in the water farther from the probe than they are (30). For needles 6 cm from the probe, the difference in indicated position is about 3 mm. Warming the water to 30°C reduces the difference at 6 cm to just over 1 mm (30). Warming the water to higher than 40°C can damage some probes and so should not be attempted without checking the probe's specifications. This test should be performed whenever the template might misalign with its intended position. Some transducer/stepper systems are designed more robustly than others. Performing this test at frequent intervals when the equipment is new constitutes part of commissioning and establishing the reliability of the system.

The last part of the report considers the import of the image information into the treatment-planning computer. As with all image information imported to a TPS, the commissioning and subsequent QA assess whether the image information is accurately reproduced through the importation process.

All of the tests discussed compare images of test objects with some expected location on the image. Performing these tests is not as easy as it seems. The image of a very small object takes on the shape of a crescent that becomes larger as the distance from the probe increases, as in Figure 10.6. Artifacts, particularly reverberations, additionally make it difficult to determine the point to assign as the location of the image.

- *QA for ultrasound used to guide tandem insertion for gynecological brachytherapy.* This application mostly uses ultrasound units called from the radiology department. A brachytherapy practice that performs a large number of cervical and intact-uterine cancer treatments may maintain its own unit. Either way, the units are the conventional hand-held devices, and for this discussion are assumed to be covered by the QA program for the hospital or clinic. Other than assuring adequate images, no additional QA is required.

- *QA for ultrasound used to establish target depth for skin cancers.* The units for this application run at a higher frequency than standard units to give finer resolution. The higher frequency reduces the depth of penetration, but because the target depth is usually only 3 to 5 mm, penetration is not an issue. The two important characteristics for this measurement are that the imaging contrast adequately images the difference between cancer and normal tissue and that indicated distances reflect true distances. Although both of these should be checked through regular imaging QA, because these are not usual units, they may not be included in a facility's routine imaging QA program. Moreover, commercially available test phantoms do not have the necessary objects and patterns.

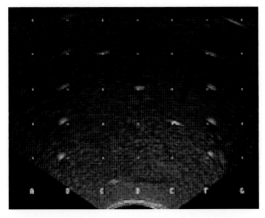

FIGURE 10.6 A test of the coincidence between the indicated template holes, as seen by the rectangular dot array, and the image of two needles inserted through an actual hole in the template, for a transrectal ultrasound unit. The transducer and needles are submerged in warm water. Notice that the images of the needles form crescents rather than dots.

Contouring

In the analysis of potential failure in intensity-modulated radiotherapy, Task Group 100 of the AAPM found that most of the highest-risk steps involve contouring the target, and the hazard likely applies to brachytherapy also (7). Errors in this function are extremely difficult to detect in later stages of the process. Even assuming that the radiation oncologist performing the contouring has the appropriate training in contouring for the treatment site, the process certainly deserves QA, although providing a check of the contours often proves challenging. Possible methods include:

- *Review by a second radiation oncologist.* In a practice with more than one radiation oncologist, cases could receive independent review. This might take the form of a Tumor Board or a casual consultation.

- *Review by a medical physicist or dosimetrist.* This option requires that the reviewing medical physicist or dosimetrist be trained and experienced in evaluating targets in various sites. It would not be expected that they could know the target in individual patients, since that would require reviewing the patient's entire history and imaging studies as well as performing the history and physical, and understanding what is indicated by what they find. While this is also true for a second radiation oncologist, the reviewer is likely to be able to evaluate the contours enough to ask questions through reviewing the chart and images. The physicist or dosimetrist, however, can learn enough about classes of patients to raise questions as appropriate about a contour, and that question may lead to the radiation oncologist reviewing the contour.

- *Automated review.* Commercial programs that generate suggested contours are becoming available. These programs are becoming more robust at a rapid pace.

Contouring normal tissue structures is usually less challenging than the target, but errors still can be made. There is also a higher likelihood that an erroneous normal structure contour may be detected later in the process. In many facilities, the dosimetrist or medical physicist will contour the normal structures, and the radiation oncologist will review the contouring, including a QA check in the process. If additional QA of normal-structure contouring is desired (although resources likely could be used better elsewhere), the same options are available, but with emphasis on a second person who is not a physician and an automated program.

Digitization of applicator

Many of the events reported to the U.S. Nuclear Regulatory Commission involve problems with positioning an applicator in a treatment plan (19,31). The following are some of the errors that can enter through the digitization of the dwell or source positions:

- The points used to describe the dwell positions can be backward from what the computer expects (i.e., the points might be entered from the tip to the connector when the input file specified connector to tip). This is a very difficult error to detect.

- The digitization can start at a different dwell position from that designated in the plan (shifting the dose distribution; this is particularly an issue for intraluminal applications intending to treat the middle of a long catheter in the anatomical tube.

- The interdwell step size can be entered differently than intended or changed accidentally during planning. Such an error stretches the treatment length, but in so doing reduces the dose to the area around the source track.

Each of these errors could be detected by highlighting a dwell position on the images and stepping through the successive dwells.

Another class of errors involves the source going to a different location than intended:

- The distance or length specification can be wrong, resulting in the treatment being delivered to the wrong location. This type of error, by far, is the most common error in reported HDR brachytherapy events. These errors often originate during measurement of the length of the source-track channel with a device as shown in Figure 10.7. The device has a cable with a capsule on one end to simulate the source, with the other end attached to a scale. Sometimes the capsule becomes bent and catches at a junction (for example, between the transfer tube and a catheter) instead of going to the end of the source channel. Such errors shift the dose distribution toward the treatment unit by tens of centimeters. This error cannot be found by study of the dwell pattern on the images, as the length has no connections with the image coordinates. For many applications, simply comparing the measured

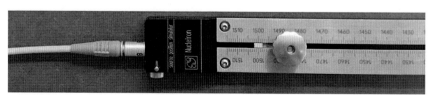

FIGURE 10.7 Source position simulator used to measure the length to the first possible dwell position in an applicator.

length with the expected range will uncover an error in measurement. For routine interstitial cases, however, catheters may be cut to arbitrary lengths, in which case there would be no expected value. When using a length measurement device to determine the first dwell position for several of the units, some extra distance must be added because the check cable or the source cable moves a few millimeters past the first dwell position. Not giving a margin to accommodate this extra distance will result in the unit detecting a blockage when the cable hits the end of the applicator.

- Another problem that occurs repeatedly is the use of transfer tubes of the wrong length. If the incorrect transfer tubes are too short, the treatment unit is likely to detect the error during the check-cable run as the cable hits the end of the applicator. Transfer tubes that are erroneously long, however, will not be detected during the check-cable run, resulting in the dose being delivered considerably nearer the unit than intended.

Both of these classes of errors could be detected by imaging just before treatment using a marker cable that would follow the path of the source from the connector that plugs into the front of the treatment unit through the distal-most dwell position. Such images would uncover any length issues.

Rigid applicators are sometimes positioned using a library description of the applicator. In such an approach, the dwell positions would be checked during commissioning of the library, but the applicator for the library must be registered with the patient images. Such a registration is usually very simple for radiographs, particularly if a marker cable was in the applicator when the images were made. The registration becomes slightly more difficult for CT images, mostly because of the axial uncertainly due to window width. Registration on MRI can be challenging for all the reasons discussed in the section *"Quality management for MRI guidance."*

Errors in the registration should be obvious if they are significant enough to pose dosimetric problems, but in a hurried environment, poor alignment might be missed. A second person intentionally evaluating the quality of the registration should suffice to catch an error.

Dose calculation parameters

Assuming that the TPS has undergone comprehensive commissioning, the most common errors in the input of dose-calculation parameters involve the source strength. This is true for HDR or LDR sources. One of the most common errors is a mix-up of source strength in air-kerma strength and activity, and the switch goes in both directions. For the dose calculation, the TPS may expect the source strength in a particular unit, whereas

the operator enters it in different units. An alternative scenario occurs by entering the source strength for the wrong patient.

For HDR units, the error comes during assay of a new source in a well chamber and entry into the TPS. An error at this point propagates into the same amount of error in all patients planned from the time of the erroneous entry until discovery of the error. Prevention of errors of this nature, or other assay and entry errors, is best addressed by establishing a routine verification check of new-source commissioning, preferably by a second qualified person.

For permanent LDR sources, the errors in source strength may also happen during input into the treatment-planning computer, or during source ordering. If ordered verbally, the wrong strength could be said accidentally or heard incorrectly owing to many possible causes. Transmitting the order in written copy (for example, by attachment to an e-mail or by fax) prevents the verbal failures. The possibility of transcription errors remains. A verification check of the source strength as part of a planning QA can intercept many possible errors. These checks can use a nomogram or predictive equations that have been validated for the particular practice by testing on a set of patients (32–34).

QUALITY ASSURANCE OF THE TREATMENT PLAN

QA for treatment plans has always been an important part of the physicist's role. A good and efficient QA program for treatment plan and delivery is extremely important and necessary for quality and safety in the treatments. Intracavitary and interstitial treatment plans often have different goals for the dose distribution: the former usually projects dose through a volume with few source tracks, resulting in a large dose gradient from the sources to the edge of the target, whereas the latter usually tries for uniformity in the treatment volume.

Verification of length

The length often becomes a more critical parameter for intracavitary treatments than for interstitial treatments. Intracavitary treatments usually use few catheters, frequently one to three. An erroneous length in one alters much of the dose distribution. With interstitial implants, a shift in one catheter alters the dose distribution locally, but usually does not make a large difference in the overall dose distribution. Of course, a systematic error in all the catheter lengths shifts the whole distribution for either an intracavitary or an interstitial application. The measurement of the treatment length has been discussed in several earlier sections because of its importance in correct treatment and the varied ways that errors in length can enter the process. Verification of the length in the treatment plan, maintaining a record of these lengths, and verifying the recorded length with the planned and programmed length before each treatment forms the follow-up to its correct measurement.

Appropriateness of application

The prescription provides the evaluation criteria for appropriateness of the plan. The prescription includes not only the dose and dose uniformity across the target but also the volume-based dose limits to the normal tissue structures. The plan, of course, should satisfy the prescribed criteria. However, between the applicator geometry and the patient's anatomy, for some treatments satisfying all criteria may prove impossible. The choices in these cases include accepting a higher dose to normal structures, compromising on the target dose—or some of both—or attempting to reposition the applicator. Many cases use several insertions, so lowering the dose in a fraction with a less-than-desired distribution may be recoverable with later applications. If the mismatch between applicator and anatomy is too great, the treatment may call for a different application approach, perhaps with the addition of some interstitial needles.

Target coverage

The most common tool for evaluation of target coverage is the cumulative dose volume histogram (DVH). An indication of target coverage comes from measures such as the $_{CTV}V_{95\%}$, which is the fractional volume of the clinical target volume, CTV, covered by 95% of the prescribed dose. Similarly, the $_{CTV}D_{95\%}$ indicates the dose, either absolute in gray or as a percentage of the prescription dose, that covers 95% of the CTV. While these quantities are the same for external-beam therapy, in those cases they usually apply to the planning target volume, PTV. Indeed, PTV may also be used in brachytherapy. When planning an implant, establishing a PTV as a volumetric expansion around a CTV often serves to ensure adequate placement of needles around a target to allow target coverage during optimization. Once needles have been placed, the plan may be optimized on the CTV directly. Exceptions include multifraction interstitial implants where the needles may shift along the needle axis and positioning QA measures cannot ensure placement identical to the original. A similar situation may obtain with a uterine tandem, which may slip slightly between imaging and treatment. In both cases, a prescription may use a PTV expanded only in the direction of the applicator axis to ensure coverage of the CTV. Figure 10.8(A) shows an interstitial, post-tylectomy breast implant dose distribution in two sample planes, and Figure 10.8(B) displays the DVH for the plan.

High-dose volume

In any brachytherapy treatment plan, the tissue around the radioactive source will receive very high doses. Large dose inhomogeneities are an inherent part of intracavitary insertions. Developing the plan includes being mindful of the tolerances of all the structures receiving dose. By distributing the source material through the volume, an interstitial implant can better control the extent of the high-dose volume. Rules from the classic systems can help minimize this volume, for example, by following the Paris guidelines with catheters equidistant to one another with separations based on the implant geometry (35). While optimizing the dose distribution, great care should be taken to distribute the "high-dose volumes" (150% isodose line and greater) among as many dwell positions as possible rather than to a few, and this balancing usually takes the form of minimizing variations among neighboring dwell times or source strengths. A rule of thumb for interstitial implants is not to let two adjacent 150% isodose surfaces coalesce or touch each other, although in practice this rule often expands to three. A "good" or "optimal" implant with adequate catheters facilitates maintenance of this rule. The rule is related to the maximum significant dose, MSD, which is the highest isodose surface where dose coalesces around more than one needle or source track. A companion concept is the maximum contiguous dose, MCD, which is the highest valued isodose surface that encompasses all the source positions (36). In general, the MSD should remain less than 150% of the MCD (37,38).

Uniformity

One measure of the uniformity of dose distribution in a brachytherapy implant is termed the *dose homogeneity index* (DHI), defined as (39)

$$\mathrm{DHI} = (_{CTV}V_{100\%} - {}_{CTV}V_{150\%}) / (_{CTV}V_{100\%}) \qquad [4]$$

The ideal value for DHI would be 1.0, which is realistically impossible because of the hot spots around each dwell position. Part of the concept is that doses above 150% of the prescription dose provide no increased therapeutic value but can lead to increased toxicity. So, the useful volume is just that raised to the prescribed dose. Additionally, the formula is based on the prescribed dose as the $D_{100\%}$. For intracavitary applications where the base of the isodose values is the dose to a reference point, such as point A, $D_{100\%}$ may actually refer to a dose that is some percentage of that reference point dose. Such a practice, though

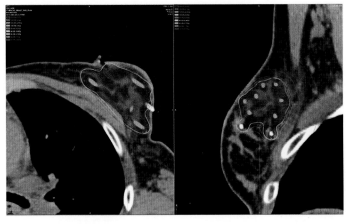

FIGURE 10.8 (A) A dose distribution for interstitial treatment of a posttylectomy breast shown in transverse and sagittal planes. (B) The dose volume histogram for the dose distribution in Figure 10.8(A). The prescribed dose is 3.4 Gy/fraction giving V95% of 95% and D95% of 3.23 Gy.

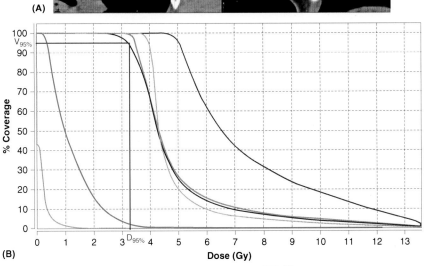

(B)

Dose for BreastIST CT F × 1

——— **Skin (1)**
4449.26 ml, Max Dose: 4.69 Gy, Min Dose: 0.00 Gy
Mean Dose: 0.14 Gy, SD: 0.24 Gy

——— **Chest wall (3)**
83.28 ml, Max Dose: 12.17 Gy, Min Dose: 0.00 Gy
Mean Dose: 1.22 Gy, SD: 0.81 Gy

——— **GTV (5)**
4.03 ml, Max Dose: 13.60 Gy, Min Dose: 3.46 Gy
Mean Dose: 4.83 Gy, SD: 1.48 Gy

——— **CTV (6)**
43.74 ml, Max Dose: 13.60 Gy, Min Dose: 2.18 Gy
Mean Dose: 4.86 Gy, SD: 1.93 Gy

——— **V 150% (8)**
13.73 ml, Max Dose: 13.60 Gy, Min Dose: 3.49 Gy
Mean Dose: 7.50 Gy, SD: 2.49 Gy

——— **V 100.0 % (9)**
54.59 ml, Max Dose: 13.60 Gy, Min Dose: 2.37 Gy
Mean Dose: 4.96 Gy, SD: 1.97 Gy

historically common, can cause confusion and should be left to history.

Conformality

Target volume and the volume covered by the 100% isodose surface, V_{100}, should be as conformal as possible. Mathematically, a conformality index (CI) can be defined as (40)

$$CI = \frac{Target\ Volume \cap V_{100}}{Target\ Volume \cup V_{100}}$$ [5]

The CI can be calculated as (41,42)

$$CI = \left(\frac{_{CTV}V_{100\%}}{V_{100\%}} \right) \left(\frac{_{CTV}V_{100\%}}{_{CTV}V} \right)$$

(all volumes absolute, e.g., in cm)   [6]

In an ideal implant, CI should equal 1.0, indicating perfect conformance between the 100% isodose surface and the target volume. As explained earlier, a DVH of the brachytherapy implant is necessary to generate the V_{100} and the volume of CTV covered and not covered by the 100% isodose line. The first factor in the equation evaluates

Table 10.3 Values for the Variables in Eq. [3] Used for Checking the Total Time in a Treatment Plan for an Intracavitary Balloon-Catheter Treatment for HDR Sources Using ^{192}Ir (44) and ^{60}Co (45), and the Xoft Electronic Brachytherapy Source (46)

Variable	Name	Value for Isotopic HDR Sources	Value for the Xoft Electronic Brachytherapy Sources
Λ	Dose rate constant [cGy/µGy m^2]	1.11 for ^{192}Ir 1.09 for ^{60}Co	0.709
S_k	Air-kerma strength [µGy m^2 h^{-1}]	From the source assay corrected for decay	From the source assay, multiplying the calibration factor for a model 6711 iodine seed by 1.78 and correcting for decay
r	Radius of the balloon + 1 cm [cm]	As per patient plan	As per patient plan
$g(r)$	Radial dose function	1.006 for ^{192}Ir For ^{60}Co: 0.976 for $r_{balloon}$ = 1.5 cm 0.968 for $r_{balloon}$ = 2.0 cm 0.960 for $r_{balloon}$ = 2.5 cm	0.544 for $r_{balloon}$ = 1.5 cm 0.470 for $r_{balloon}$ = 2.0 cm 0.411 for $r_{balloon}$ = 2.5 cm

how efficiently the dose distribution is placed in the target, whereas the second considers the coverage of the target.

Dwell time or source strength check

Remote-afterloaders utilize the stepping source technology, which enables the planner to maximize the dose uniformity, while minimizing the implant volume needed to adequately cover the target volume. Such flexibility creates a challenge for verification of the optimized calculations, with practical manual calculation techniques taking only a few minutes and at the same time detecting significant errors. Commonly, variations of greater than 5% in external-beam treatments are felt to potentially compromise outcomes. Whereas the accuracy of brachytherapy treatments likely falls at about this level, clearly there is a need for a quick method to verify the accuracy of an optimized plan.

Das et al (43) proposed a check for ^{192}Ir applications with

$$\text{Time [s]} = \frac{\text{Prescribed Dose [Gy]} \cdot K\left[U \cdot s \cdot Gy^{-1}\right] \cdot \text{PTV V}_{100\%}^{2/3} [cm^{2/3}] \cdot EC}{S_K[U]} \quad [7]$$

where EC is the elongation correction, equal to

$$EC = 1 + 0.06\left(\frac{\text{Longest Dimension}}{\text{Shortest Orthogonal Dimension}} - 1\right)^{1.26} \quad [8]$$

The parameter K assumes the values:

- K = 1.267 × 10^5 U·s·Gy$^{\wedge(-1)}$ for a single source track
- K = 1.182 × 10^5 U·s·Gy$^{\wedge(-1)}$ for two or three source tracks, and
- K = 0.928 × 10^5 U·s·Gy$^{\wedge(-1)}$ for four or more source tracks.

While Das et al explicitly considered checks for HDR implants, the same equations could be used for temporary LDR implants.

For electronic brachytherapy as well as isotopic HDR approaches, use Eq. [9]

$$\text{Time [s]} = \frac{\text{Prescribed Dose [Gy]} \cdot r^2}{S_K \cdot \Lambda \cdot g(r)} \quad [9]$$

with the values in Table 10.3.

For low-energy sources such as those used for permanent implants, the desired strength depends on the treatment techniques, and QA checks of the source strength can best be achieved through comparison with a large number of previous cases, based on implant size and shape. In a facility without a long history of similar cases, practitioners should check with the instructors with whom they trained to find the expected values for source strength.

REFERENCES

1. Zietman A, Palta J, Steinberg M. *Safety Is No Accident: A Framework for Quality Radiation Oncology and Care.* Fairfax, VA: American Society for Radiation Oncology; 2012.

2. Thomadsen B. *Achieving Quality in Brachytherapy.* London, UK: Taylor & Francis; 2000.

3. Mayadev J, Dieterich S, Harse R, et al. A failure mode and effects analysis for gynecological

high-dose-rate brachytherapy. *Brachytherapy.* 2015;14(6):866–875.

4. Giardina M, Castiglia F, Tomarchio E. Risk assessment of component failure modes and human errors using a new FMECA approach: application in the safety analysis of HDR brachytherapy. *J Radiol Prot.* 2014;34(4):891–914.

5. Damato AL, Lee LJ, Bhagwat MS, et al. Redesign of process map to increase efficiency: reducing procedure time in cervical cancer brachytherapy. *Brachytherapy.* 2015;14(4):471–480.

6. Sayler E, Eldredge-Hindy H, Dinome J, et al. Clinical implementation and failure mode and effects analysis of HDR skin brachytherapy using Valencia and Leipzig surface applicators. *Brachytherapy.* 2015;14(2):293–299.

7. Huq S, Fraass B, Dunscombe P. The report of Task Group 100 of the AAPM: application of risk analysis methods to radiation therapy quality management. *Med Phys.* 2016;43(7):4209–4262.

8. Thomadsen B, Dunscombe P, Ford E, et al. *Quality and Safety in Radiotherapy: Learning the New Approaches in Task Group 100 and Beyond.* Madison, WI: Medical Physics; 2013.

9. National Council on Radiation Protection and Measurements. *A Handbook of Radioactivity Measurements Procedures: With Nuclear Data for Some Biomedically Important Radionuclides: Recommendations of the National Council on Radiation Protection and Measurements.* Bethesda, MD: National Council on Radiation Protection and Measurements; 1984.

10. Altshuler B, Pasternack B. Statistical measures of the lower limit of detection of a radioactivity counter. *Health Phys.* 1963;9:293–298.

11. Nath R, Anderson L, Jones D, et al. *Specification of Brachytherapy Source Strength: Report of AAPM Task Group No. 32.* New York, NY: American Institute of Physics; 1987.

12. Nath R, Anderson L, Meli J, et al. Code of practice for brachytherapy physics: report of the AAPM Radiation Therapy Committee Task Group No. 56. *Med Phys.* 1997;24(10):1557–1598.

13. Kubo HD, Glasgow GP, Pethel TD, et al. High-dose rate brachytherapy treatment delivery: report of the AAPM Radiation Therapy Committee Task Group No. 59. *Med Phys.* 1998;25(4):375.

14. American College of Radiology. www.acr.org.

15. Erickson BA, Demanes DJ, Ibbott GS, et al. American Society for Radiation Oncology (ASTRO) and American College of Radiology (ACR) practice guideline for the performance of high-dose rate brachytherapy. *Int J Radiat Oncol Biol Phys.* 2011;79(3):641.

16. Thomadsen BR, Erickson BA, Eifel PJ, et al. A review of safety, quality management, and practice guidelines for high-dose-rate brachytherapy: executive summary. *Pract Radiat Oncol.* 2014;4(2):65.

17. Venselaar JLM, Perez-Calatayud J, eds. *A Practical Guide to Quality Control of Brachytherapy Equipment.* 1st ed. Brussels, Belgium: ESTRO; 2004.

18. DeWerd L, Jursinic P, Kitchen R, et al. Quality assurance tool for high-dose rate brachytherapy. *Med Phys.* 1995;22:435–440.

19. U.S. Nuclear Regulatory Commission. *The U.S. Nuclear Regulatory Commission's Advisory Committee on Medical Uses of Isotopes Reviews Medical Events Involving Radioactive Materials Annually at Its Fall Meeting.* Washington, DC: U.S. Nuclear Regulatory Commission. www.nrc.gov/reading-rm/doc-collections/acmui.

20. Nath R, Bice W, Butler W, et al. AAPM recommendations on dose prescription and reporting methods for permanent interstitial brachytherapy for prostate cancer: report of Task Group 137. *Med Phys.* 2009;36(11):5310–5322.

21. Lin P-JP, Beck TJ, Borras C, et al. *Specification and Acceptance Testing of Computed Tomography Scanners: Report of Task Group 2 Diagnostic X-Ray Imaging Committee.* College Park, MD: American Institute of Physics; 1993. AAPM Report 39.

22. Judy PF, Balter S, Bassano D, et al. *Phantoms for Performance Evaluation and Quality Assurance of CT Scanners: Report 1 or the Diagnostic Radiology Committee Task Force on CT Scanner Phantoms.* Chicago, IL: American Association of Physicists in Medicine; 1977.

23. Mutic S, Palta J, Butker E, et al. Quality assurance for computed-tomography simulators and the computed-tomography-simulation process: report of the AAPM Radiation Therapy Committee Task Group No. 66. *Med Phys.* 2003;30(10):2762–2792.

24. Bissonnette J-P, Balter P, Dong L, et al. Quality assurance for image-guided radiation therapy utilizing CT-based technologies: a report of the AAPM TG-179. *Med Phys.* 2012;39(4):1946–1963.

25. Price R, Axel L, Morgan T, et al. Quality assurance methods and phantoms for magnetic resonance imaging: report of AAPM Nuclear Magnetic Resonance Task Group No. 1. *Med Phys.* 1990;17(2):287–295.

26. Och J, Clark G, Sobol W, et al. Acceptance testing of magnetic resonance imaging systems: report of Task Group No. 6, AAPM Nuclear Magnetic Resonance Committee. *Med Phys.* 1992;19(1):217–229.

27. Goodsitt M, Carson P, Witt S, et al. Real-time B-mode ultrasound quality control test procedures: report of AAPM Ultrasound Task Group No. 1. *Med Phys.* 1998;25(8):1385–1406.

28. Lin P-JP, Rauch P, Balter S, et al. *Functionality and Operation of Fluoroscopic Automatic Brightness Control/Automatic Dose Rate Control Logic in Modern Cardiovascular and Interventional Angiography Systems: A Report of AAPM Task Group 125, Radiography/Fluoroscopy Subcommittee.* College Park, MD: American Association of Physicists in Medicine; 2012.

29. Hellebust T, Kirisits C, Berger D, et al. Recommendations from Gynaecological (GYN) GEC-ESTRO Working Group: considerations and pitfalls in commissioning and applicator reconstruction in 3D image-based treatment planning of cervix cancer brachytherapy. *Radiother Oncol.* 2010;96(2):153–160.

30. Pfeiffer D, Sutlief S, Feng W, et al. AAPM Task Group 128: quality assurance tests for prostate brachytherapy ultrasound systems. *Med Phys.* 2008;35(12):5471–5489.

31. U.S. Nuclear Regulatory Commission. *NRC Information Notice 2013–16: Importance of Verification of Treatment Parameters for High Dose-Rate Remote Afterloader Administrations.* Washington, DC: U.S. Nuclear Regulatory Commission; 2013.

32. Lafata KJ, Bushe H, Aronowitz JN. A simple technique for the generation of institution-specific nomograms for permanent prostate cancer brachytherapy. *J Contemp Brachytherapy.* 2014;6(3):293–296. doi:10.5114/jcb.2014.45582.

33. Pujades MC, Camacho C, Perez-Calatayud J, et al. The use of nomograms in LDR-HDR prostate brachytherapy. *J Contemp Brachytherapy.* 2011;3(3):121–124. doi:10.5114/jcb.2011.24817.

34. Aronowitz JN, Michalski JM, Merrick GS, et al. Optimal equations for describing the relationship between prostate volume, number of sources, and total activity in permanent prostate brachytherapy. *Am J Clin Oncol.* 2010;33(2):164–167. doi:10.1097/COC.0b013e31819d3684.

35. Pierquin B, Marinello G. *A Practical Manual of Brachytherapy.* Wilson F, Erickson B, Cunningham J, trans-ed. Madison, WI: Medical Physics; 1997.

36. Neblett D, Syed AMN, Puthawala AA, et al. An interstitial implant technique evaluated by contiguous volume analysis. *Endocurietherapy/Hyperthem Oncol.* 1985;1:213–221.

37. Thomadsen BR, Shahabi S, Buchler DA. Differential loadings of brachytherapy templates. *Endocurietherapy/Hyperthermia Oncol.* 1990;6:197–202.

38. Thomadsen BR. *Achieving Quality in Brachytherapy.* London, UK: Taylor & Francis; 2000.

39. Wu A, Ulin K, Sternick ES. A dose homogeneity index for evaluating ^{192}Ir interstitial breast implants. *Med Phys.* 1988;15(1):104–107.

40. Das RK, Patel R. Breast interstitial implant and treatment planning. In: Thomadsen B, Rivar M, Buttler W, eds. *Brachytherapy Physics.* 2nd ed. Madison, WI: Medical Physics; 2005.

41. van't Riet A, Mak AC, Moerland MA, et al. A conformation number to quantify the degree of conformality in brachytherapy and external beam irradiation: application to the prostate. *Int J Radiat Oncol Biol Phys.* 1997;37(3):731–736.

42. Baltas D, Kolotas C, Geramani K, et al. A conformal index (COIN) to evaluate implant quality and dose specification in brachytherapy. *Int J Radiat Oncol Biol Phys.* 1998;40(2):515–524.

43. Das RK, Bradley KA, Nelson IA, et al. Quality assurance of treatment plans for interstitial and intracavitary high-dose rate brachytherapy. *Brachytherapy.* 2006;5(1):56–60.

44. Papagiannis P, Angelopoulos A, Pantelis E, et al. Dosimetry comparison of ^{192}Ir sources. *Med Phys.* 2002;29(10):2239–2246.

45. Perez-Calatayud J, Facundo B, Rupak K, et al. Dose calculation for photon-emitting brachytherapy sources with average energy higher than 50 keV: full report of the AAPM and ESTRO HEBD working group. *Med Phys.* 2012;39(5):2904–2929.

46. Rivard MJ, Davis SD, DeWerd LA, et al. Calculated and measured brachytherapy dosimetry parameters in water for the Xoft Axxent x-ray source: an electronic brachytherapy source. *Med Phys.* 2006;33(11):4020–4032.

11 Quality Considerations in Proton and Particle Therapy

Brian Winey, Benjamin Clasie, and Yuting Lin

INTRODUCTION

Quality management programs in proton and particle therapy share the same goal with photon therapy: to deliver a prescribed radiation dose to the prescribed target while sparing normal tissue as accurately, precisely, and efficiently as possible. Both particle and photon therapies use a similar framework for quality management, consisting of activities such as commissioning, routine and patient-specific quality assurance (QA), process design, and human resources. Differences in processes, tools, and techniques arise, however, owing to the unique properties of the Bragg peak. A more subtle issue, but one that is equally important for accurate calibration of particle beams, is the impact of linear energy transfer (LET) on the measurement device. In this chapter, we describe the differences in QA considerations in particle therapy, owing to the Bragg peak and the impact of LET on the measurement device, compared with photon therapy.

COMMISSIONING

Commissioning in proton and particle therapy systems has similar goals and procedures as photon therapy (see Chapter 7). These include tuning machine parameters, measuring the machine performance, tuning treatment planning system parameters, and checking the accuracy of the beam models.

Commissioning of a proton or particle machine includes calibrations and/or characterization of dose, depth-dose, off-axis profiles, field size, source-to-axis distance, mechanical isocenter, imaging system, alignment of radiation field with the imaging system, and delivery of test plans (1–3).

Primary differences with photon therapies during machine commissioning are the Bragg peak and the commissioning of variables that affect the particle beam depth, which must be tuned during commissioning (1,3–6).

Because the depth of a Bragg peak in a water phantom or patient is energy dependent, proton and particle therapy accelerators and the nozzle produce beam energies that are customized for each patient, usually with energies between 0 and 250 MeV, with increments as small as 1 MeV. For systems that change energies before or within the beam line (i.e., excluding systems that change energies within the nozzle), the beam line is tuned to transport each beam momentum that will be used. To properly deliver the correct beam energy to patients, a machine commissioning data set should account for the multiple variables in the accelerator, beam line, and/or nozzle that affect the beam energy in a patient.

Lateral profile measurements for particle beams are typically performed with ion chambers or ion chamber arrays (7,8). Other studies have analyzed film, scintillation screens, and diodes for lateral profiles (9–12). Lateral profiles have less LET variability, which allows for solid-state devices to be employed more reliably. Depth doses are more challenging because of the variability of LET with depth, which can result in quenching with solid-state detectors, and the sharp distal penumbra of the Bragg peak. Parallel-plate ion chambers of varying diameters are typically used for depth-ionization curves. Small corrections can be applied to obtain depth-dose distributions. Some treatment planning systems (TPSs) require central axis depth doses for small fields and single pencil beams. Measurements of such beams are subject to volume averaging. In these scenarios, small-diameter Markus chambers are utilized. When an integrated depth dose is desired (i.e., dose integrated in the plane perpendicular to the beam), larger plane parallel chambers can be utilized. For a central axis depth dose for a broad field, a small-diameter chamber can be utilized. Multilayer ion chambers (MLICs) with small, large, or adjustable diameter-sensitive volumes can also be utilized. There are reports of solid-state detectors being used for depth doses with appropriate corrections for quenching (13–15).

Methods for absolute calibrations of particle beams are detailed in IAEA TRS 398 and ICRU 78 (16,17). Absolute dose calibrations in these protocols use a water phantom with uniform dose delivered that is wide enough for lateral dose equilibrium, including the halo dose, which has a large lateral range that can exceed 5 cm depending upon the energy of the beam (18,19). Many centers select a range and modulation combination representative of an average clinical treatment, with a field size large enough to guarantee dose equilibrium at the ionization chamber. Typical correction factors are applied, and proton centers calibrate against a cobalt-60 source with a kQ, Q0 correction derived from Monte Carlo as a function of the residual range at the point of measurement. kQ, Q0 corrects for the response of the ionization chamber to equal dose delivered by radiation of quality Q to the reference radiation of quality Q0. It can be measured using a calorimeter or calculated by Bragg–Gray theory. As with photon therapy centers, the Imaging and Radiation Oncology Core (IROC) can provide an absolute calibration verification check by means of mail-order optically stimulated luminescent dosimeter (OSLD).

All proton and particle therapy facilities perform dose calculations with 3D CT data. Unlike photon therapy, which can directly use the attenuation coefficient (Hounsfield units) information from the CT data, particle therapy must use the particle stopping power of the materials for energy degradation and dose deposition. To convert Hounsfield units into particle stopping power, each CT device used for patient imaging and dose calculations must be commissioned, typically utilizing an electron density phantom with inserts representing materials with well-defined stopping powers. Another common method employs a stoichiometric calculation to determine the stopping power from the tissue compositions (20–23). The CT density to stopping power calculation can introduce the largest systematic error in particle therapy range calculations (24).

Commissioning passive scattering systems

Passively scattered particle fields employ one or two scattering devices to spread a beam with several mm radius to a beam with radius >12 cm. The scatterers are shaped and constructed of varying Z materials to produce as flat a beam as possible (25). Because there is a dependency of scattering power on energy, passively scattered systems have multiple sets of scattering devices for different ranges of beam energies.

Passive scattering systems are dependent upon the position of the particle beam when entering the scattering system. All clinical particle systems employ beam monitoring systems to ensure that the particle beam is positioned correctly upon the scattering system in real time. When commissioning a passively double scattered system, the output of the system is dependent upon each range and modulation combination, owing to the change in scattering

cross section, energy absorption, and beam modulator thickness. There is currently no analytical method to model the output of a passively scattered particle beam, which necessitates large amounts of commissioning data for various range and modulation combinations. There are empirical models that are fit to the commissioning data (26) for each scatterer combination as a function of range and modulation. Alternatively, some particle therapy facilities calibrate each passively scattered field individually.

Commissioning scanning systems

A scanning delivery system employs scanning magnets instead of scatterers to broaden the treatment region of the particle beam. Thus, the system can be considered simpler for commissioning measurements owing to the reduction of devices intercepting the beam and the use of universal properties of protons to model the pencil beam delivery. Proton accelerators mounted outside of a rotating gantry system may require gantry-dependent tunes of the beam line to keep the pencil beam positioned correctly with a small and circular profile at isocenter. Scanning system commissioning must include measurements of the spot profiles as a function of energy and gantry angle, but many treatment planning systems do not allow the additional variable of gantry angle dependency of the spot profile.

A scanning system must be capable of precisely, accurately, and reproducibly delivering pencil beams with a specific ellipticity, size, energy, position, and dose. Commissioning measurements must include validation of these beam properties, the performance during nonnominal events, and verification that the machine log files can accurately reconstruct the dose delivered.

A typical issue encountered with many of the more recent scanning systems is the high instantaneous dose rate of the scanning delivery system. Ionization chambers can suffer from recombination effects when measuring particle therapy beams with high instantaneous dose rates. There are multiple studies that have determined which detectors and biases can be reliably employed for particle therapy systems with particularly high dose rates (8,27).

Dose algorithms

After the collection and entry of commissioning data into the treatment planning system, there are multiple proposed methods to commission a dose algorithm (3,5,6,28–32). Traditionally, analytic dose engines based upon a pencil beam algorithm were employed (33). For homogeneous phantoms, the pencil beam algorithms are reliable with some corrections for nuclear interactions (33). The limitations of the pencil beam algorithm are most pronounced in heterogeneous materials and regions in the patient. To more accurately model the dose in heterogeneous regions and capture the nuclear interactions, Monte Carlo dose engines are becoming more popular. More recently, it has been proposed to use calculated monoenergetic peaks as the basis of the dose algorithm and fit these fundamental peaks to commissioning data (30,34).

Regardless of the dose algorithm, the commissioning of the treatment planning system always employs the delivery of test plans to a phantom. Additionally, many centers check TPS dose calculations against Monte Carlo.

Small fields and pencil beams

For particle therapy depth dose measurements, an important distinction is required between integrated (IDD) and percent depth dose (PDD). For small passive scattered fields or a single particle pencil beams, a large area parallel detector will measure an IDD, integrated over the lateral dose profile. Some treatment planning systems require an IDD, whereas other systems require a central axis PDD. The distinction is most pronounced when the lateral scatter contribution increases with small fields and at larger depths. In these cases, the Bragg peak can disappear because it is spread laterally with depth in the phantom (35–37). If the IDD device is large enough to capture the entire lateral penumbra, the measurement will still display the Bragg peak even though the dose along the central axis no longer displays the common Bragg peak characteristics (Figure 11.1). Heavier ions such as carbon are less affected by scatter interactions, and the Bragg peak remains observable for small fields.

ROUTINE QUALITY ASSURANCE

Daily, monthly, and annual QA is very similar to that for photon therapy, consisting of constancy checks, isocentricity, beam flatness and symmetry, and absolute dosimetry. Passively scattered system QA is more similar to that for photons because of the reduced complexity of the delivered dose profiles, and the capability of delivering large, uniform fields without scanning. Because scanning systems can deliver more complicated dose patterns, regular QA must be capable of measuring the spot profiles and positions. Vendors and institutions have designed scanning patterns that allow for efficient delivery of one or few energy layers capable of testing the spot position, size, and energy utilizing planar detector arrays (Figure 11.2). Routine checks in scanning also ensure that the real-time nozzle feedback signals are operating normally and interlocks are enabled.

The largest difference with photon therapy is the routine measurement of the particle beam energy and Bragg peak or peaks. The measurements can be accomplished with parallel plate ionization chambers or Markus chambers scanned through a water phantom or an MLIC. MLIC devices can acquire an entire Bragg peak without the need to scan a point chamber or integrate charge collected over multiple Bragg peaks. The calibration of the output and the layer spacing of the MLIC require tandem measurements with an ionization chamber measurement.

PATIENT-SPECIFIC QUALITY ASSURANCE

Patient-specific QA requires large time and personnel commitments in proton therapy centers. Many centers have opened only recently. In these newer centers, the experience with the treatment delivery tools and the number of patients treated is relatively limited and not sufficient to provide confidence in procedures and beam delivery systems. More thorough and frequent measurements are therefore required. Even in centers with longer experience

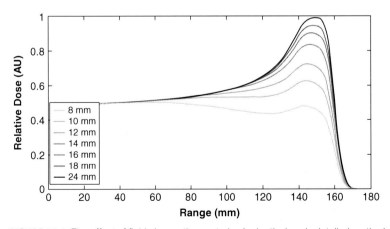
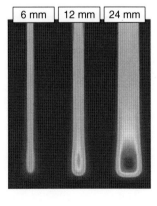

FIGURE 11.1 The effect of field size on the central axis depth dose is detailed on the left, with a planar view of the dose distribution on the right. All fields have the same range and modulation. As the field size decreases, the multiple coulomb scatter affects the central axis dose distribution, even reducing the pronounced Bragg peak commonly observed in proton and particle therapy. The reduction of the Bragg peak due to scatter is less significant in heavier ions that have fewer scatter interactions.

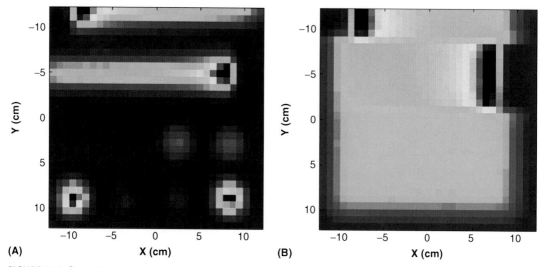

FIGURE 11.2 Scanning patterns are tailored to the specific arrangement of detectors and phantom material, as shown in (A) and (B). (A) shows line scans and spots that check the beam position, width, and individual dose per pencil beam. (B) shows a 2-dimensional scanning pattern that is sensitive to the depth-dose distribution in the top half of the image and the dose uniformity in the lower half of the image.

and large numbers of patients treated, there are often new developments, including the introduction of scanning systems, newer treatment planning systems, newer beam control systems, and the general rapid development of clinical particle therapy.

Patient-specific quality assurance for passive scattering systems

Passive scattering has been deployed for decades in some institutions, and the resulting experience with patient-specific QA has resulted in two common measurement techniques. Many centers routinely measure the output of patient

treatment fields with a single ionization chamber at one or a few depths, relying upon the other routine dosimetry tests to verify the field uniformity, flatness, and symmetry. It has also been proposed to develop an empirical output model based on commissioning measurements of treatment fields representing the array of range, modulation, and field sizes to be used in the clinic (26).

The patient-specific hardware that provides lateral (apertures) and distal (range compensators) (Figure 11.3) shaping of the beam is measured against the planning system requested hardware. The verification of the hardware can be performed with automated measuring devices such as laser scanning systems, or manually with calipers or calibrated tools.

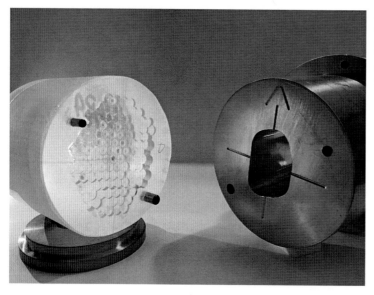

FIGURE 11.3 A range compensator on the left uses plastic to conform the proton fields to the distal edge of the target, and the aperture on the right conforms the proton fields to the lateral edges of the target.

Patient-specific quality assurance for scanning systems

There are various implementations of scanned beam particle therapy, from uniform scanning to intensity-modulated proton therapy (IMPT), which does not limit dose heterogeneity per field. For all varieties of scanned beam delivery, the beam delivery is dynamic, with active feedback in the nozzle to verify the spot position, size, and dose. Each spot is modeled in a treatment planning system and specified through the treatment plan, which is transferred to the treatment delivery system and subject to translations into machine parameters. The treatment delivery system requires the translation of spot energy, position, and dose into magnet parameters, energy at the exit of the accelerator or energy selection system, and scanning magnet current and timing settings. Hence, a patient-specific QA procedure involves verifying that the treatment planning system has properly modeled the absolute dose and dose distribution during treatment delivery, specifically the combination of spot energies, positions, doses, and gantry angles. QA measurements include verifying that the treatment delivery system has correctly translated the planned spot properties into a delivered dose distribution.

Intensity-modulated radiation therapy (IMRT) can only alter the two-dimensional fluence of the photon treatment beam, but proton beam scanning can alter the three-dimensional fluence of individual treatment beams. An ideal patient dosimetry check would allow for accurate and rapid three-dimensional dose measurements for each of the treatment beams. The best current technology allows

multiple two-dimensional planar measurements. All institutions currently utilizing scanning delivery perform multiple 2D measurements. Typically, this is accomplished with planar array detectors positioned at multiple depths, to assess as closely as possible the three-dimensional dose distribution. The need for multiple experimental set-ups greatly increases the time required for scanning patient-specific QA (Figure 11.4).

Quality assurance with Monte Carlo

Given the large amount of work detailed in the earlier two sections regarding the QA of patient-specific treatment fields, current clinical implementations that have been described fail to verify the delivery in the actual patient. Monte Carlo calculations are employed by some institutions to validate the treatment planning system dose calculation utilizing the patient CT information (38–41). Recently, some centers have begun to incorporate the machine log files into the secondary dose calculation, similar to IMRT QA techniques (42–49), in an attempt to reproduce more directly what has been delivered by the machine in the patient.

PROCESS DESIGN

One key to improving quality in a radiation therapy facility is reducing variation in processes between facilities and within a facility (50). Photon technology has become more uniform with the consolidation of modern treatment delivery devices, treatment delivery modalities, and image guidance, enabling the application of a consistent treatment

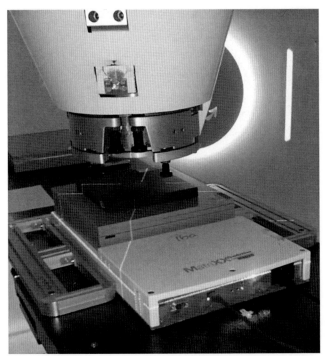

FIGURE 11.4 Measurement of the absolute dose and dose distribution with a planar array of ionization chambers in the MatriXX detector (IBA-Dosimetry GmbH). Phantom material is arranged on the detector to simulate energy loss within the patient.

process to most patients. In particle therapy, there are a wide variety of technical and process parameters that can result in wider variations. These include Hounsfield unit (HU) to stopping power conversion, artifact correction, commissioning techniques, manual imaging and registration techniques, patient-specific apertures and range compensators, different snouts, different measurement techniques and tools, and QA protocol variation. The variable processes employed at each proton or particle therapy facility complicate the comparison of quality data, credentialing for clinical trials, and generation of protocol consensus for clinical trials and QA. With the swell of new proton therapy centers opening and the consolidation of technology toward image-guided, scanning proton therapy, there will be more consensus and international protocol development to reduce the current procedural variations.

HUMAN RESOURCES

Particle therapy does not share the large community of mostly similar technologies, as in photon therapy. The American Association of Physicists in Medicine (AAPM) is currently working on several proton-specific QA protocols; for example, TG-185 on the commissioning of proton therapy systems and TG-224 on proton therapy machine QA. However, currently published QA reports in the AAPM Task Group library are all related to imaging, brachytherapy, and photon or electron therapy. It is left to individual facilities to adapt these photon procedures to each particular particle therapy machine. Furthermore, implementing change is a time-consuming process, and changes usually cannot be transferred easily between facilities. Creating and implementing a quality framework in this environment becomes a large departmental effort and, consequently, more resources must be devoted to quality in a particle therapy facility. The recommended staffing level of a particle facility should be expanded to accommodate an appropriate quality management program. Such a program should include an expert responsible for safety within the facility, careful oversight by a QA committee, and medical physicists to design and maintain specialized QA procedures.

FUTURE DEVELOPMENTS

The future of proton and particle therapy QA is actively progressing in two primary directions: consensus protocols and patient-specific QA.

The AAPM is currently developing multiple proton-specific QA documents. The formation of general consensus documents should ease the development of new proton therapy centers and increase the safety of patient treatments. There is a consolidation of some treatment delivery techniques and increasing understanding of credentialing specifications, which will produce more robust clinical outcome data for the benchmarking of proton therapy. The addition of modern three-dimensional image guidance in proton therapy centers will also increase the reliability of the clinical outcome data and further allow for the utilization of Bragg peak data in patient treatments.

There remains a large need for more efficient yet robust patient-specific QA when treating with scanning beams. Multiple vendors and research groups are actively working toward a more efficient and three-dimensional QA method.

Even with all of this work regarding patient-specific QA, there remains no clinical option for in vivo dosimetry, as is available for photon therapy. Portal dosimetry is not an option because protons have no exit dose to measure and the fluence is optimized in three dimensions. At present, uncertainties of proton and particle therapy delivery, such as range uncertainty (24,38,51), are typically incorporated into treatment planning with the use of margins or robust treatment planning optimization. Many range uncertainties, specifically due to motion, deformation, patient set-up, and tissue heterogeneities, could be reduced or eliminated with accurate and precise in vivo QA, with the goal of increasing the therapeutic ratio of particle therapy. Multiple studies have presented methods to assess the three-dimensional dose, including PET, MR, prompt gamma, and diodes (52–71). In their current forms, none of these technologies is unable to precisely (<1 mm) determine the dose distribution in the patient. The technology may develop into precise and clinically useful tools in the future and allow for more accurate assessment of the location of Bragg peaks in the patient, reducing the uncertainties prevalent in current proton therapy.

REFERENCES

1. Engelsman M, Lu HM, Herrup D, et al. Commissioning a passive-scattering proton therapy nozzle for accurate SOBP delivery. *Med Phys.* 2009;36:2172–2180.

2. Paganetti H. *Proton Therapy Physics.* Boca Raton, FL: CRC Press; 2011.

3. Gillin MT, Sahoo N, Bues N, et al. Commissioning of the discrete spot scanning proton beam delivery system at the University of Texas M. D. Anderson Cancer Center, Proton Therapy Center, Houston. *Med Phys.* 2010;37:154–163.

4. Koch N, Newhauser W. Virtual commissioning of a treatment planning system for proton therapy of ocular cancers. *Radiat Prot Dosimetry.* 2005;115:159–163.

5. Meier G, Besson R, Nanz A, et al. Independent dose calculations for commissioning, quality assurance and dose reconstruction of PBS proton therapy. *Phys Med Biol.* 2015;60(7):2819–2836.

6. Paganetti H, Jiang H, Lee SY, et al. Accurate Monte Carlo simulations for nozzle design, commissioning and quality assurance for a

proton radiation therapy facility. *Med Phys.* 2004;31:2107–2118.

7. Arjomandy B, Sahoo N, Ding X, et al. Use of a two-dimensional ionization chamber array for proton therapy beam quality assurance. *Med Phys.* 2008;35:3889–3894.

8. Lin L, Kang M, Solberg TD, et al. Use of a novel two-dimensional ionization chamber array for pencil beam scanning proton therapy beam quality assurance. *J Appl Clin Med Phys.* 2015;16:5323.

9. Piermattei A, Miceli R, Azario L, et al. Radiochromic film dosimetry of a low energy proton beam. *Med Phys.* 2000;27(7):1655–1660.

10. Vatnitsky SM. Radiochromic film dosimetry for clinical proton beams. *Appl Radiat Isot.* 1997;48:643–651.

11. Vatnitsky SM, Schulte RW, Galindo R, et al. Radiochromic film dosimetry for verification of dose distributions delivered with proton-beam radiosurgery. *Phys Med Biol.* 1997;42:1887–1898.

12. Zhao L, Newton J, Oldham M, et al. Feasibility of using PRESAGE® for relative 3D dosimetry of small proton fields. *Phys Med Biol.* 2012;57:N431–N443.

13. Fidanzio A, Azario L, De Angelis, et al. A correction method for diamond detector signal dependence with proton energy. *Med Phys.* 2002;29:669–675.

14. Goma C, Andreo P, Sempau J. Spencer-Attix water/medium stopping-power ratios for the dosimetry of proton pencil beams. *Phys Med Biol.* 2013;58:2509–2522.

15. Koehler AM. Dosimetry of proton beams using small silicon diodes. *Radiat Res Suppl.* 1967;7:53–63.

16. International Atomic Energy Agency. *Technical Reports Series No. 398: Absorbed Dose Determination in External Beam Radiotherapy: An International Code of Practice for Dosimetry Based on Standards of Absorbed Dose to Water.* Vienna, Austria: International Atomic Energy Agency; 2001.

17. *Prescribing, Recording and Reporting Proton-Beam Therapy.* Oxford, UK: Oxford University Press; 2007.

18. Gottschalk B, Cascio EW, Daartz J, et al. On the nuclear halo of a proton pencil beam stopping in water. *Phys Med Biol.* 2015 Jul 21;60(14):5627-5654. doi: 10.1088/0031-9155/60/14/5627. Epub 2015 Jul 6.

19. Lin L, Huang S, Kang M, et al. Technical note: validation of halo modeling for proton pencil beam spot scanning using a quality assurance test pattern. *Med Phys.* 2015;42:5138.

20. Oden J, Zimmerman J, Bujila R, et al. Technical note: on the calculation of stopping-power ratio for stoichiometric calibration in proton therapy. *Med Phys.* 2015;42(9):5252–5257.

21. Schneider U, Pedroni E, Lomax A. The calibration of CT Hounsfield units for radiotherapy treatment planning. *Phys Med Biol.* 1996;41:111–124.

22. Schneider U, Pemler P, Besserer J, et al. Patient specific optimization of the relation between CT-Hounsfield units and proton stopping power with proton radiography. *Med Phys.* 2005;32(1):195–199.

23. Yang M, Zhu XR, Park PC, et al. Comprehensive analysis of proton range uncertainties related to patient stopping-power-ratio estimation using the stoichiometric calibration. *Phys Med Biol.* 2012;57(13):4095–4115.

24. Paganetti H. Range uncertainties in proton therapy and the role of Monte Carlo simulations. *Phys Med Biol.* 2012;57:R99–R117.

25. Gottschalk B. On the scattering power of radiotherapy protons. *Med Phys.* 2010;37:352–367.

26. Kooy HM, Schaefer M, Rosenthal S, et al. Monitor unit calculations for range-modulated spread-out Bragg peak fields. *Phys Med Biol.* 2003;48:2797–2808.

27. Lorin S, Grusell E, Tilly N, et al. Reference dosimetry in a scanned pulsed proton beam using ionisation chambers and a Faraday cup. *Phys Med Biol.* 2008;53:3519–3529.

28. Li Y, Zhu RX, Sahoo N, et al. Beyond Gaussians: a study of single-spot modeling for scanning proton dose calculation. *Phys Med Biol.* 2012;57(4):983–997.

29. Seco J, Clasie B, Partridge M. Review on the characteristics of radiation detectors for dosimetry and imaging. *Phys Med Biol.* 2014;59:R303–R347.

30. Slopsema RL, et al. Development of a golden beam data set for the commissioning of a proton double-scattering system in a pencil-beam dose calculation algorithm. *Med Phys.* 2014;41(9):091710.

31. Zheng Y, Ramirez E, Mascia A, et al. Commissioning of output factors for uniform scanning proton beams. *Med Phys.* 2011;38:2299–2306.

32. Zhu XR, Poenisch F, Lii F, et al. Commissioning dose computation models for spot scanning proton beams in water for a commercially available treatment planning system. *Med Phys.* 2013;40:041723.

33. Hong L, Goitein M, Bucciolini M, et al. A pencil beam algorithm for proton dose calculations. *Phys Med Biol.* 1996;41(8):1305–1330.

34. Clasie B, Depauw N, Fransen M, et al. Golden beam data for proton pencil-beam scanning. *Phys Med Biol.* 2012;57:1147–1158.

35. Das IJ, Paganetti H. *Principles and Practice of Proton Beam Therapy*. Madison, WI: Medical Physics; 2015.

36. Daartz J, Engelsman M, Paganetti H, et al. Field size dependence of the output factor in passively scattered proton therapy: influence of range, modulation, air gap, and machine settings. *Med Phys.* 2009;36:3205–3210.

37. Fontenot JD, Newhauser WD, Bloch C, et al. Determination of output factors for small proton therapy fields. *Med Phys.* 2007;34:489–498.

38. Schuemann J, Dowdell S, Grassberger C, et al. Site-specific range uncertainties caused by dose calculation algorithms for proton therapy. *Phys Med Biol.* 2014;59:4007–4031.

39. Paganetti H. Monte Carlo simulations will change the way we treat patients with proton beams today. *Br J Radiol.* 2014;87:20140293.

40. Grassberger C, Daartz J, Dowdell S, et al. Quantification of proton dose calculation accuracy in the lung. *Int J Radiat Oncol Biol Phys.* 2014;89:424–430.

41. Testa M, Schumann J, Lu HM, et al. Experimental validation of the TOPAS Monte Carlo system for passive scattering proton therapy. *Med Phys.* 2013;40(12):121719.

42. Agnew CE, King RB, Hounsell AR, et al. Implementation of phantom-less IMRT delivery verification using Varian DynaLog files and R/V output. *Phys Med Biol.* 2012;57:6761–6777.

43. Burman C, Chui CS, Kutcher G, et al. Planning, delivery, and quality assurance of intensity-modulated radiotherapy using dynamic multileaf collimator: a strategy for large-scale implementation for the treatment of carcinoma of the prostate. *Int J Radiat Oncol Biol Phys.* 1997;39:863–873.

44. Calvo-Ortega JF, Teke T, Moragues S, et al. A Varian DynaLog file-based procedure for patient dose-volume histogram-based IMRT QA. *J Appl Clin Med Phys.* 2014;15:4665.

45. Eckhause T, Al-Hallaq H, Ritter T, et al. Automating linear accelerator quality assurance. *Med Phys.* 2015;42:6074.

46. Fan J, Li J, Chen L, et al. A practical Monte Carlo MU verification tool for IMRT quality assurance. *Phys Med Biol.* 2006;51:2503–2515.

47. Litzenberg DW, Moran JM, Fraass BA. Verification of dynamic and segmental IMRT delivery by dynamic log file analysis. *J Appl Clin Med Phys.* 2002;3:63–72.

48. Rangaraj D, Zhu M, Yang D, et al. Catching errors with patient-specific pretreatment machine log file analysis. *Pract Radiat Oncol.* 2013;3:80–90.

49. Stell AM, Li JG, Zeidan OA, et al. An extensive log-file analysis of step-and-shoot intensity modulated radiation therapy segment delivery errors. *Med Phys.* 2004;31:1593–1602.

50. Pawlicki T, Mundt AJ. Quality in radiation oncology. *Med Phys.* 2007;34:1529–1534.

51. Liebl J, Paganetti H, Zhu M, et al. The influence of patient positioning uncertainties in proton radiotherapy on proton range and dose distributions. *Med Phys.* 2014;41:091711.

52. Espana S, Paganetti H. The impact of uncertainties in the CT conversion algorithm when predicting proton beam ranges in patients from dose and PET-activity distributions. *Phys Med Biol.* 2010;55:7557–7571.

53. Grogg K, Zhu X, Min CH, et al. Feasibility of using distal endpoints for in-room PET range verification of proton therapy. *IEEE Trans Nucl Sci.* 2013;60:3290–3297.

54. Knopf A, Parodi K, Bortfeld T, et al. Systematic analysis of biological and physical limitations of proton beam range verification with offline PET/CT scans. *Phys Med Biol.* 2009;54:4477–4795.

55. Kraan AC. Range verification methods in particle therapy: underlying physics and Monte Carlo modeling. *Front Oncol.* 2015;5:150.

56. Min CH, Zhu X, Grogg K, et al. A recommendation on how to analyze in-room PET for in vivo proton range verification using a distal PET surface method. *Technol Cancer Res Treat.* 2015;14:320–325.

57. Min CH, Zhu X, Winey BA, et al. Clinical application of in-room positron emission tomography for in vivo treatment monitoring in proton radiation therapy. *Int J Radiat Oncol Biol Phys.* 2013;86:183–189.

58. Parodi K, Bortfeld T, Haberer T. Comparison between in-beam and offline positron emission tomography imaging of proton and carbon ion therapeutic irradiation at synchrotron- and cyclotron-based facilities. *Int J Radiat Oncol Biol Phys.* 2008;71:945–956.

59. Parodi K, Paganetti H, Shih HA, et al. Patient study of in vivo verification of beam delivery and range, using positron emission tomography and computed tomography imaging after proton therapy. *Int J Radiat Oncol Biol Phys.* 2007;68:920–934.

60. Zhu X, El Fakhri G. Proton therapy verification with PET imaging. *Theranostics.* 2013;3:731–740.

61. Zhu X, Espana S, Daartz J, et al. Monitoring proton radiation therapy with in-room PET imaging. *Phys Med Biol.* 2011;56:4041–4057.

62. Verburg JM, Riley K, Bortfeld T, et al. Energy- and time-resolved detection of prompt gamma-rays for proton range verification. *Phys Med Biol.* 2011;58:L37–L49.

63. Verburg JM, Seco J. Proton range verification through prompt gamma-ray spectroscopy. *Phys Med Biol.* 2014;59(23):7089–7106.

64. Verburg JM, Shih HA, Seco J. Simulation of prompt gamma-ray emission during proton radiotherapy. *Phys Med Biol.* 2012;57:5459–5472.

65. Verburg JM, Testa M, Seco J. Range verification of passively scattered proton beams using prompt gamma-ray detection. *Phys Med Biol.* 2015;60:1019–1029.

66. Yuan Y, Andronesi OC, Bortfeld TR, et al. Feasibility study of in vivo MRI based dosimetric verification of proton end-of-range for liver cancer patients. *Radiother Oncol.* 2013;106:378–382.

67. Knopf AC, Parodi K, Paganetti H, et al. Accuracy of proton beam range verification using post-treatment positron emission tomography/computed tomography as function of treatment site. *Int J Radiat Oncol Biol Phys.* 2011;79(1):297–304.

68. Lu HM. On measuring depth-dose distribution of range-modulated proton therapy fields. *Med Phys.* 2006;33:236–238.

69. Lu HM. A point dose method for in vivo range verification in proton therapy. *Phys Med Biol.* 2008;53:N415–N22.

70. Lu HM. A potential method for in vivo range verification in proton therapy treatment. *Phys Med Biol.* 2008;53:1413–1424.

71. Testa M, Min CH, Verburg JM, et al. Range verification of passively scattered proton beams based on prompt gamma time patterns. *Phys Med Biol.* 2014;59:4181–4195.

12 | Quality Assurance and Verification of Treatment

Bernard L. Jones and Moyed Miften

INTRODUCTION

Importance of patient-specific quality assurance

In radiotherapy, the components of the treatment delivery system are periodically tested to ensure adequate function. In this model, each component of the process (such as multileaf collimator, jaws, couch, output calibration, dose calculation, and image-guidance system) is analyzed to ensure that it is functioning within tolerance. These tolerances are set at a level that translates to accurate treatment delivery (1). After the completion of daily, monthly, or annual quality assurance (QA), one is confident that the delivery machine will accurately deliver a reference dose of radiation to a reference object such as a diode array, or ion chamber in solid water.

Clinically, each patient receives a unique prescription, which specifies the tumorcidal dose to the target and the dose limits to the surrounding normal tissue. Because the treatment management of each patient is unique, the process to generate the treatment plan for that prescription is also unique. Assuming the existence of a robust, periodic QA program, the treatment machine is expected to carry out the radiation delivery instructions within specified tolerances. The process of patient-specific QA verifies that these instructions will satisfy the prescription. In other words, patient-specific QA consists of those tests ensuring that, for this unique treatment plan, the proper dose will be delivered as planned, both to the tumor and to organs at risk.

The verification of treatment in a patient-specific manner applies to all modalities of radiation therapy; external beam therapy with photons, electrons, or protons; brachytherapy; and other procedures such as interoperative radiation therapy. This chapter focuses mostly on external beam therapy with photons, although many of the concepts are more generally applicable. In-depth discussions of other modalities can be found in Chapter 10 (brachytherapy) and Chapter 11 (proton therapy).

Sources of uncertainty

In modern radiation therapy, the majority of accidents arise from human factors, such as therapist error, failure to follow policies/procedures, or errors in treatment planning, commissioning, data transfer, and treatment delivery (2–4). Although errors can arise at any step in the process, the most common errors occur during manual human involvement (4), such as connecting the channels in a high-dose rate (HDR) brachytherapy remote afterloader, placing treatment accessories such as bolus or spoiler, or typing treatment objectives/optimization parameters into the treatment planning system. For a further discussion of errors and risk in the process of treatment planning and simulation, see Chapter 9 in this text.

The complexities involved with the delivery of intensity-modulated radiation therapy (IMRT) add additional uncertainties, which in terms of treatment planning include the following: multileaf collimator (MLC) leaf end modeling, MLC tongue-and-groove effect, leaf/collimator transmission, penumbra modeling, compensator systems, output factors, head backscatter, dose calculation grid size, off-axis profiles, and heterogeneity corrections. Accurate IMRT treatment planning system (TPS) beam modeling is essential to reduce the uncertainties associated with the TPS planning process and, consequently, to ensure good agreement between calculations and measurements when performing patient-specific verification QA (5,6). Spatial and dosimetric uncertainties of the delivery systems also have effects on IMRT dose distribution delivery accuracy. These uncertainties include: MLC leaf position errors, MLC leaf speed, gantry rotational stability, table motion stability, and beam stability. In addition, differences and limitations in the design of the MLC and accelerators, including the treatment head design, as well as the age of the accelerator/equipment, can have an impact on the accuracy of IMRT delivery techniques (5,6).

Objectives of patient-specific quality assurance

Broadly, the purpose of patient-specific QA is to ensure both the fidelity and the safety of patient treatment. This is accomplished by avoiding errors (ranging from those of mild severity to catastrophic errors), but also by serving as an opportunity for process improvement. A plan that passes all tests can be used for treatment, but a plan that fails a given test is an opportunity to examine why that failure occurred and how the process can be improved. As such, it can be useful to define the test thresholds (e.g., IMRT QA gamma thresholds) to flag a given percentage of plans for further review.

Broadly, a patient-specific QA program should answer the following:

1. Does the treatment plan match the physician intent?

2. Is the dose calculation correct?

3. Is the patient being treated according to the treatment plan?

In the years following the Therac-25 accidents, clinical accelerators received a radical overhaul with respect to systems and software engineering (7). As the amount of manual involvement radiotherapy has decreased, so too has the risk of many common errors (8). While modern accelerators are not infallible, the many redundant hardware and software interlocks have resulted in a landscape where most errors can be traced to human factors (4). In treatments with little manual involvement of the therapists, dosimetrists, and physicists, a "Systems QA" approach is typically employed. In this paradigm, the function of each piece within the process is tested separately, and the output of that piece is validated. With these treatments (such as 3D, IMRT, or stereotactic body radiation therapy [SBRT]), there is a great deal of complexity up front in the treatment planning and testing phase; in the context of a robust periodic QA system (e.g., according to TG-142 (1)), testing each component separately (such as secondary MU calculation, secondary plan check, and pretreatment IMRT QA) is well suited to catching the majority of errors. However, in treatments with more manual involvement, it is more common to utilize a "Process QA" approach. In modalities such as brachytherapy, total body irradiation (TBI), or total skin electrons (TSE), the planning process is less complex; however, there are a number of human factors involved in delivering the proper treatment. In these situations, patient-specific QA includes verifying that all steps of the treatment have taken place correctly (e.g., checklists), in addition to other checks. There is considerable work within the radiotherapy physics community to develop a more comprehensive "Process" approach that encompasses all aspects of QA, such as the forthcoming report of the American Association of Physicists in Medicine (AAPM) Task Group 100 (9), and in time, Process QA may supplant Systems QA as the dominant paradigm.

Regardless of the approach to patient-specific QA, the process will generally involve the following:

1. A review of the treatment plan, data transfer, and plan parameters by an independent physicist not involved in creation of the plan.

2. Secondary dose calculation or measurement.

3. Pretreatment review.

PHYSICIST PLAN REVIEW

Each treatment plan should be reviewed by a medical physicist before the start of treatment. The physicist should not have been involved in the creation of the plan, in order to bring an independent perspective to the review. Physicist plan review is recommended in a wide array of publications and practice guidelines, such as the AAPM Task Group 40 Report (10), American College of Radiology (ACR) Practice Guidelines (11), and the American Society for Radiation Oncology (ASTRO) safety white papers for stereotactic radiosurgery (SRS), HDR, and IMRT treatment (12–14). The purpose of the review is to ensure that the treatment plan will perform as specified in the physician's prescription, as well as to check for errors in the treatment planning process. In a review of more than 4,000 incidents reported to a multi-institutional incident learning database, physicist plan review was found to be the most effective QA check in clinical practice, as it was capable of detecting more than 60% of the errors reported (15).

TG-40 describes in detail the specific parameters that should be checked during the physicist plan review (10). In general, the review should verify that the prescription is complete, that it is signed by the physician, and that the plan reflects the most current version of the prescription. The review should also verify that the plan agrees with the prescription, including patient name and identification, anatomical site, technique, modality, energy, target dose, and normal tissue dose constraints. The review should also include a "sanity check," which verifies that the plan is consistent with the physicist's prior clinical experience. For instance, are the dose constraints reasonable, does the prescription make sense (e.g., 78,000 cGy vs. 7,800 cGy), are the hot and cold spots reasonable, and are the dose volume histogram (DVH) values consistent with prior plans for this site? The review should also verify the integrity of the data transfer from the TPS to the treatment management system (TMS). This should be performed by checking relevant treatment plan parameters (e.g., for external beam: wedges, compensators, bolus, source-to-surface distance [SSD], gantry angle, collimator rotation, couch position/angle, field size, etc., or for HDR: dwell positions, dwell time, etc.). Finally, the review should include a verification of the initial dose calculation. Physics plan and chart review are the subject of an upcoming AAPM Task Group report, TG-275, due out in 2017.

PLAN DOSE VERIFICATION

Calculation methods

For external beam therapy, the monitor unit (MU)/timer calculation should be verified by a secondary dose calculation (8). This is typically carried out using a point dose calculation to a point in a low-gradient, high-dose region away from significant heterogeneities. For simple treatment scenarios (e.g., rectangular fields), this calculation could be performed manually using physics data tables. For more complex scenarios (e.g., irregular fields), this calculation is often performed using a secondary software calculation. The methodology of the calculation check should be as independent as achievable from the primary calculation. If automated data transfer is used, the validity of derived parameters (such as blocked equivalent squares or radiologic depths) should be examined by the physicist. Action thresholds should be set for the point dose difference between the primary and the secondary calculations based on the confidence in the accuracy of the secondary calculation (8). In practice, this threshold is generally on the order of 5%, but depends on the observed agreement during commissioning between the primary and the secondary dose calculations.

In addition to the secondary dose calculation, it is often useful to perform a "sanity check" of the treatment plan by comparing it with plans from similar past patients. For instance, in permanent-implant low-dose rate (LDR) brachytherapy of the prostate, one can check that the number and activity of seeds is similar to those in previous cases with roughly the same prostate volume.

Measurement methods

Measurements can be used alongside secondary dose calculations for simple treatment scenarios, and are strongly recommended for more complex/high-dose treatments such as IMRT or stereotactic radiosurgery (SRS)/SBRT (11,12). In vivo dosimetry is also a useful tool for verifying dose, especially in procedures such as high dose-per-fraction electron treatments with custom blocking, treatment using bolus, or special procedures such as TBI or TSE. In these cases, the dose in a high-dose/low-gradient region at the surface (beneath bolus, if used) is measured using thermoluminescent dosimeters, optically stimulated luminescent dosimeters, or diodes. The World Health Organization (WHO) identifies in vivo dosimetry as a "high-impact" intervention capable of detecting errors in treatment planning, calculation, and delivery (3).

PATIENT-SPECIFIC INTENSITY-MODULATED RADIATION THERAPY QUALITY ASSURANCE

Measurement methods

The most common and most widely recommended method for IMRT dose verification is to perform measurements of the delivered dose. Patient-specific QA measurements verify not only the accuracy of dose calculation, but also the integrity of data transfer from the TPS to the TMS. Patient-specific measurements are recommended by ACR/ASTRO practice guidelines (11), and the ASTRO safety white papers regarding SRS/SBRT and IMRT note the potential pitfalls of removing the measurement component from the IMRT QA program (12,14).

To calculate the reference dose for the measurements, the fields used for the patient's dose delivery are transferred onto the measurement phantom and recalculated. Measurements are generally performed on 2D devices such as electronic portal imaging devices (EPIDs), detector arrays (either diodes or ion chambers), or a combination of film and ion chamber. For these 2D devices, the most common measurement geometries in clinical practice are (a) true composite (TC), (b) perpendicular field-by-field (PFF), and (c) perpendicular composite (PC) (16). In the TC method, all beams are delivered using the actual MUs, gantry/collimator/couch angles, and jaw/leaf positions from the patient treatment plan. In TC delivery, the measurement includes inaccuracies from all treatment parameters and gravity effects, and the resulting dose distribution is roughly equivalent to the dose that will be delivered in the patient. However, in view of the variety of gantry angles that are generally involved, the angular dependence of the measurement device must be carefully considered. In perpendicular methods, the radiation fluence is always perpendicular to the 2D measuring device. For devices placed on the couch, the gantry angles are set to 0 degree; otherwise, the device must rotate with the gantry (either by mounting the device to the gantry or having the device automatically rotate to compensate). In PFF, a separate measurement is performed for each field, whereas for PC, the dose is integrated across all fields. PFF prevents the averaging of errors in PC analysis, and may thus reveal potential errors in treatment delivery. However, the review of QA results should be thorough because a number of studies have shown that the correlation between IMRT QA metrics and clinical dose differences is a challenging QA process (17–21).

Verification metrics

Comparing two distributions is a nontrivial task: dose difference maps can yield hundreds or thousands of points, and this information must be distilled in a few values in order to judge the acceptability of a plan. The analysis is further complicated by the fact that it must consider both the differences in dose and the spatial uncertainties in dose delivery. Imagine a 10 cm × 10 cm field that delivers a uniform dose of 200 cGy. To check this plan, the field is delivered to film, and this dose distribution is compared with the dose calculated by the TPS. The simplest metric to evaluate this delivery is the dose difference; at each point in the distribution, what is the absolute difference between the calculated and the measured dose? If the linac output was 2% low on the day of measurement, the dose difference within the field would record a difference of 4 cGy, and one would likely judge this plan acceptable. However, imagine a spatial shift in the field of a few millimeters. In this case, misalignment of the steep dose gradients at the edge of the field would result in a very large absolute dose difference. This delivery would likely fail the dose difference test despite the fact that a small spatial shift in dose is likely clinically acceptable. In IMRT, the dose distribution is often extremely inhomogeneous, and thus metrics to evaluate the acceptability of a plan must also include some criteria for spatial differences. This is accomplished through the distance-to-agreement (DTA) test (22), which is calculated by finding the closest point in the evaluated dose distribution with the same dose as the reference point.

The dose difference test is excellent at interpreting differences in regions of shallow dose gradient, while the DTA test performs well in areas of high dose gradient. Harms et al (22) developed the "composite test," whereby a point in the distribution passes if it meets either the dose difference or DTA criteria. Low et al (23,24) developed this concept by generalizing the composite test, introducing a parameter called γ. In this formalism, the dose and distance scales are renormalized by dividing them by the dose and DTA criteria, respectively. In this renormalized space, γ is calculated for each point in the dose distribution as the minimum distance to the reference distribution. Because the dose and distance axes are renormalized relative to the dose and DTA criteria, a value of γ between 0 and 1 indicates an overall difference that is less than those criteria (pass), whereas values greater than 1 indicate failure.

There are several important practical considerations when applying γ for clinical use. The choice of the normalization point affects the scale of the dose difference results, which in turn affects the sensitivity of the test to detect relevant errors at different dose levels. For instance, if the results are globally normalized to a point in the high-dose region, the tolerance in critical structures may be less stringent; however, applying a local normalization at each point may make the dose accuracy requirements in lower-dose areas unrealistic, when the contributions of leakage and scatter are more pronounced. The spatial resolution of dose measurement also has an impact on γ results, because the error in γ depends on the local dose gradient, the spatial resolution, and the magnitude of the DTA criterion. Finally, when interpreting γ results, one should not ignore the spatial distribution of failing points, but should consider the clinical impact of the dose errors detected by the test.

Recommendations for intensity-modulated radiation therapy quality assurance measurements

The forthcoming report of AAPM Task Group 218 makes the following general recommendations regarding IMRT QA measurements:

TC delivery should be used if the angular dependence of the IMRT QA device is not a factor (e.g., if the effect is negligible or if the effect is accounted for). Otherwise, measurements should be performed using PFF delivery. Analysis should be performed in absolute dose mode (rather than relative dose) using global normalization. The normalization point should be in a high-dose, low-gradient region of the dose distribution, and the dose threshold should be selected to exclude low-dose areas with little clinical relevance.

Tolerance and action limits should be set in each clinic on the basis of institutional experience of the specific treatment delivery modes in use. If the plan fails the action limit, the most important factor for the physicist to consider is the spatial distribution of failing points. If these points lie in regions of little clinical importance, the plan may be clinically acceptable; however, if the failing points are within the target structure or critical structures, the physicist should follow the corrective actions outlined later. The physicist can also use tighter γ passing criteria to examine the QA results more closely. For instance, tighter criteria could be used to detect subtle regional errors or to test whether errors are systematic for a certain treatment machine, tumor site, or treatment technique. Tighter tolerance criteria can also be used to examine dose in areas where the critical structure tolerance is a small percentage of the maximum dose. If the results consistently fail to meet the tolerance limits (but are above the action limits), the IMRT treatment process should be thoroughly investigated for systematic problems.

Corrective actions

In a well-designed IMRT QA program, some treatment plans will not pass these tolerance limits and/or action limits. When encountering a failure, the medical physicist should investigate the potential reasons for the IMRT QA failure. The forthcoming report of Task Group 218 specifies that the following should be checked with respect to each system in the order given:

Set-up and beam

- Check correctness of measurement phantom set-up, plan version received by the TMS, QA plan generation, dose per fraction, and data transfer to IMRT QA verification software.

- Verify machine parameters on the day of measurement, such as beam flatness, symmetry, and output.

- Check calibration of the measurement device, detector size (and spacing) with respect to the size of the IMRT fields, and the value of the global dose normalization point.

Intensity-modulated radiation therapy quality assurance software

- Check the handling of the plan and measured data by the IMRT QA verification software, the values used for dose and DTA tolerance, dose threshold, and the registration of the two dose distributions.

Multileaf collimator

- Review results of other IMRT QA measurements, MLC leaf tolerances (such as speed, position, acceleration), tongue-and-groove effects, beam profile data (both for collimator- and MLC-defined fields), dynamic leaf gap data, MLC leaf transmission, and jaw tracking.

Treatment planning system

- Review the amount of modulation and the number of small segments in the plan, the total number of MUs, minimum MU numbers, the minimum segment size, and the dose calculation grid size (for non–Monte Carlo algorithms) or the variance setting (for Monte Carlo algorithms).
- Analyze TPS modeling accuracy for small fields and characterization of the leaf-parameters in the TPS.

If the IMRT verification plan fails and there is more complex modulation than normal in a clinical practice, the planner should consider replanning the IMRT case and attempt to achieve the planning objectives with less complex intensity patterns.

Novel methods for patient-specific intensity-modulated radiation therapy quality assurance

Although patient-specific IMRT QA measurements using the γ metric are the most widely used, there are several other methods that satisfy the same needs. These methods typically require additional calculations using the phantom-measured dose, and attempt to relate deficiencies in IMRT delivery or calculation back to the dose within the patient. In the Forward Calculation algorithm, the fluence map measured from the linac is used as input in a forward dose calculation algorithm that reconstructs the 3D dose in the patient geometry (25,26). The measurement data can be from an EPID (27), 2D diode or 2D chamber arrays (25,28,29), or a rotating phantom with an embedded 2D array (30). Additionally, similar results can be calculated from patient transmission data on a per-fraction basis, allowing for QA of every treated fraction (27,31,32). In Plan Dose Perturbation, the difference between the calculated and measured dose within the phantom is

used to perturb the clinical dose distribution in the patient geometry (20,21,33–35).

There are also methods for patient-specific QA that do not involve measurement. In some methods, an independent fluence-based dose calculation is used to verify the clinical plan (36). In other methods, the accuracy of delivery is calculated through analysis of treatment log files (37). These files record the positions of the gantry, jaws, MLC leaves, and so on, throughout treatment delivery. These positions can be used to calculate beamlets at each point in time, which are then summed to calculate a fluence map for this delivery. This 2D fluence map can then be compared with the expected fluence map using traditional IMRT QA tools (e.g., γ) (37). These fluence maps can also be used to recompute the dose in the patient geometry using the original calculation algorithm (38), or independent algorithms such as Monte Carlo (39,40). Some authors propose a combination of these approaches (both a separate MU calculation and log file analysis) as an alternative to traditional measurement-based IMRT QA (41).

TREATMENT VERIFICATION

Patient position

Prior to delivery of radiation, the position of the patient should be verified with respect to the intended radiation delivery. In external beam, pretreatment localization images (such as cone-beam CT or 2D planar kV or MV images) and/or portal images using the treatment beams should be acquired and compared with the reference images from the treatment plan (14). In all modalities, the immobilization devices used should also be reviewed.

Process review

Before treating the first fraction, a final review of the treatment process should occur. In general, this review should verify (a) patient identification, (b) review and approval of the treatment plan by physician/physicist, (c) proper patient set-up, and (d) that the treatment to be delivered matches the plan (12,42). In particular, the checks should focus on potential sources of human error, such as the placement of treatment accessories (bolus, spoiler, immobilization devices, afterloader transfer tubes, etc.).

Checklists are one potential tool to accomplish this, as they serve the critical role of helping to reduce errors resulting from human-related factors. Checklists are discussed in the AAPM *Medical Physics Practice Guideline* 4.a (43). Checklists are recommended for use in IMRT (14), SRS/SBRT (12), and brachytherapy (13,44), because they have been shown to be effective in reducing human error for complex processes. Because processes, procedures, and roles of personnel vary between institutions, each group should design checklists suited to its individual workflow. Sample checklists can be found in the practice guidelines for IMRT (14), image-guided radiation therapy (IGRT) (45), SRS/SBRT (12), and HDR brachytherapy (46).

Ongoing review

The fidelity of treatment should be reviewed periodically. This can be accomplished in several ways. In non-IGRT treatments, localization images can be acquired and reviewed periodically to ensure the accuracy of treatment delivery, whereas in IGRT treatments, it is recommended that thresholds be placed on imaging shifts above which the daily set-up must be reviewed by a physicist or physician (45). The SSD for each treatment field can be measured on a weekly basis to monitor changes in patient anatomy (e.g., weight loss) that would affect the accuracy of dose calculation. Dose measurements are also useful in monitoring the accuracy of treatment, such as periodic in vivo dosimetry or exit dosimetry with the portal imager (47). As with the initial plan check, the progress of treatment can be reviewed by physicists on a weekly basis to ensure continuous adherence of the treatment plan to the physician intent.

SUMMARY

Modern radiation therapy devices are extremely precise machines that are tested periodically to ensure function. However, radiation treatment planning and delivery is still a manual process that includes many individualized aspects that differ for each patient. By testing the individualized aspects of each patient's treatment plan, patient-specific QA plays a key role within a broader quality management system. Patient-specific QA serves to ensure that each patient receives treatment according to the physician's intent, that the dose calculation is correct, and that treatment proceeds according to the treatment plan. Additionally, the patient-specific QA process provides an opportunity for the physicist to examine the particular aspects of nearly every treatment plan, providing an avenue for analysis of subpar plans and processes that can lead to further improvements.

REFERENCES

1. Klein EE, Hanley J, Bayouth J, et al. Task Group 142 report: quality assurance of medical accelerators. *Med Phys.* 2009;36(9):4197–4212.

2. Dansereau R. *Misadministrations-Event Summaries and Prevention Strategies.* Troy, NY: State of New York Department of Health; 2010:2010–2011.

3. Barton M, Shafiq J. *Radiotherapy Risk Profile: Technical Manual.* Geneva, Switzerland: World Health Organization, Radiotherapy Safety Team within the World Alliance for Patient Safety; 2008.

4. Marks LB, Jackson M, Xie L, et al. The challenge of maximizing safety in radiation oncology. *Pract Radiat Oncol.* 2011;1(1):2–14.

5. LoSasso T, Chui C-S, Ling CC. Comprehensive quality assurance for the delivery of intensity modulated radiotherapy with a multileaf collimator used in the dynamic mode. *Med Phys.* 2001;28(11):2209–2219.

6. Alber M, Mijnheer B, Georg D, et al. *Guidelines for the Verification of IMRT.* Brussels, Belgium: ESTRO; 2008.

7. Leveson NG, Turner CS. An investigation of the Therac-25 accidents. *Computer.* 1993;26(7):18–41.

8. Stern RL, Heaton R, Fraser MW, et al. Verification of monitor unit calculations for non-IMRT clinical radiotherapy: report of AAPM Task Group 114. *Med Phys.* 2011;38(1):504–530.

9. Huq MS, Fraass BA, Dunscombe PB, et al. A method for evaluating quality assurance needs in radiation therapy. *Int J Radiat Oncol Biol Phys.* 2008;71(1):S170–S173.

10. Kutcher GJ, Coia L, Gillin M, et al. Comprehensive QA for radiation oncology: report of AAPM Radiation Therapy Committee Task Group 40. *Med Phys.* 1994;21:581–612.

11. Hartford AC, Galvin JM, Beyer DC, et al. American College of Radiology (ACR) and American Society for Radiation Oncology (ASTRO) practice guideline for intensity-modulated radiation therapy (IMRT). *Am J Clin Oncol.* 2012;35(6):612–617.

12. Solberg TD, Balter JM, Benedict SH, et al. Quality and safety considerations in stereotactic radiosurgery and stereotactic body radiation therapy: executive summary. *Pract Radiat Oncol.* 2012;2(1):2–9.

13. Thomadsen BR, Erickson BA, Eifel PJ, et al. A review of safety, quality management, and practice guidelines for high-dose-rate brachytherapy: executive summary. *Pract Radiat Oncol.* 2014;4(2):65–70.

14. Moran JM, Dempsey M, Eisbruch A, et al. Safety considerations for IMRT: executive summary. *Med Phys.* 2011;38(9):5067–5072.

15. Ford EC, Terezakis S, Souranis A, et al. Quality control quantification (QCQ): a tool to measure the value of quality control checks in radiation oncology. *Int J Radiat Oncol Biol Phys.* 2012;84(3):e263–e269.

16. Nelms BE, Simon JA. A survey on planar IMRT QA analysis. *J Appl Clin Med Phys.* 2007;8(3):76–90.

17. Kruse JJ. On the insensitivity of single field planar dosimetry to IMRT inaccuracies. *Med Phys.* 2010;37(6):2516–2524.

18. Nelms BE, Zhen H, Tomé WA. Per-beam, planar IMRT QA passing rates do not predict clinically relevant patient dose errors. *Med Phys.* 2011;38(2):1037–1044.

19. Stasi M, Bresciani S, Miranti A, et al. Pretreatment patient-specific IMRT quality assurance: a correlation study between gamma index and patient clinical dose volume histogram. *Med Phys.* 2012;39(12):7626–7634.

20. Carrasco P, Jornet N, Latorre A, et al. 3D DVH-based metric analysis versus per-beam planar analysis in IMRT pretreatment verification. *Med Phys.* 2012;39(8):5040–5049.

21. Zhen H, Nelms BE, Tome WA. Moving from gamma passing rates to patient DVH-based QA metrics in pretreatment dose QA. *Med Phys.* 2011;38(10):5477–5489.

22. Harms WB, Low DA, Wong JW, et al. A software tool for the quantitative evaluation of 3D dose calculation algorithms. *Med Phys.* 1998;25(10):1830–1836.

23. Low DA, Harms WB, Mutic S, et al. A technique for the quantitative evaluation of dose distributions. *Med Phys.* 1998;25(5):656–661.

24. Low DA, Dempsey JF. Evaluation of the gamma dose distribution comparison method. *Med Phys.* 2003;30(9):2455–2464.

25. Boggula R, Lorenz F, Mueller L, et al. Experimental validation of a commercial 3D dose verification system for intensity-modulated arc therapies. *Phys Med Biol.* 2010;55(19):5619–5633.

26. Renner WD, Norton KJ, Holmes TW. A method for deconvolution of integrated electronic portal images to obtain fluence for dose reconstruction. *J Appl Clin Med Phys.* 2005;6(4):22–39.

27. Wu C, Hosier KE, Beck KE, et al. On using 3D γ-analysis for IMRT and VMAT pretreatment plan QA. *Med Phys.* 2012;39(6):3051–3059.

28. Van Esch A, Depuydt T, Huyskens DP. The use of an aSi-based EPID for routine absolute dosimetric pre-treatment verification of dynamic IMRT fields. *Radiat Oncol.* 2004;71(2):223–234.

29. Nakaguchi Y, Araki F, Maruyama M, et al. Dose verification of IMRT by use of a COMPASS transmission detector. *Radiol Phys Technol.* 2012;5(1):63–70.

30. Stathakis S, Myers P, Esquivel C, et al. Characterization of a novel 2D array dosimeter for patient-specific quality assurance with volumetric arc therapy. *Med Phys.* 2013;40(7):0717311–0717315.

31. Wendling M, Louwe RJW, McDermott LN, et al. Accurate two-dimensional IMRT verification using a back-projection EPID dosimetry method. *Med Phys.* 2006;33(2):259–273.

32. Wendling M, McDermott LN, Mans A, et al. A simple backprojection algorithm for 3D in vivo EPID dosimetry of IMRT treatments. *Med Phys.* 2009;36(7):3310–3321.

33. Olch AJ. Evaluation of the accuracy of 3DVH software estimates of dose to virtual ion chamber and film in composite IMRT QA. *Med Phys.* 2012;39(1):81–86.

34. Nelms BE, Opp D, Robinson J, et al. VMAT QA: measurement-guided 4D dose reconstruction on a patient. *Med Phys.* 2012;39(7):4228–4238.

35. Opp D, Nelms BE, Zhang G, et al. Validation of measurement-guided 3D VMAT dose reconstruction on a heterogeneous anthropomorphic phantom. *J Appl Clin Med Phys.* 2013;14:70–84.

36. Georg D, Stock M, Kroupa B, et al. Patient-specific IMRT verification using independent fluence-based dose calculation software: experimental benchmarking and initial clinical experience. *Phys Med Biol.* 2007;52(16):4981.

37. Litzenberg DW, Moran JM, Fraass BA. Verification of dynamic and segmental IMRT delivery by dynamic log file analysis. *J Appl Clin Med Phys.* 2002;3(2):63–72.

38. Schreibmann E, Dhabaan A, Elder E, et al. Patient-specific quality assurance method for VMAT treatment delivery. *Med Phys.* 2009;36(10):4530–4535.

39. Teke T, Bergman AM, Kwa W, et al. Monte Carlo based, patient-specific RapidArc QA using linac log files. *Med Phys.* 2010;37(1):116–123.

40. Luo W, Li J, Price RA Jr, et al. Monte Carlo based IMRT dose verification using MLC log files and R/V outputs. *Med Phys.* 2006;33(7):2557–2564.

41. Sun B, Rangaraj D, Boddu S, et al. Evaluation of the efficiency and effectiveness of independent dose calculation followed by machine log file analysis against conventional measurement based IMRT QA. *J Appl Clin Med Phys.* 2012;13(5):3837.

42. Viswanathan AN, Beriwal S, Jennifer F, et al. American Brachytherapy Society consensus guidelines for locally advanced carcinoma of the cervix: Part II: high-dose-rate brachytherapy. *Brachytherapy.* 2012;11(1):47–52.

43. Jaffray DA, Langen KM, Mageras G, et al. Safety considerations for IGRT: executive summary. *Pract Radiat Oncol.* 2013;3(3):167–170.

44. de los Santos LEF, Evans S, Ford EC, et al. Medical Physics Practice Guideline 4.a: development, implementation, use and maintenance

of safety checklists. *J Appl Clin Med Phys.* 2015;16(3):37–59.

45. Nath R, Anderson LL, Meli JA, et al. Code of practice for brachytherapy physics: report of the AAPM Radiation Therapy Committee Task Group No. 56. *Medical Phys.* 1997;24(10):1557–1598.

46. Kubo HD, Glasgow GP, Pethel TD, et al. High dose-rate brachytherapy treatment delivery: report of the AAPM Radiation Therapy Committee Task Group No. 59. *Med Phys.* 1998;25(4):375–403.

47. Kirby MC, Williams PC. The use of an electronic portal imaging device for exit dosimetry and quality control measurements. *Int J Radiat Oncol Biol Phys.* 1995;31(3):593–603.

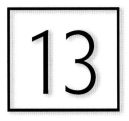

13 Plan Quality: The Good, the Bad, and the Ugly

Kevin L. Moore

THE UGLY TRUTH ABOUT PLAN QUALITY

Any characterization of treatment plans as *ugly* might sound a bit hyperbolic, yet most clinicians have encountered such plans and, unfortunately, patients have in fact been treated with such plans. Another characterization of this phenomenon could be a *blunder*, defined in Merriam-Webster as "a gross error or mistake resulting usually from . . . ignorance or carelessness." The human element as the source of a blunder is unavoidable in this definition, and can thus be distinguished from several well-documented errors (1) in radiotherapy that, at least initially, could be sourced to other mechanisms, such as software glitches, data transfer errors, or hardware malfunctions. Figure 13.1 shows a real-world instance of an ugly treatment plan, wherein two organs-at-risk (OARs) were not appropriately spared when the human planner was performing the intensity-modulated radiation therapy (IMRT) optimization (see dotted lines on the dose volume histogram [DVH]). It was, thankfully, caught before the patient was treated, and an improved final treatment plan was created (solid lines on the DVH). In most instances, treatment planning blunders are not of this magnitude, although assessing the frequency and severity of treatment plan quality deficiencies is not at all easy; this is discussed in more detail later in this chapter.

Classifying treatment plan quality blunders is instructive, as the spectrum of preventative actions depends strongly on the source of the errors. For this we consider three categories of planning blunders: errors of commission (performing the wrong action), errors of omission (failing to perform a required action), and errors of ignorance (lack of understanding of proper actions). Generally, errors of omission and ignorance are more easily prevented through automated measures

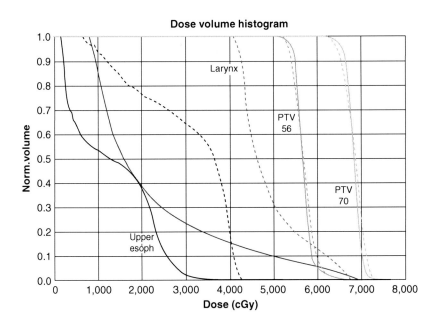

Dose volume histogram

FIGURE 13.1 An example of a treatment planning blunder in head-and-neck IMRT *(dotted lines)*, where the optimization process failed to avoid the larynx and upper esophagus. This ugly plan was reviewed and approved for treatment, but luckily was identified as suboptimal before the patient was treated. When a replan *(solid lines)* was developed, the delivered dose to these two organs-at-risk was reduced substantially, with no cost to the coverage of the PTVs.

and/or standardized quality checks, whereas errors of commission are more difficult to automate. For example, manual or automated checks can quite easily detect whether an OAR is either empty or not present (error of omission), but it is significantly harder to detect whether a clinical target volume (CTV) has been incorrectly contoured by the physician (error of commission). In Table 13.1, some examples of plan quality blunders are presented, including both manual preventative measures and potentially automated preventative measures.

In an attempt to classify the ugly plan presented in Figure 13.1, it would seem that this cannot be identified as an error of either omission or ignorance, as the OARs were correctly contoured and included in the plan optimization. Thus, this planning blunder must be sourced back to an error of commission, wherein the erroneous action was the use of inappropriate optimization objectives that allowed far more dose than necessary to be delivered to these OARs in the initial plan. Standard quality assurance (QA) for treatment planning workflows include both a physician and a physicist review of candidate treatment plans before treatment (11), but, of course, this falls into the manual preventative measures column of Table 13.1, and, unfortunately in this case, the on-screen physician review failed to detect the suboptimal nature of the initial treatment plan. When IMRT began in the mid-1990s, such a blunder could perhaps have been identified as an error of ignorance, but after 20 years of collective experience with inverse-optimized planning, we cannot claim complete ignorance of what is possible with IMRT.

Such an extreme case is almost certainly the exception, and yet the reader is encouraged to pause and consider just how often such a case could have been delivered to patients in your clinic. Although nearly all clinical scenarios have multiple plan quality criteria and cannot be distilled down to a single number, as a thought experiment one can posit a theoretical axis of plan quality whereby plans can be scored from catastrophic and dangerous (leftmost side of Figure 13.2) to fully optimal with respect to limits of the radiation delivery method used (rightmost side of Figure 13.2). Now consider that every plan ever delivered at your clinic will reside somewhere on this axis, and looking at all of them in aggregate will form a frequency histogram. If this distribution could be known, clinicians could quantify the probability that any given plan might be fatally flawed and institute quality control measures accordingly. With the exception of a handful of studies that will be discussed later in this chapter, clinicians typically do not know what the actual distribution of plan quality is in their own clinic. Radiotherapy is, quite regrettably, in a state where no one knows how widespread plan quality deficiencies are in clinical practice, nor the degree to which these quality deficits negatively impact patient care.

The quantitative tools that could query large pluralities of patient treatments to generate a true picture of the plan quality distribution in Figure 13.2 are not yet available to most clinicians. However, there are methods that, were they put into the hands of clinicians, could not only illuminate the distribution of plan quality from retrospective samples (*without QC curve* in Figure 13.2), but also fundamentally alter the shape of the distribution itself through true quantitative quality control tools (*with QC curve* in Figure 13.2).

The remainder of this chapter focuses on such methods of knowledge-based treatment plan quality control—that is, combating the problem of errors in plan optimization that lead to bad and ugly plans—but the reader is encouraged to consult the references in the last column of Table 13.1 for literature on tools to address the other types of planning errors.

Table 13.1 Examples and Categorization of Treatment Planning Blunders

Type of Radiotherapy Planning Blunder	Examples	Manual Preventative Measures	Automated Preventative Measures
Errors of commission	• Contouring errors • Fusion errors • Prescription errors • Inappropriate beam energy • Poorly optimized plan	• Pretreatment physics review • Peer review (chart rounds)	• Autocontouring checks (2–5) • Library search • Knowledge-based plan quality control (6,7)
Errors of omission	• OARs not contoured • OARs not included in optimization	• Checklists • Peer review (chart rounds)	• Templates • Autocontouring (2,3) • Reporting tools (8–10)
Errors of ignorance	• Wrong assumptions (e.g., integrity of CT scan) • Dose calculation errors • Previous treatment not accounted for	• Pretreatment physics review	• Reporting tools (8–10)

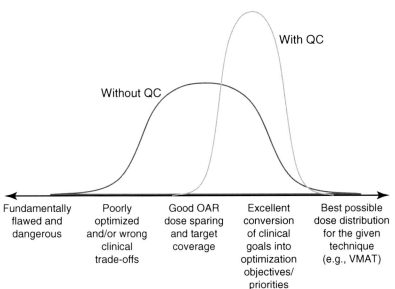

FIGURE 13.2 Cartoon view of clinical plan quality distributions with and without quality control measures.

FROM QUALITATIVE TO QUANTITATIVE PLAN QUALITY ASSESSMENTS

The treatment plan quality problem can be attributed to a number of factors: the anatomic variations between patients, the complexity of clinical goals, the paucity of quantitative metrics to judge the optimality of a given plan, and, of course, the subjectivity and relative experience of the humans involved in the planning process. As explored in many of the other chapters in this book, human error is the vexing source of many critical failure modes in clinical radiotherapy, and treatment plan quality deficiencies are no exception. A fundamental tenet of treatment plan quality control is to remove, to as large a degree as possible, the reliance of plan quality assessments on subjective human experience. To accomplish this, one *must* be able to make accurate quantitative predictions of plan quality metrics on a patient-specific basis, and so the question now turns to how such quantitative predictions are made.

Some plan quality metrics are universal across patients and are well suited as immutable constraints on some aspects of plan quality. Examples of such instances are the specification of the minimum allowable coverage criteria on a target volume (e.g., $V_{95\%} \geq 95\%$ (12)) or a hard constraint on a serial organ (e.g., Cord $D_{\max} \leq 45$ Gy). Such specifications form the core of radiotherapy protocol guidelines such as those found at the National Cancer Institute (NCI) cooperative groups (13). However, it must be clearly stated that not all dosimetric goals should be set at the same value for all patients. There are numerous clinical examples, but one storied and instructive case study is the parotid gland in head-and-neck cancer. There is a factor of three difference between

the region of highest dose response for the parotid gland (20–30 Gy (14–17)) and the therapeutic dose response curve of head-and-neck tumors (60–70 Gy (18)), and yet the advent of IMRT has allowed in-field dose gradients to be tuned to such a degree that salivary function can be preserved in cases that would be impossible with 3D-CRT (19). The planner is thus presented with the ability to effect a broad range of final mean doses to the parotid gland, and the "optimal" value is not constant between patients. On one end of the spectrum, sparing the parotid gland too much at the expense of clinical target coverage is highly undesirable, as evidenced by the increased risk of local failures observed under such a planning strategy (20). On the other end of the spectrum, it is trivially possible to insufficiently spare the parotid gland with IMRT planning by failing to create any negative dose gradient across the parotid gland, that is, in the 3D-CRT limit of opposed lateral fields. Given that salivary flow is a smooth inverse function of dose (15,16), a reasonable planning specification for a parotid gland could be written "as low as possible without losing target coverage," and yet this does not advance one's knowledge of what the mean dose to the parotid gland should be for any particular patient.

This ignorance of what is possible for any given patient clearly has a cost. In Moore et al (6), a simple mathematical model was developed from a plurality of previous cases that allowed a patient-specific prediction of mean dose based on the geometric overlap of a parotid gland with the planning target volume, with approximately ±10% accuracy. The effect of incorporating this prediction into the IMRT planning process was dramatic (Figure 13.3), resulting in significantly lowered and much less variable mean doses delivered patient-to-patient.

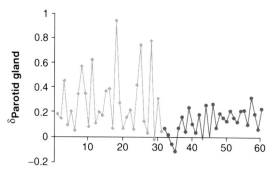

FIGURE 13.3 Washington University implemented a knowledge-based quality control tool for head-and-neck IMRT, observing significant reductions in excess parotid gland dose and reduced variability between treatment planners. The predictive model for parotid gland mean dose, developed through a model-based analysis of prior clinical treatment plans, gave a prediction for the mean dose (D_{pred}) that could be compared with the observed mean dose (D_{mean}). The parameter $\delta = (D_{mean} - D_{pred})/D_{pred}$ quantified the percentage by which the clinical treatment plans exceeded the model predictions. Diamonds and circles represent head-and-neck treatment plans before and after the clinical implementation of the quality control (QC) tool, respectively. (*Source*: From Ref. (6). Moore KL, Brame RS, Low DA, et al. Experience-based quality control of clinical intensity-modulated radiotherapy planning. *Int J Radiat Oncol Biol Phys.* 2011;81:545–551.) With permission.

This reduction in variability is not merely an academic matter; the patients planned before the model-driven feedback were at much higher risk of incurring salivary complications based on the aforementioned parotid gland dose response curve (6).

The means by which patient-specific predictions are obtained follows from the root cause of the dosimetric variation itself. In most cases, patients are planned according to standardized *clinical* goals determined entirely by the staging of their disease, meaning that the only predominant difference between one patient and another is their unique anatomy. The understanding of the degree to which a radiotherapy plan can or cannot meet a set of clinical goals for a given patient thus follows directly from the geometric properties of that patient's underlying anatomy. Although this is simply stated and quite intuitive, this confounding element is the primary reason behind the plan quality variations observed in the clinical practice of IMRT.

The remedy for this lack of clarity is to construct some predictive apparatus that quantifiably connects patient anatomy to expected dosimetry, and like all other scientific endeavors, the best guide for all numerical predictions is careful observation of controlled experimental data and a theoretical framework that allows for accurate future predictions. For radiotherapy clinicians, the obvious source of this data would be previously treated patients who shared the same clinical goals. If there were anatomic quantities that were strongly predictive of output dosimetry, we would need only plot several patients on these axes, as in the diagrammatic representation in Figure 13.4. As the geometric variable(s) for new patients can be computed irrespective of whether a plan has yet been generated, plotting the data on these axes can facilitate a knowledge-based prediction for the new case via two possible strategies. A similar patient (or patients) could be identified who shares similar geometric variables, an approach that could be characterized as a *knowledge-based library search*. Another approach to utilizing the data cast on these axes would be to develop some curve fit to the data, which could be characterized as a *knowledge-based model* that converts some geometric variable(s) X to some output dosimetric variable(s) Y via some functional relationship F, that is, $Y_{predicted} = F(X)$.

Returning to the primary goal of this chapter, which is to describe how to identify and eliminate treatment planning blunders from clinical practice, either the knowledge-based library approach or the knowledge-based modeling does much to advance this goal. Should a candidate plan differ greatly from either the matched plan in the library search or the model-predicted value, this could trigger a closer evaluation of whether the difference is "legitimate" (plan is truly optimal and the discrepancy is due to other factors) or is truly a blunder (plan is suboptimal and can be further improved). Both strategies have advantages and disadvantages associated with their use, which are summarized in Table 13.2.

Ultimately, the use of prior experience to inform future cases depends most strongly on the correlative power of the chosen geometric variable(s) to the dosimetric quantity of interest *in the absence of plan*

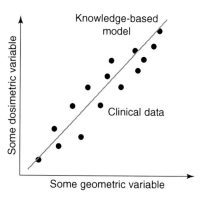

FIGURE 13.4 Cartoon picture of generating knowledge-based predictions for future patients based on observed correlations between anatomical geometry and dosimetric variables.

Table 13.2 Advantages and Disadvantages of Library Search Versus Model-Based Dosimetric Prediction Methodologies

	Advantages	Disadvantages
Knowledge-based library approach	• Possibly more robust regarding unknown geometric variables • Intuitive and independent of any mathematical framework • Can construct patient-mixing framework to increase accuracy of predictions (7)	• Plan quality of matched plan(s) is critical • Libraries could be difficult to transfer between institutions • Cannot extrapolate to unobserved regions of geometric space
Knowledge-based model approach	• Less susceptible to individual plan quality • Models are easily transferred between institutions • Can extrapolate to unobserved regions • Error estimations possible from aggregate model performance	• Chance of overfitting • Could mask unknown important geometric variables • Unknown predictive power in unobserved regions

quality variations; that is, how accurately the geometric quantities explain the observed dosimetric variations if all suboptimal plans have been eliminated. The reader would be readily forgiven for balking at this statement as a logical Catch-22, whereby plan quality deficiencies must be eliminated before one could develop the means to construct a quantitative plan quality control system to eliminate plan quality deficiencies. This is a core problem facing knowledge-based methods that purport to identify suboptimal treatment plans, and the quantification of aggregate plan quality deficiencies is the problem to which we must now turn our attention.

HOW BAD AND HOW OFTEN? QUANTIFYING THE FREQUENCY AND CLINICAL SEVERITY OF SUBOPTIMAL PLANS WITH KNOWLEDGE-BASED PREDICTIONS

Returning now to the theoretical plan quality distribution of Figure 13.2, we consider how one might answer the key question of ascertaining the nature of the distribution from a sample of *N* patients' treatment plans, that is, quantifying the frequency and clinical severity of suboptimal plans in clinical practice. One instructive example from the literature provides a hint at the question of the frequency of suboptimal plans, alternatively interpreted as quantifying the variation in plan quality due to less-than-ideal treatment plan development. In Nelms et al (21), the authors provided a single prostate patient's data set (simulation CT and contouring structure set) to the community as part of the ROR plan challenge, an annual contest whereby entrants attempt to achieve the highest possible plan quality metric (PQM) score according to a specified combination of DVH-based target and organ metrics. Upon analysis of the more than 125 submitted cases, the authors ultimately

reported the following: "There is a large inter-planning variation in plan quality defined by a quantitative PQM score that measures the ability of the planner to meet very specific plan objectives. Plan quality was not statistically different between different treatment planning systems or delivery techniques and was not correlated to metrics of plan complexity. Certification and education demographics, experience, and confidence level of the planner were not good predictors of plan quality." Figure 13.5 shows the observed distribution of PQM scores, exhibiting an extremely wide variance across the submitted cases. That the treatment planning system and delivery technique were *not* correlated with PQM score provides evidence that the limitation in achieving high-quality plans is not the fault, at least in this case, of the tools at the disposal of the planners. Although this study was limited to a single patient's data set and was unable to ascertain any specific factors that correlated with suboptimal plan submission, the breadth of plan quality variations in normal clinical practice could be reasonably inferred to be quite large given the very reasonable assumption that the individuals submitting contest submissions were a self-selected group who presumably thought their plans were good enough to warrant submission to a plan quality contest.

Bookending this study are several investigations, drawn from multi-institutional clinical trials, correlating the failure to meet dosimetric protocol constraints with worsened outcome (22–25). The outcomes tracking and centralized quality assurance of these trials provide strong evidence that buttresses the intuition that large deviations from clinical quality parameters really do subvert patient outcome, and yet these studies were unable to provide an answer to the question of whether any of the protocol-noncompliant cases could actually have been made to be compliant through better planning.

A knowledge-based methodology of collecting previous patients and developing sufficiently accurate dosimetric

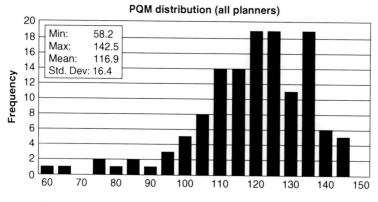

PQM distribution (all planners)

Min:	58.2
Max:	142.5
Mean:	116.9
Std. Dev:	16.4

FIGURE 13.5 Direct observation of a wide plan quality distribution based on 125 separate planners' treatment plans for a single prostate data set. The plan quality metric (PQM) score was calculated according to a specified combination of DVH-based target and organ metrics. (*Source*: From Ref. (21). Nelms BE, Robinson G, Markham J, et al. Variation in external beam treatment plan quality: an inter-institutional study of planners and planning systems. *Pract Radiat Oncol.* 2012;2:296–305.)

predictions does have the ability to address both the frequency and the clinical severity aspect of the plan quality problem. Focusing on one specific knowledge-based modeling strategy, we can examine how making accurate patient-specific DVH predictions could accomplish this. In Appenzoller et al (26), a knowledge-based method is described whereby parametric models are developed on the basis of the correlation of expected dose to the minimum distance from a voxel to the planning target volume (PTV) surface. A three-parameter probability distribution function (PDF) was used to model iso-distance OAR subvolume dose distributions. The knowledge-based DVH models were obtained by fitting the evolution of the PDF with distance, yielding accurate organ-specific models that make DVH predictions based on the synthesized experience of the training set. Figure 13.6 depicts the comparison of a predicted DVH to a candidate clinical DVH, putting into sharp relief the potential of accurate DVH predictions for plan quality control. Depending on the component (e.g., V_x) or derivative element (e.g., equivalent uniform dose [EUD] (27)) of the DVH that matters clinically, a comparison of the predicted dosimetric value against the candidate plan's value gives immediate quantitative feedback (within the accuracy of the DVH prediction) as to whether and by how much a plan could be improved.

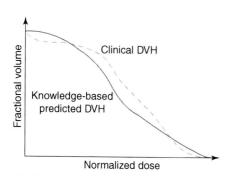

FIGURE 13.6 Comparing candidate plan DVH (*dotted line*) with a knowledge-based predicted DVH (*solid line*).

With this model-building and plan quality scoring apparatus, the elucidation of the plan quality distribution becomes a matter primarily of finding a properly representative data set. In Moore et al (28), parametric knowledge-based model DVH predictions were brought to bear on a multi-institutional clinical trial to directly assess the frequency and clinical severity of suboptimal treatment planning on a large scale: The Radiation Therapy Oncology Group (RTOG) 0126 protocol, *A Phase III Randomized Study of High Dose 3DCRT/IMRT Versus Standard Dose 3DCRT/IMRT in Patients Treated for Localized Prostate Cancer.* Briefly, this work examined high-dose IMRT patients (79.2 Gy prescription dose in 44 fractions), and after using knowledge-based DVH prediction models (26) to eliminate other plan quality indices as problematic, the study ultimately focused on grade 2+ late rectal toxicities as the primary plan quality marker. Using an outcomes-validated Lyman–Kutcher–Burman (LKB) model for the normal tissue complication probability (NTCP) for late rectal toxicities (29), comparisons between clinical and model-predicted DVHs yielded the absolute excess risk (actual NTCP – predicted NTCP) from suboptimal planning: 94/219 (42.9%) had ≥5% excess risk, 20/219 (9.1%) had ≥10% excess risk, and 2/219 (0.9%) had ≥15% excess risk. The results of this study definitively demonstrated that poor-quality IMRT planning frequently put protocol patients at substantial and unnecessary risk of normal tissue toxicities. The excess risks were directly found to be unnecessary, as the validated LKB model quantified the potential risk reductions and replanning demonstrated the achievability of this reduction without compromise of target structures or other OARs. The characterization of +4.7% average excess risk as "substantial" requires context, to which two key points of comparison are available from Michalski et al (30). On the high-dose arm of RTOG 0126, at median follow-up of 3 years, patients treated with 3D-CRT had a 22.0% cumulative incidence of grade 2+ GI toxicity, whereas IMRT patients had a 15.1% cumulative incidence (*P* = .039). A 4.7%

risk reduction in the IMRT group rate might have cut the incidence by nearly a third. Further, the predicted 4.7% risk reduction is on a par with the toxicity rate difference between 3D-CRT and IMRT of 22.0% to 15.1% = 7.1%, implying that quality-controlled IMRT planning could have yielded nearly as much clinical benefit as uncontrolled IMRT planning offered over 3D-CRT (Figure 13.7).

It is highly likely that, at least for the time period from which the plans were drawn (2003–2008), this study is representative of the plan quality variations present in the general population. Given the types of institutions that participate in national trials and the efforts expended to meet protocol requirements, it is plausible that the plan quality variations in this work actually underestimate the variability in wider clinical practice. The observed quality variations in this study hint, troublingly, at potentially larger variations in sites where the spread between the prescription dose and organ tolerances is even wider, for example, the aforementioned case of parotid glands in head-and-neck cancer. Further investigations into plan quality variation distributions in different disease sites and larger clinical data sets will likely expand as knowledge-based tools become more widely available.

AUTOMATED PLANNING WITH KNOWLEDGE-BASED DOSE PREDICTIONS

Of course, the promise of knowledge-based plan quality control is not just a quantification of clinical plan quality

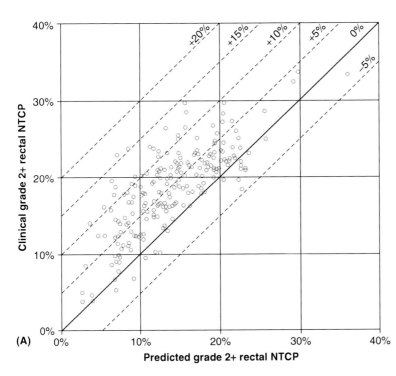

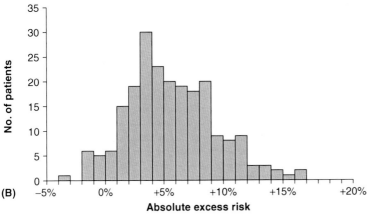

FIGURE 13.7 Secondary study on RTOG 0126 quantified excess risk of late rectal complication due to suboptimal IMRT planning. (A) Scatter plot shows knowledge-based prediction of NTCP versus the actual treated plans' NTCP. (B) Frequency histogram of the same data shows a mean excess risk of 4.7% ± 3.9% and represents the largest and most institutionally diverse measurement of plan quality variations to date. (*Source*: From Ref. (28). Moore KL, Schmidt R, Moiseenko V, et al. Quantifying unnecessary normal tissue complication risks due to suboptimal planning: a secondary study of RTOG 0126. *Int J Radiat Oncol Biol Phys.* 2015;92:228–235.)

variations, but an entire reshaping of the distribution itself (Figure 13.2). With objective dosimetric predictions for individual patients, it is an easily logical step to move from knowledge-based quality control (comparing a candidate plan with the knowledge-based prediction) to fully automated *knowledge-based planning* (KBP), whereby the dosimetric predictions are directly incorporated into the plan optimization process. The utility of this can be readily seen by a reconsideration of the ugly plan in Figure 13.1, where the only plausible explanation for these dangerous OAR DVHs is that inappropriate DVH objectives and/or weights were entered into the IMRT optimization engine. Had knowledge-based DVH predictions resembled closely the final plan's solid DVH curves available, and had the IMRT optimization objectives been based on these, the inferior plan (dotted DVHs) would not have resulted. There are several means by which knowledge-based DVH predictions are used to automate the generation of the discrete DVH-based IMRT objectives (8,31–33), including one commercial offering (34) at the time of publication. Knowledge-based DVH prediction models are necessary but not sufficient for such automated KBP, as the estimated curves have to be converted to DVH objectives and priority weights. Here we see a two-fold layering to any automated KBP schema, whereby the DVH prediction algorithm (the "model") must be sufficiently accurate and the relative weighting of the generated DVH-based objectives have to be properly calibrated against each other (the autoplanning "routine"). The independent validation of both the models and the autoplanning routines is a critical step, and several approaches have been presented in the literature (26,28,33–36), by setting aside a sizeable number of retrospectively collected patients from the model training set and then applying the DVH estimation models and autoplanning routines to these "new" patients to confirm that the output of the autoplanning system is in line with previous experience. The process of applying a trained dose prediction model to a set of unseen validation patients is the primary protection against overfitting and, assuming the validation set contains predominantly high-quality plans, quantifies the uncertainty in the model's dose metric prediction. If the plans in the validation set have unknown quality, the incorporation of some replanning endeavor will be required to separate whether prediction inaccuracies are true model uncertainty or should be ascribed to plan quality variations.

QUIS CUSTODIET IPSO CUSTODES? (WHO WILL GUARD THE GUARDS THEMSELVES?)

If knowledge-based automated planning is supposed to protect clinicians and patients from suboptimal plans, how can we be certain that it is performing this task flawlessly in all cases? To explore the implications of this question, as a thought experiment we can envision a knowledge-based automated planning system for an arbitrary disease site, an arbitrary delivery technique, and a set of several dosimetric plan quality indices of interest. For every plan quality index, we can consider three quantities:

- D_{optimal}—The optimum dose value for the plan quality index, taking into account the delivery technique and the necessary trade-offs of this metric against the other plan quality indices

- $D_{\text{model}} \pm \delta D_{\text{model}}$—The knowledge-based model prediction for the plan quality index, including some error bounds quantifying the precision of the prediction

- D_{autoplan}—The resultant value of the plan quality index upon use of the knowledge-based autoplanning routine to generate a deliverable plan with the given delivery technique

It must be noted that D_{optimal} is never actually known for all metrics. The closest we might get to discovering D_{optimal} for all the quality metrics in an individual case would be to go through something like the multiuser planning contest that generated the distribution in Figure 13.5. The highest scoring plan could be reasonably assumed to approach D_{optimal} for each of the multiple planning criteria, but of course, such a process is not possible in normal clinical practice. Table 13.3 examines a theoretical instance of three OAR quality indices with comparisons for D_{optimal}, $D_{\text{model}} \pm \delta D_{\text{model}}$, and D_{autoplan} in each dose metric.

With D_{optimal} unknown, it is not obvious how to determine whether any of a particular plan's quality metrics might be falling victim to one of the error types, nor how this will be limited. Of the two error types, "false negatives" may be the most concerning, as these would represent precisely the inadequate dose sparing that knowledge-based planning is designed to mitigate. This consideration makes the quantitative assessment of the model uncertainty δD_{model} all the more critical, and although Table 13.3 utilized a standard deviation to describe the model error, other quantifications (such as box-and-whisker plots examining the full range of observed model prediction variation) can also be valuable quantitative feedback to the clinician as to how far the model prediction might deviate.

In addition to normal and expected model prediction variation, there is the matter of geometric outliers, that is, patients whose anatomy lies outside the observed range of geometric variables in whatever space has been used to train the knowledge-based system. This can be envisioned by a new patient taking a geometric variable value to the left or to the right of all of the training data in the cartoon picture of Figure 13.4. One must then consider whether the knowledge-based model can be legitimately extrapolated to this as-yet unobserved value or, if a knowledge-based library approach is used, how to

Table 13.3 Example of a Set of Dosimetric Plan Quality Metrics and How Knowledge-Based Model Predictions and Autoplans Might Compare With the Fully Optimal Values

	$D_{optimal}$ (Gy)	$D_{model} \pm \delta D_{model}$ (Gy)	$D_{autoplan}$ (Gy)	Error Type	Consequence
Dose metric #1	32.4	32.6 ± 0.7	32.8		
Dose metric #2	23.8	26.1 ± 2.3	26.0	False-negative	OAR underspared, plan is suboptimal with respect to this metric
Dose metric #3	11.0	9.3 ± 0.8	9.4	False-positive	OAR overspared, targets or other OARs are compromised, plan is suboptimal owing to incorrect trade-off

δD_{model} is expressed here as a standard deviation, but could be represented by any statistics from the application of the model to an established validation set. The first dose metric is an example of normative behavior where the model prediction closely approximates the ideal value, and the autoplan result closely follows this. The second dose metric is an example of a "false-negative" error, whereby the model prediction overestimates by a significant margin the truly optimal value, resulting in a final plan value that is not as low as possible for the associated organ. The third dose metric is an example of a "false-positive" error, whereby the model prediction is significantly lower than the truly optimal value, and the resultant plan value forces an inappropriate trade-off to achieve this erroneously aggressive value.

match this patient to the existing database. To complicate things further, all modern knowledge-based systems (31,33,37) utilize a set of geometric inputs comprising a multivariable space that is not readily visualized, so a mechanism to identify outliers in a multidimensional space (38) will be required to understand the degree to which an individual observation is within the range of or outside the geometric variation in the training data. The user's response to identification of a geometric outlier should be one of caution and heightened skepticism, not only with regard to the values of the model's dosimetric prediction but to the model uncertainty estimates as well. In these instances, extra scrutiny of the autoplanning routine's output is a necessity, up to and including manual adjustment of the optimization parameters in a replanning effort to ensure that the resultant plan is not readily improved in any of the plan quality dimensions. It would be advisable to both retain the KBP result to compare against the replan(s) and to incorporate some reporting system (10,36) that can quickly analyze all quality metrics together in case one was improved at the expense of another.

The imperative to continually expand the breadth and accuracy of KBP routines finally brings us to the notion of knowledge-based model maintenance. As geometric outliers are discovered in the course of normal clinical practice, it would be highly advantageous to incorporate new information into updated models and improved autoplanning routines. Unlike the treatment planning system (TPS) beam models used for dose calculation that are rarely (if ever) changed after commissioning, the merging of new patient plans into the knowledge-based

models is readily accomplished by retraining the system with an expanded patient pool. Besides the inclusion of geometric outlier patients to broaden the dynamic range of the knowledge-based predictions, it is entirely possible to continually add high-quality plans, perhaps even filtering out training plans that appear inferior to the quality distribution within the training sample itself. The difficulties of this value proposition lie in the bookkeeping aspects of keeping track of several models and in the concern that the model output may drift to a new state, thus inadvertently driving the clinical trade-offs in an undesirable direction. The latter worry can be substantially alleviated by maintaining a large and constant validation pool of patients to which separate models can be applied. The performance of differing models can be assessed on the aggregation of the many PQMs across a constant plurality of patients, so any unintended consequences of adjustment of the training pool on the model's performance should be transparent and easily discovered.

CONCLUSIONS

Although this chapter has focused on knowledge-based dose predictions as a potential solution to the problem of plan quality variations, it is notable that knowledge-based techniques would still remain susceptible to several of the radiotherapy planning blunders listed in Table 13.1. Without the addition of further safety measures, for example, it is easy to see how prescription errors, contouring errors, and dose calculation errors could still propagate through the planning process even if KBP reduces or eliminates the chance of highly suboptimal plans being generated. As should be clear from a survey of the other chapters in this book, a modern quality and safety apparatus must include a portfolio of checks and redundant quality systems to ensure consistently optimal behavior. We should go into the future with strong optimism that the rate of "ugly" and "bad" plans will decrease, although it will take quite some time to automate all treatment sites and for these systems to become ubiquitous.

REFERENCES

1. Bogdanich W. Radiation offers new cures, and ways to do harm. *New York Times*. January 23, 2010.

2. Chen H-C, Tan J, Dolly S, et al. Automated contouring error detection based on supervised geometric attribute distribution models for radiation therapy: a general strategy. *Med Phys*. 2015;42:1048–1059.

3. Chao KC, Bhide S, Chen H, et al. Reduce in variation and improve efficiency of target volume delineation by a computer-assisted system using a deformable image registration approach. *Int J Radiat Oncol Biol Phys*. 2007;68:1512–1521.

4. Han X, Hibbard LS, O'Connell NP, et al. Automatic segmentation of parotids in head and neck CT images using multi-atlas fusion. *Med Image Anal*. 2010:297–304.

5. Moore CS, Liney GP, Beavis AW. Quality assurance of registration of CT and MRI data sets for treatment planning of radiotherapy for head and neck cancers. *J Appl Clin Med Phys*. 2004;5:25–35.

6. Moore KL, Brame RS, Low DA, et al. Experience-based quality control of clinical intensity-modulated radiotherapy planning. *Int J Radiat Oncol Biol Phys*. 2011;81:545–551.

7. Wu B, Ricchetti F, Sanguineti G, et al. Patient geometry-driven information retrieval for IMRT treatment plan quality control. *Med Phys*. 2009;36:5497–5505.

8. Yang D, Moore KL. Automated radiotherapy treatment plan integrity verification. *Med Phys*. 2012;39:1542–1551.

9. Yang D, Wu Y, Brame RS, et al. Technical note: electronic chart checks in a paperless radiation therapy clinic. *Med Phys*. 2012;39:4726–4732.

10. Olsen LA, Robinson CG, He GR, et al. Automated radiation therapy treatment plan workflow using a commercial application programming interface. *Pract Radiat Oncol*. 2014;4:358–367.

11. Kutcher GJ, Coia L, Gillin M, et al. Comprehensive QA for radiation oncology: report of AAPM Radiation Therapy Committee Task Group 40. *Med Phys*. 1994;21:581–618.

12. Moore KL, Brame RS, Low DA, et al. Quantitative metrics for assessing plan quality. *Semin Radiat Oncol*. 2012;22:62–69.

13. Scoggins JF, Ramsey SD. A national cancer clinical trials system for the 21st century: reinvigorating the NCI cooperative group program. *J Natl Cancer Inst*. 2010;102:1371–1371.

14. Beetz I, Schilstra C, van der Schaaf A, et al. NTCP models for patient-rated xerostomia and sticky saliva after treatment with intensity modulated radiotherapy for head and neck cancer: the role of dosimetric and clinical factors. *Radiot Oncol*. 2012;105:101–106.

15. Moiseenko V, Wu J, Hovan A, et al. Treatment planning constraints to avoid xerostomia in head-and-neck radiotherapy: an independent test of quantec criteria using a prospectively collected dataset. *Int J Radiat Oncol Biol Phys*. 2012;82:1108–1114.

16. Deasy JO, Moiseenko V, Marks L, et al. Radiotherapy dose–volume effects on salivary gland function. *Int J Radiat Oncol Biol Phys*. 2010;76:S58–S63.

17. Houweling AC, Philippens MEP, Dijkema T, et al. A comparison of dose–response models for the parotid gland in a large group of head-and-neck cancer patients. *Int J Radiat Oncol Biol Phys*. 2010;76:1259–1265.

18. Halperin EC, Brady LW, Wazer DE, et al. *Perez & Brady's Principles and Practice of Radiation Oncology*. Philadelphia, PA: Lippincott Williams & Wilkins; 2013.

19. Nutting CM, Morden JP, Harrington KJ, et al. Parotid-sparing intensity modulated versus conventional radiotherapy in head and neck cancer (parsport): a phase 3 multicentre randomized controlled trial. *Lancet Oncol*. 2011;12:127–136.

20. Cannon DM, Lee NY. Recurrence in region of spared parotid gland after definitive intensity-modulated radiotherapy for head and neck cancer. *Int J Radiat Oncol Biol Phys*. 2008;70:660–665.

21. Nelms BE, Robinson G, Markham J, et al. Variation in external beam treatment plan quality: an inter-institutional study of planners and planning systems. *Pract Radiat Oncol*. 2012;2:296–305.

22. Peters LJ, O'Sullivan B, Giralt J, et al. Critical impact of radiotherapy protocol compliance and

quality in the treatment of advanced head and neck cancer: results from TROG 02.02. *J Clin Oncol.* 2010;28:2996–3001.

23. Fitzgerald TJ. What we have learned: the impact of quality from a clinical trials perspective. *Semin Radiat Oncol.* 2012;22:18–28.

24. Abrams RA, Winter KA, Regine WF, et al. Failure to adhere to protocol specified radiation therapy guidelines was associated with decreased survival in RTOG 9704—a phase III trial of adjuvant chemotherapy and chemoradiotherapy for patients with resected adenocarcinoma of the pancreas. *Int J Radiat Oncol Biol Phys.* 2012;82:809–816.

25. Fairchild A, Straube W, Laurie F, et al. Does quality of radiation therapy predict outcomes of multicenter cooperative group trials? A literature review. *Int J Radiat Oncol Biol Phys.* 2013;87:246–260.

26. Appenzoller LM, Michalski JM, Thorstad WL, et al. Predicting dose-volume histograms for organs-at-risk in IMRT planning. *Med Phys.* 2012;39:7446.

27. Niemierko A. Reporting and analyzing dose distributions: a concept of equivalent uniform dose. *Med Phys.* 1997;24:103–110.

28. Moore KL, Schmidt R, Moiseenko V, et al. Quantifying unnecessary normal tissue complication risks due to suboptimal planning: a secondary study of RTOG 0126. *Int J Radiat Oncol Biol Phys.* 2015;92:228–235.

29. Michalski JM, Gay H, Jackson A, et al. Radiation dose-volume effects in radiation-induced rectal injury. *Int J Radiat Oncol Biol Phys.* 2010;76:S123–S129.

30. Michalski JM, Yan Y, Watkins-Bruner D, et al. Preliminary toxicity analysis of 3-dimensional conformal radiation therapy versus intensity modulated radiation therapy on the high-dose arm of the Radiation Therapy Oncology Group 0126 prostate cancer trial. *Int J Radiat Oncol Biol Phys.* 2013;87:932–938.

31. Wu B, McNutt T, Zahurak M, et al. Fully automated simultaneous integrated boosted–intensity modulated radiation therapy treatment planning is feasible for head-and-neck cancer: a prospective clinical study. *Int J Radiat Oncol Biol Phys* 2012;84(5):e647–e653.

32. Zhang X, Li X, Quan EM, et al. A methodology for automatic intensity-modulated radiation treatment planning for lung cancer. *Phys Med Biol.* 2011;56:3873–3893.

33. Zhu X, Ge Y, Li T, et al. A planning quality evaluation tool for prostate adaptive IMRT based on machine learning. *Med Phys.* 2011;38:719–726.

34. Tol JP, Delaney AR, Dahele M, et al. Evaluation of a knowledge-based planning solution for head and neck cancer. *Int J Radiat Oncol Biol Phys.* 2015;91:612–620.

35. Shiraishi S, Tan J, Olsen LA, et al. Knowledge-based prediction of plan quality metrics in intracranial stereotactic radiosurgery. *Med Phys.* 2015;42:908–917.

36. Li N, Carmona R, Sirak I, et al. Validation of a knowledge based automated planning system in cervical cancer as a clinical trial quality system. *Int J Radiat Oncol Biol Phys.* 2015;93(3):S40.

37. Moore K, Appenzoller L, Tan J, et al. Clinical implementation of dose-volume histogram predictions for organs-at-risk in IMRT planning. *J Phys Conf Ser.* 2014;489:012055.

38. Frank EG. Procedures for detecting outlying observations in samples. *Technometrics.* 1969;11:1–21.

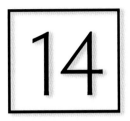

Special Procedures and Equipment

H. Harold Li, Michael B. Altman, and H. Omar Wooten

STEREOTACTIC RADIOSURGERY AND GAMMA KNIFE

Management of benign, functional, and metastatic intracranial lesions has been accomplished through the use of single-fraction stereotactic radiosurgery (SRS), or hypofractionated stereotactic radiation therapy (SRT). Linear accelerator-based SRS methods are becoming increasingly popular with the continuous improvement in multileaf collimator (MLC) technology, which yields increasingly narrow leaves capable of field shapes that mimic the traditional linac-based SRS cones in field sizes of 0.5 to 1.0 cm. Linac-based SRS offers the advantage of versatility. The larger field sizes and narrower leaves allow clinicians to use the same machine to treat extracranial disease using both conventional and hypofractionated techniques. Such systems are more often accompanied by onboard kV imaging capabilities for image-guided radiation therapy.

Each incremental improvement of linac-based SRS technology is still compared against the original method of intracranial SRS, the Leksell Gamma Knife platform (1,2). Developed by neurosurgeon Lars Leksell in 1950, the Gamma Knife SRS uses a hemispherical array of cobalt-60 sources all focused upon a common isocenter (3). A stereotactic frame, rigidly affixed to the patient's skull, registers to the couch, and serves as the stereotactic coordinate system used to compute the couch coordinates required to place the isocenter at specific positions within the tumor. The Gamma Knife Perfexion (Elekta, AB Stockholm, Sweden) comprises an integrated system that includes (a) the treatment unit housing 192 cobalt-60 sources arranged in eight azimuthal "sectors," (b) the precision-controlled stereotactic couch and frame mount, (c) the treatment console unit, and (d) the GammaPlan treatment planning system (4). The Perfexion provides 4, 8, and 16 mm collimation to individual sectors automatically, as specified by the planner. Figure 14.1 shows a typical process for a Gamma Knife Perfexion treatment at the St. Louis Gamma Knife Center at Barnes-Jewish Hospital.

Compared with most external beam radiation therapy techniques, Gamma Knife procedures have several unique features: (a) the entire treatment process is time compressed, with simulation-to-completion of treatment times ranging between 2 and 4 hours depending on the complexity of the target, the prescription dose, and the activity of the sources; and (b) single-fraction treatments make quality of the highest importance.

The Gamma Knife Perfexion (GKP) comprises an integrated treatment delivery unit, control console, and treatment planning system. Although the manufacturer performs the installation, clinical commissioning and establishment of quality assurance (QA) in accordance with Nuclear Regulatory Commission (NRC) license requirements are the responsibility of the authorized medical physicist. QA procedures for Gamma Knife have been published (5), and an example of daily QA procedures prior to a treatment session are provided in the appendix. The remainder of this section focuses on ensuring the quality of a clinical Gamma Knife (GK) Perfexion treatment.

The application of secondary (quality control) checks of the data used to create a treatment plan is one step in guaranteeing the high quality of any process. An example of redundant checks for GKP treatments would be the skull measurements obtained immediately following frame placement. These measurements are acquired at intervals around the skull and may be used by the system to determine the depths of treatment for each cobalt-60 source. After importing CT or MRI data, one can visualize the estimated surface relative to the actual surface as determined by the imaging.

Typically, both CT and MRI images are used for GK treatment planning. Although the MRI images provide excellent soft-tissue contrast for delineating targets and normal structures, MRI images are subject to distortions arising from variability in the magnetic field. Therefore, quality of treatment is enhanced if a CT is available. The CT is rigidly registered to the MRI data sets, providing greater spatial accuracy. Some intracranial targets, such as punctate metastases and trigeminal nerves, can be quite small (< 3 mm in diameter), requiring images with a minimum slice thickness of 1 mm. The image quality for all imported data

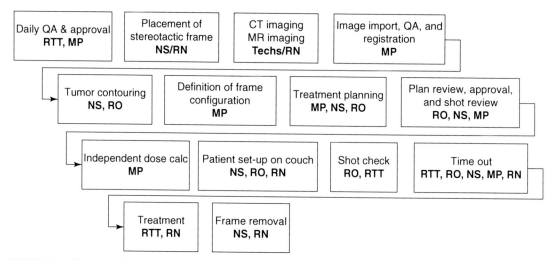

FIGURE 14.1 Clinical workflow for a typical Gamma Knife Perfexion treatment at the St. Louis Gamma Knife Center. MP, medical physicist; NS, neurosurgeon; RN, nurse; RO, radiation oncologist; RTT, radiation therapist.

sets should be assessed, noting regions of excessive motion and reconstruction artifacts and distortion. Upon importing images, the stereotactic coordinate system can be automatically determined by identifying the fiducials. The maximum distances between the fiducials on imaging, and the expected position, are provided by the treatment planning system and should be less than 1.0 mm, especially in the regions of the target(s). Should the fiducial error exceed 1.0 mm, rigid registration to the CT is highly recommended. If the CT fiducial error exceeds tolerance, additional investigation may be required, as the CT scan and reconstruction parameters may have to be adjusted. Fusions should be reviewed by either the radiation oncologist or the neurosurgeon before contouring, and should include side-by-side comparison of key anatomical landmarks, such as the basilar artery, auditory nerves, and gyri and sulci near the target regions. Contouring of targets and organs-at-risk (OARs) should be reviewed by the radiation oncologist and neurosurgeon before planning. For situations with multiple data sets, multiplanar review of the contours superimposed on each data set ensures that structures not visible on all data sets are properly accounted for. Multiplanar review can be used to identify any issues with end-capping. Target matrices comprising 10,000 calculation points should be placed around each target and should have the minimum size possible that allows for visualization of some of the 25% to 30% isodose line.

Although the features of any particular plan's dose distribution will be specific to that plan (e.g., size of hotspot, degree of gradient near OARs), Gamma Knife treatment plans are typically judged using conformity and gradient indices. A conformity index of 1.3 for simple cases to 2.0 for complex targets is generally indicative of good quality (1). Independent dose computation is a well-established QA principle in external beam radiation therapy, and various tools for Gamma Knife planning have also been developed, such as reference (6).

Minimization of process variability is a key aspect of ensuring high quality, and although local clinical procedures will vary, the list of items provided in the appendix, if implemented and adapted to the local clinic, can result in a consistent process in treating intracranial lesions with the Gamma Knife Perfexion.

MAGNETIC RESONANCE IMAGE–GUIDED RADIATION THERAPY (MR-IGRT)

The ability of MR imaging to visualize soft tissues has proved useful for SRS, but multimodality imaging is increasingly used to treat other anatomical sites. Registration of MR images with CT has proven useful for fractionated intracranial, head and neck, thorax, breast, abdomen, pelvis, and extremity radiation therapy treatments.

Over the past decade, there has been increasing interest in using MR images not only for target delineation during treatment planning, but also for daily localization. MR-IGRT has been in development by a number of groups. The first commercially available MR-IGRT device was developed by ViewRay (ViewRay, Inc., Oakwood, OH) and clinically implemented at Washington University in St. Louis, with the first patient receiving treatment in January 2014 (7).

The ViewRay device comprises a three-headed cobalt-60 radiation therapy system and a 0.35-T MR imaging system. The device acquires fast MR images for patient localization and sagittal MRI images simultaneously during RT beam delivery. Motion tracking software tracks tumors and anatomy in real time. ViewRay's integrated treatment planning and delivery systems are specifically designed for on-treatment adaptive treatment delivery, allowing imaging, recontouring, reoptimization, and delivery of a new plan within minutes without moving the patient.

Adaptive treatments began at Washington University in September 2014.

This technology being new, a detailed consensus of machine QA procedures is still in development. However, the NRC has issued guidance for daily, weekly, monthly, and annual QA tasks (8). In summary, daily QA tests include verifying the functionality of audiovisual equipment, door interlocks, and in-room monitors. Image quality and output are tested by scanning a phantom and ionization chamber, verifying key dimensions, and delivering a known dose to the chamber. Weekly QA tests include MLC field shape and source position verification. Monthly QA tests include more detailed versions of the daily QA tests, gantry and MLC mechanical accuracy verification, and radiation and MRI isocenter coincidence. Annually, detailed dosimetric verifications (output factors, percent depth dose, and absolute calibration) are performed in addition to MLC and couch mechanical tests. A complete list of NRC-required QA tests may be found in the NRC's license guidance (8). Three-dimensional and intensity-modulated radiation therapy (IMRT) treatments are delivered with three cobalt-60 heads capable of simultaneous irradiation, each of which is equipped with a 30 leaf-pair MLC.

Li et al (9) described the development of a program for patient-specific QA for ViewRay IMRT using measurements and log file analysis techniques. Measurements include ionization chamber measurements in a square water-equivalent phantom, 3D diode array with a central ionization chamber, and radiographic film. For 102 ionization chamber measurements, a mean difference of $0.0\% \pm 1.3\%$ between measured and expected values was reported. The mean gamma pass rate (3% dose difference, 3 mm distance to agreement) was $94.6\% \pm 3.4\%$ for 30 radiographic film measurements and $98.9\% \pm 1.1\%$ for 34 3D diode array measurements. Log file analysis and 3D dose reconstruction using the log file data showed similar agreement with reference treatment plans.

The ability of the ViewRay system to deliver IMRT treatment plans was further investigated by Wooten et al (10), who conducted end-to-end treatment procedures using the AAPM Task Group 119 reference data. Ionization chamber, film, and 3D diode array measurements showed excellent agreement relative to expected values, and relative to the results of the TG-119 participant clinics. In a separate study, Wooten et al (11) compared the treatment plan quality of cobalt-60 IMRT with linac IMRT for 33 patients treated with the ViewRay device. For all patients in this study, backup linac plans were created using normal clinical workflow and procedures, and were approved for treatment. ViewRay treatment plans demonstrated similar planning target volume (PTV) coverage and similar OAR mean doses above 20 Gy. The lower cobalt-60 beam energies resulted in slightly greater PTV heterogeneity and larger volumes of tissue receiving 25% of prescription dose.

STEREOTACTIC BODY RADIATION THERAPY

The majority of patients treated with stereotactic body radiation therapy (SBRT) are those with lung, liver, and spinal tumors. SBRT delivers large doses in a few fractions, which results in a high biological effective dose. The safety and quality issues surrounding SBRT are well described in a number of documents (12,13). This section presents a highlight of the central points.

Commissioning

Small field data acquisition

Owing to the small size of the fields employed, output factor, percentage depth dose, and profile measurements require the use of small detectors. AAPM TG 101 recommends the use of a dosimeter with an active area of 1 mm^2 or less. It is important to verify positional accuracy of the dosimeter to ensure that measurement occurs at the intended position(s). In addition, volume averaging effect may cause additional measurement artifacts, such as underestimation of the output factors and overestimation of the penumbrae. Therefore, it is a good practice to compare measurements with various detectors (for example, diode, ionization chamber and film) and to compare against published data from other institutions.

Heterogeneity calculation

Accurate dose calculation in heterogeneity is challenging in situations where the target is surrounded by low-density tissue such as the lungs, as a result of transient electronic disequilibrium and increased lateral electron range. Algorithms that account for 3D scatter integration, such as convolution/superposition, should be used for dose calculation. Depth dose and profile measurements should be measured using ionization chamber and film positioned within an inhomogeneous phantom consisting of lung-equivalent materials embedded within solid water.

Immobilization and four-dimensional computed tomography

Management of respiratory motion is a critical aspect of SBRT planning and delivery of moving tumors. A number of techniques have been developed to account for tumor motion, either by minimizing respiratory motion via immobilization (e.g., abdominal compression, breath hold techniques) or by accounting for physiologic tumor motion via tracking or gating the beam-on time to a particular phase of the respiratory cycle. For example, abdominal compression works by limiting diaphragmatic excursion and thus the breathing-induced motion of the tumor. The efficacy of the selected immobilization system to reduce intrafraction tumor motion should be thoroughly evaluated. The set-up efficiency and patient's comfort level should also be evaluated.

Acquisition and use of four-dimensional computed tomography (4DCT) is a widely used technique to measure anatomical motion during quiet respiration. 4DCT accuracy should be evaluated by scanning a phantom with hidden targets of known geometry mounted on a 4D motion platform programmed with representative respiratory waves, either computer generated or from the patient. The reconstructed 4DCT images using amplitude- or phase-binning algorithms can then be compared against ground truth in terms of range, phase, trajectory, shape, and volume. The accuracy of the 4DCT-derived internal target volume from all or selected phases using maximum intensity projection should also be evaluated.

In-room imaging

Onboard image guidance utilizing volumetric techniques such as cone beam CT (CBCT) is indispensable for SBRT localization. Automatic online registration of CBCT and planning CT utilizes either rigid bony structures or soft tissue information or both. Registration accuracy with various sizes of the selected region of registration should be evaluated using phantoms with hidden targets, especially for targets that have a large variation in size and/or location compared with that at simulation. Automatic couch shifts should be measured against known values.

End-to-end test

It is essential to recognize that commissioning SBRT involves more than just ensuring that individual equipment works properly. The whole treatment chain must be tested, from simulation to localization and delivery. In addition, commissioning is also essential for establishing baseline parameters for quality control and improvement programs and processes. The end-to-end tests can be accomplished in-house with various commercial phantoms available. Alternatively, and in addition, independent verification of the whole process can be accomplished by utilizing a phantom delivery service such as that provided by the IROC-H.

Patient-specific considerations

Daily stereotactic body radiation therapy-specific quality assurance

Daily QA should be performed to verify the basic functionality and safe operation of the delivery and imaging equipment. For onboard imaging, collision interlocks should be tested to be functional, imaging and treatment coordinate coincidence should be within 1 mm, and repositioning accuracy using 2D/2D or 3D/3D match and automatic couch movement should be within 1 mm (14).

Target delineation

Accurate target delineation often requires multimodality imaging including CT, MRI, and PET. As a result of often differing imaging positions, deformable image registration is needed. Registration accuracy should be carefully reviewed slice by slice. Even for the best available deformable image registration techniques, error or uncertainty could amount to a few millimeters, which should be considered for target volume contouring. If the internal target volume (ITV) approach is used for lung tumor delineation, additional efforts should be made if the tumor is in the neighborhood of structures that have similar Hounsfield numbers (for example, chest wall or diaphragm). The clinician needs to review all phases of the 4DCT data set to assure that no portion of the tumor is missed.

Treatment planning

Noncoplanar beams or arcs with couch kick are commonly used to create a conformal dose distribution. For static fields, field aperture size and shape should correspond nearly identically to the projection of the PTV in the beam's eye view (i.e., zero margins). For lung tumors with IMRT, it is necessary to set a minimum dose objective on the ITV in order to achieve the desired hot spot in the GTV/ITV region. For arc delivery, collimator rotations are needed in order to prevent the tongue-and-groove effect from being along the same lines as the arc goes around the patient. Note that potential patient collision with the treatment device should be checked in the treatment room using the expected treatment couch coordinates with the immobilization device in place. Average CT or helical CT should be used for dose calculation. Maximum intensity projection (MIP) CT should not be used for dose calculation. Conformality of PTV coverage should be evaluated and recorded using conformity index as described in ICRU Report No. 83.

Patient-specific dosimetry quality assurance

SBRT IMRT should be performed in a composite way using high-resolution dosimeters, such as film. The ionization chamber should be used in the same phantom to assure correct absolute dose. Machine delivery log files may be analyzed against indented delivery sequences and fluence. 2D or 3D array dosimeters may also be used in addition to film measurements. Gamma analysis based on TG-119 recommendations should be performed. Many centers use 3% dose error global and 3 mm distance to agreement. Tighter tolerances—for example, 2% dose error local and 2 mm distance to agreement—should also be used to better identify potential limitations of either planning, delivery, or dosimetry techniques. The forthcoming AAPM TG-218 will have more recommendations, and further discussion can be found in Chapter 12.

For static fields, verification can be accomplished using an independent calculation program to assure correct monitor units. The calculation point should be selected to be in the center of the tumor to assure sufficient charge particle equilibrium.

Localization

Prior to treatment, CBCT should be acquired and registered with planning CT either automatically or manually. Alignment should be based on soft tissue or fiducials, but one should verify that bony anatomy is reasonable. The shifts should be reviewed and approved by the physician. Additional orthogonal kV fluoroscopy should be performed to confirm the localization of the tumor. If the target is not visible, static images should be taken to assure that no gross errors exist based on bony anatomy. If gating, target or fiducial should be inside the PTV when the beam is on. Where needed, kV fluoroscopy using one of the treatment beams should be performed to achieve a final confirmation of the treatment geometry. It is important to verify that couch coordinates do not change in between beams, as for some beams, the therapists have to move the couch to be able to get the gantry to where it has to go.

TOTAL BODY IRRADIATION

Total body irradiation (TBI) is frequently used as part of the conditioning regimen for hematopoietic stem cell transplant. In conjunction with chemotherapy, TBI is useful for eradicating residual malignant or genetically disordered cells and for immunosuppression prior to subsequent transplantation.

Commissioning

The goal of TBI is to deliver as uniform and accurate a dose as possible to the entire body. Because large variations in geometry and tissue density exist throughout the patient's body, dose delivery within ±10% of the prescription dose is standard, although higher dose deviations confined to smaller volumes, particularly in the extremities, are acceptable. Many centers use opposing anterior and posterior fields with the patient standing upright. Alternatively, patients can be irradiated with lateral fields in a sitting or partly reclining position. This approach is usually better tolerated by patients, but presents additional dosimetric challenges that must be addressed to improve dose uniformity. In addition, bone marrow transplantation protocols have strict time constraints. Therefore, a backup TBI system is important to assure the timing of successive fractions once the patient begins a course of TBI. If the primary system is unavailable, a fully commissioned backup TBI system must be available to complete the remaining treatment.

Absolute dose calibration of the large TBI field should be performed at the TBI treatment distance using water-equivalent phantoms of a minimum size of $40 \times 40 \times 40$ cm^3. The effects of both patient and room scatters are thus accounted for because the same conditions are used for calibration and treatment. Note that the tray at the linear accelerator head for holding compensating filters and the beam spoiler in front of the patient to increase skin dose must be in place in the dose calibration. Tissue-phantom ratios should be measured in the same set-up for a wide range of patient thicknesses of up to 60 cm to account for both large-size and pediatric patients.

Patient-specific quality assurance

Patient thickness measurements should be obtained at the prescription point (often at the level of the umbilicus) and at other points of interest for dose calculations and homogeneity determinations, such as head, neck, midmediastinum, midlung, pelvis, knee, ankle, and so on. Appropriate compensator thicknesses for different body parts should be determined to achieve the desired 10% dose homogeneity. Note that the thickness at the prescription point should be measured at the treatment position and verified at the first fraction.

Patients receiving TBI are normally not rigidly immobilized, and the compensator material is usually mounted at some distance from the patient, such as at the head of the linear accelerator. Therefore, a simple one-dimensional compensator constructed of lead, copper, or brass is adequate to even out the thickness variation from head to toe. If compensators are positioned in the head and neck region, care should be taken not to underdose the shoulders by shifting the compensator too far inferiorly. For the AP/PA technique, patient height should be measured to determine the appropriate source-to-patient distance to fit the patient within the field with sufficient margin around the patient (usually >5 cm). Best practice is for a medical physicist to be present at the first fraction of treatment. In vivo dosimetry should be used to assess dose delivery accuracy, homogeneity, and consistency.

For lung or other organ blocking, a simulation is required in the treatment position. Lung blocks can be designed on megavoltage radiographs generated by a linear accelerator with the patient in an upright position. Reference points for block placement at the time of treatment should be marked on the patient's body for reproducibility, which should be verified for each fraction. For the lateral technique, the arm can be used to shield the lungs. Care must be taken to cover the lung with the arm. For pediatric patients, the arm may not be large or thick enough to sufficiently cover the entire lung, for which additional saline bags may be used. Very young children who require anesthesia or careful lung/kidney shielding should be treated lying on the floor, with the gantry pointing downward and with the scatter screen and blocks placed above the patient.

TOTAL SKIN ELECTRON THERAPY

Total skin electron therapy (TSET) is an effective treatment for cutaneous T-cell lymphomas. Of the many techniques to deliver TSET, the most common is the modified Stanford technique, which typically uses two electron beams angled approximately 20° above and below the horizontal plane while the patient holds six different standing positions.

Commissioning

Percentage depth dose and absolute output should be measured in the total-skin-electron mode using a parallel plate chamber with a 1 cm thick plastic screen in place. Absolute output is the machine output at actual treatment distance (3–4 m) with the gantry at 90° (or 270°). Plastic screen serves as both an energy degrader and a scatterer. The screen increases the angular spread of the electrons, thereby causing them to hit the patient at a more oblique angle. This effectively decreases the penetration of the electrons, allowing for a more superficial depth dose and a more uniform deposition of dose across the skin. Note that stopping power ratio difference between a 1 m SSD electron beam and a degraded 3 m SSD electron beam can be as large as 10%, which can be obtained from the AAPM TG-21 report. Output variation with differing scatter-to-surface distance should also be measured. The output for the 12 treatment beams together (six directions and two gantry angles each direction) should be measured for monitor unit (MU) calculation in conjunction with the output data at gantry 90°. Decoupling output calibration into two steps will help establish baseline values for the future periodic QA. Vertical profile should be verified using film placed on the surface of a phantom. Note that the 50% off-axis ratio lies outside the edge of the light field so there is a gap between the edges of the respective light fields when properly abutted.

Patient-specific quality assurance

TSET's challenge is to treat the entire skin surface as evenly as possible. Dose homogeneity depends on patient position. Therefore, reproducing the positions of the Stanford technique is critical. Areas that could be underdosed (e.g., inframammary folds, gluteal folds, axilla, perineum, soles) should be monitored using thermoluminescent dosimeters (TLDs) or optically stimulated luminescent dosimeters (OSLDs). External eye shields should be used to protect the cornea and lens, in addition to shielding the nails of the hands and feet.

RADIOPHARMACEUTICALS

Preparation and equipment

In the United States, radiopharmaceuticals are predominantly classified as byproduct material according to Code of Federal Regulations Title 10 Part 20 (10 C.F.R. pt. 20), and are thus regulated by the NRC (15). As such, they must be included in a hospital's/clinic's license with associated authorized users (AUs) and authorized medical physicists (AMPs). Aside from inclusion on the license,

additional equipment, staffing, and space considerations must be made.

Re-entrant ionization chambers ("well chambers") or other related types of devices will be needed to take measurements of the radioactive material (RAM) itself, as well as to perform wipe test measurements (16); the latter of these will also require alcohol wipes (or similar) and containers for the wipes to perform measurements. A survey meter (ionization or scintillator) and Geiger counter will also be required. Disposable gowns, gloves, footwear, head coverings, and mouth and eye protection should be available to all staff working with RAM. Absorbent and/ or disposable sheeting/covering is recommended for all surfaces in rooms where RAM is prepared and measured ("hot labs"), as well as any rooms where patients will be staying during or after RAM administration, including bathrooms or other facilities that patients may use. Cleaning agents, especially those that foam and have greater absorption and do not easily run, as well as disposable towels and garbage containers, can be useful for managing spills. Depending on the type, form, and radioisotope of the radiopharmaceutical used, an array of shields will be necessary, either full-body or half-body lead shields to protect radiation workers and others when interacting with a patient who is being or has been administered a radiopharmaceutical, leaded glass shields to protect the body and face of workers when preparing or administering radiopharmaceuticals, lead shields or boxes for containing equipment or RAM storage, or shields for administration (such as syringe shields) to protect the hands of radiation workers delivering a drug through an IV. Each specific radiopharmaceutical may also come with or require a specialized set of delivery equipment and shielding based on vendor specifications (16). Additional equipment (syringes, vials, sterile water) may be needed for certain radiopharmaceuticals that require clinics to draw a patient-specific dose from a larger stock.

Dedicated hot lab space with access restricted to pertinent staff is required for measurement, preparation, and/or storage of radiopharmaceuticals; proper signage is required on doors to such spaces. Additional storage spaces for RAM can be designated with proper access restriction and signage. Rooms where patients must be kept before release should be carefully selected so that proper shielding, isolation, and signage can be maintained to protect other patients, hospital workers, and the general public. A log of visitors and time spent with radioactive patients can also be useful to minimize exposure of workers and/or guests. Cleaning agents and absorbent sheeting/covering, as described earlier for use in hot labs, may be required to address any potential spills or other contamination.

Commissioning

Ultimately, a proper quality and safety program for a given radiopharmaceutical is dependent on the agent itself. The first step in commissioning a radiopharmaceutical is coordinating among physicians, physics, relevant additional hospital personnel, the radiopharmacy, and/or the drug vendor to establish the needed equipment and recommended procedures for delivering a given drug. These discussions can help establish what dose levels are needed for a given drug and how many patients might be expected for treatment, data that can inform what is added to the license. A procedure should then be created that includes all the steps needed (including designating the personnel responsible) for determining the needed dose, ordering the dose, preparing the space for patient arrival, receiving the drug, preparing the drug, delivering the dose to the patient, determining whether and when the patient can be released, and holding the patient until release. Local regulatory agencies may provide rules as to when the patient may be released and/or provided with instructions for posttreatment management (17). In the United States, the NRC states that a patient must give less than 500 and 100 rem to any member of the general public for release and have instructions provided, respectively. Instructions are also given to determine the posttreatment survey readings for patients that correlate with those limits. Going forward, audits of the procedure, both periodic and just-in-time (immediately following issues or "near-miss" issues), should be performed. Practice runs of the procedure can also be performed with simulated doses and phantoms to gain comfort before the first patient delivery.

In parallel to (and as a component of) the procedure writing, dosimetric commissioning can be performed. Well chamber(s) should be traceably calibrated by sending the chamber(s) to a standards laboratory or acquiring a lab-calibrated source. A known activity source can be acquired, kept, and used to verify the functionality of the well chamber before each use. After this, for a given drug, at least one (or a couple more if possible) dose of a "known" (i.e., calibrated) activity should be ordered from a standards laboratory or by the company itself. These known doses should be similar in magnitude to a relevant patient dose, if possible; smaller doses, may be available only in some cases, or alternative radionuclides that should engender a "similar" response will be provided. Crucially, the drug should be prepared in the same vessel or form as it would be for a patient dose, owing to the highly geometric dependence of well chamber measurements; if the drug could be in multiple vessels or forms for dosing (e.g., a 5- or 10-mL syringe), all geometries should be independently analyzed. On many well chambers, a specific measurement channel can be assigned to a given RAM.

Upon receipt of the packaged RAM, it is brought to a shielded, controlled area (such as a hot lab) for storage and analysis. Before proceeding, the workspace should be surveyed with a Geiger counter to ensure that there is no contamination; contamination should be cleaned, triaged, and investigated before proceeding. The package should be inspected for damage, then wipe-tested for contamination before opening; if contamination is detected, efforts should be made to clean and/or contain the package

and areas of contact, and the transport carrier should be notified. Limits for wipe-test contamination, the need for additional measurements, and notification procedures may be specified by a local agency. In the United States 10 C.F.R. 71 and 49 C.F.R. 173 provide a table of acceptable contamination levels (dependent on whether the RAM is an alpha, beta, or gamma emitter), and require that survey meter measurements at the package surface are less than 2 mSv/hr (10 mSv/hr with specific conditions) and that the package has a transportation index (TI) less than 10 (18,19). If these conditions are not met, the carrier should be notified within 3 hours.

Once the RAM is removed from the outer packaging, the documentation included with the RAM should be inspected to ensure that it is the correct dose that was ordered, as well as to note the time and date of calibration so that the activity can be decay-corrected for time of measurement. The RAM itself is typically in a sealed shielded vessel (the "pig"), which should also be wipe-tested, as can the RAM container itself. Regulatory limits may exist for levels of acceptable contamination on the pig and/or the RAM container (such as <2,000 dpm/100 cm^2) (18). The user can attempt to clean the contaminated structures and/or contain the contamination within the hot lab. Using tongs, the RAM can be removed from the pig and measured in the well chamber; multiple measurements can be averaged to create a reading-to-activity conversion factor (additional data can be included from multiple RAMs, if available, to refine the conversion factor). After measurement, the RAM should either be stored in a shielded isolated area to decay or disposed of according to local radiation safety protocols. A Geiger counter can then be used to survey the entire work area, including the hands and/or shoe soles of any radiation workers in the hot lab during the commissioning. Any contamination should be carefully cleaned and any contaminated sheeting, pads, or cleaning equipment disposed of according to local radiation safety protocols.

Dose preparation, delivery, and patient release

When ordering a radiation dose for a patient, it is important to understand how early before treatment the vendor/radiopharmacy will need to be notified to prepare the desired dose. This information determines how early before patient treatment the dose might arrive. The package receipt and RAM assay procedure are very similar to that just described for the calibration dose, with some differences. When the package is opened, any documentation provided should be inspected to ensure that this is the correct dose for the correct patient. The predetermined reading-to-dose conversion factor is used to convert the well chamber measurement to RAM dose. This is compared with the decay-corrected RAM dose as determined from the vendor/radiopharmacy-supplied calibration certificate; some window of agreement should be applied to accept the dose for clinical use. Any variation between the two doses outside this window should be investigated, and/or the vendor/radiopharmacy should be contacted. The recorded patient RAM dose for documentation can be stated either as the vendor/radiopharmacy-supplied value (i.e., the user's measurement is a "verification" of the vendor/radiopharmacy dose) or the user's measured value (i.e., the user "trusts" his or her own measurement based on the calibration procedure).

After assay, the dose should be prepared for treatment according to the RAM-specific procedure. In addition, a measurement should be taken of the RAM in its prepared vessel, frequently at a known distance with a survey meter; this can be compared, in a similar set-up, with the RAM vessel after treatment to ensure that a sufficient amount

has been removed from the vessel. The patient can then be brought into the treatment room prepared for dose delivery. The patient is surveyed at a specified distance (typically 1 m) to obtain a pretreatment baseline. The RAM dose is administered, and the patient is surveyed at the same distance again to determine whether the dose has been delivered (i.e., the reading is above the baseline) and the patient can be released. If the reading is sufficiently high, the patient is held in the predesignated area until the readings show the patient can be released. Frequently, RAM doses will be high enough to require that instructions be provided to the patient describing how to manage as low as reasonably achievable (ALARA) principles for themselves and those they may live or consort with (17).

REFERENCES

1. Perks, JR, St George EJ, El Hamari K, et al. Stereotactic radiosurgery XVI: isodosimetric comparison of photon stereotactic radiosurgery techniques (gamma knife vs. micromultileaf collimator linear accelerator) for acoustic neuroma—and potential clinical importance. *Int J Radiat Oncol Biol Phys.* 2003;57(5):1450–1459.

2. Thomas, EM, Popple RA, Wu X, et al. Comparison of plan quality and delivery time between volumetric arc therapy (RapidArc) and Gamma Knife radiosurgery for multiple cranial metastases. *Neurosurgery.* 2014;75(4):409–418.

3. Lunsford LD, Flickinger J, Lindner G, et al. Stereotactic radiosurgery of the brain using the first United States 201 cobalt-60 source gamma knife. *Neurosurgery.* 1989;24(2):151–159.

4. Lindquist C, Paddick I. The Leksell Gamma Knife Perfexion and comparisons with its predecessors. *Neurosurgery.* 2007;61(3):130–141.

5. Maitz AH, Wu A, Lunsford LD, et al. Quality assurance for gamma knife stereotactic radiosurgery. *Int J Radiat Oncol Biol Phys.* 1995;32(5):1465–1471.

6. Mamalui-Hunter M, Yaddanapudi S, Zhao T, et al. Patient-specific independent 3D GammaPlan quality assurance for Gamma Knife Perfexion radiosurgery. *J Appl Clin Med Phys.* 2013;14(1):62–70.

7. Mutic S, Dempsey JF. The ViewRay System: magnetic resonance–guided and controlled radiotherapy. *Semin Radiat Oncol.* 2014;24(3):196–199.

8. ViewRay™ system for radiation therapy: License guidance. Nuclear Regulatory Commission. http://pbadupws.nrc.gov/docs/ML1317/ML13179A287.pdf.

9. Li HH, Rodriguez VL, Green OL, et al. Patient-specific quality assurance for the delivery of 60 Co intensity modulated radiation therapy subject to a 0.35-T lateral magnetic field. *Int J Radiat Oncol Biol Phys.* 2015;91(1):65–72.

10. Wooten HO, Rodriguez VL, Green OL, et al. Benchmark IMRT evaluation of a Co-60 MRI-guided radiation therapy system. *Radiother Oncol.* 2015;114(3):402–405.

11. Wooten, HO, Green O, Yang M, et al. Quality of intensity modulated radiation therapy treatment plans using a (60) Co magnetic resonance image guidance radiation therapy system. *Int J Radiat Oncol Biol Phys.* 2015;92(4):771–778.

12. Benedict SH, Yenice KM, Followill D, et al. Stereotactic body radiation therapy: the report of AAPM Task Group 101. *Med Phys.* 2010;37;4078–4101.

13. Solberg TD, Balter JM, Benedict SH, et al. Quality and safety considerations in stereotactic radiosurgery and stereotactic body radiation therapy: executive summary. *Pract Radiat Oncol.* 2012;2:2–9.

14. Klein EE, Hanley J, Bayouth J, et al. Task Group 142 report: quality assurance of medical accelerators. *Med Phys.* 2009;36:4197–4212.

15. Standards for protection against radiation. *Code of Federal Regulations.* Title 10, Part 20; 2015.

16. Dezarn WA, Cessna JT, DeWerd LA, et al. Recommendations of the American Association of Physicists in Medicine on dosimetry, imaging, and quality assurance procedures for 90Y microsphere brachytherapy in the treatment of hepatic malignancies. *Med Phys.* 2011;38(8):4824–4845.

17. United States Nuclear Regulatory Commission. Consolidated guidance about materials license. NUREG-1556, Vol. 9, Revision 2; 2008.

18. Packaging and Transport of Radioactive Materials. *Code of Federal Regulations.* Title 10, Part 71; 2015.

19. Shippers—general requirement for shipping and packaging. *Code of Federal Regulations.* Title 49, Part 173; 2015.

15 | Individual Patient-Based Peer Review for Photon and Proton Therapy

Genevieve M. Maquilan, Henry K. Tsai, and Hiral P. Fontanilla

INTRODUCTION

Quality assurance (QA) is an integral component of the practice of radiation oncology, involving the implementation of various patient and personnel safety measures. This chapter focuses on the individual patient-based peer review ("chart rounds"), particularly as it relates to proton therapy and highly conformal photon treatments. With the emergence of highly conformal and technically challenging treatment modalities, the role and quality of peer review have had to adapt. Additionally, there is increasing scrutiny of the use of proton therapy and other advanced technologies, and a comprehensive peer-review process serves as an important tool to document the appropriateness of treatment and multidisciplinary consensus. It can also reduce errors, cost, and improve quality of treatment.

The American College of Radiology (ACR) and American Society for Radiation Oncology (ASTRO) practice parameters for radiation oncology describe physician peer review as a typical component of a continuing quality improvement (CQI) program. The practice parameters acknowledge that the methods used for peer review are varied, but they encourage facilities to utilize the general concept of a weekly case-specific peer review, with the radiation oncologist presenting patients who recently started or will soon start treatment. They recommend that the conference be attended by radiation oncologist(s), physicist(s), dosimetrist(s), radiation therapist(s), and nursing staff. Items that should be reviewed by the other radiation oncologists in attendance should include indications for radiation therapy, target(s), dose per fraction, and total dose. Documentation of attendance and feedback given, as well as follow-up on feedback, should be completed (1).

ASTRO has published a white paper describing a prioritized list of items for peer review. Each item is assigned a priority level, with level 1 being the highest priority for peer review because of the presence of marked interpatient variations, level 2 the next highest (clinical situations for which guidelines or atlases are often available to guide decision making), and level 3 the lowest priority (clinical situations for which there is a general consensus in clinical practice and established standards). The list consists of seven items: (a) Decision to include radiation as part of treatment (level 2), (b) General radiation treatment approach (level 3), (c) Target definition (level 1), (d) Normal tissue image segmentation (level 3), (e) Planning directive (dose/volume goals/constraints for targets and normal tissues) (level 2), (f) Technical plan quality (level 2), (g) Treatment delivery, for example, patient set-up (first day is level 1, other days are level 2) (2).

These guidelines establish a framework for the physician peer-review process of patient-specific medical decisions, which is present in most practices but not standardized. A survey of peer-review QA meetings within North American academic institutions found variations in terms of whether chart rounds were conducted or not, thoroughness of discussion of each plan, frequency with which treatment changes were recommended, types of changes recommended, and the percentage of plans utilizing more advanced technologies that underwent peer review (3). Peer review was common for most external beam radiation treatments, but it was highly variable for more advanced technologies. More than 80% of the institutions surveyed in the study conducted peer review of all external beam therapy courses, but the rates were much lower for other modalities such as radiosurgery (58%) and brachytherapy (40%–47%) (3). There have

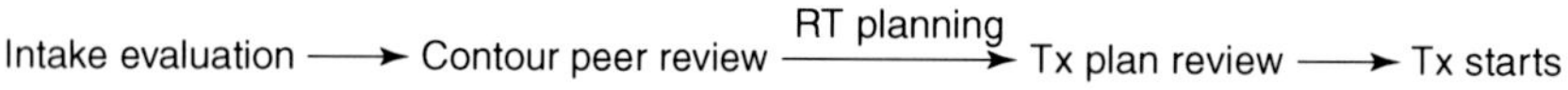

Intake evaluation ⟶ Contour peer review $\xrightarrow{\text{RT planning}}$ Tx plan review ⟶ Tx starts

FIGURE 15.1 Schematic workflow of a comprehensive prospective peer-review process.

been no reports in the literature regarding peer review of physician decisions specifically in proton therapy, although it often involves complex treatment plans and patients with uncommon clinical situations (e.g., reirradiation setting, rare histology, complex tumor locations).

Treatments with proton therapy and other advanced technologies such as stereotactic body radiation therapy (SBRT) would satisfy the definition of the level 1 priority for need for peer review under the ASTRO guidelines, as it represents treatment where there is significant controversy and lack of standard practice guidelines.

Princeton Radiation Oncology/NJ Procure Proton Therapy Center have developed a comprehensive prospective peer-review process, which we discuss here in the context of needs and challenges specific to proton treatment (4). Peer review begins at the earliest stage—at the time of referral. Cases are reviewed for appropriateness for proton therapy at daily rounds. The patient is then presented, after simulation but before treatment planning, at biweekly web-based chart rounds for review of the decision to treat, target and normal tissue contours, immobilization, treatment dose, and discussion of approach to treatment planning. After treatment planning is complete, the case is presented again, before the start of treatment, for review of the treatment plan with a focus on dose distribution, normal tissue constraints, robustness of plan, and anticipated toxicity (Figure 15.1). Recommendations made at any time in the review process are documented in a log by a dedicated member of the team and addressed by the treating physician.

In what follows, we describe strategies to integrate technology to facilitate a more timely and comprehensive review process to deliver high-quality treatment. We also discuss lessons that can be applied to develop similar programs for photon therapies, particularly in the community setting.

CHALLENGES IN THE IMPLEMENTATION OF PEER REVIEW

Various barriers are often cited as factors in preventing the institution of an effective, standardized, physician peer-review process. The aforementioned survey of North American academic institutions found that unprotected time for peer review led to decreased attendance. Additionally, the study found that the median amount of time spent on each patient was 2.7 minutes, and most of the changes that were made were ones that could be quickly reviewed. This finding suggests that the current practices for peer review are inadequate because of insufficient time dedicated to the process, often leading to omission of crucial items such as

review of target volume delineation, which would require a more in-depth examination (3). Another study of a more comprehensive "contour review" program found that the time required per patient was 8 minutes (5). An inquiry into the perspectives of Canadian radiation oncologists on peer review demonstrated that the majority of physicians recognized the benefits of peer review, but most felt the need for extra resources to implement a process of peer review into their schedules. Such resources would include designating a QA work code, assigning other health care providers to organize QA sessions, setting aside protected time, and ensuring that sufficient computer resources are available (6). We have found that biweekly rounds, with protected time for physicians, physicists, dosimetrists, and lead therapist, are feasible and lead to excellent participation by all members of the team.

The issues of physician time constraints, and the logistics of organizing a formal meeting, can be addressed with web-based applications allowing for virtual meetings and "offline" review of contours. We have used a web-based platform, with audio and visual communication, for the biweekly chart rounds that allows physicians who are off-site to participate. This can also be an important strategy for practices with multiple locations and solo practitioners in the community. For complex treatment modalities such as proton therapy, it allows experts in various locations to collaborate in peer review, further improving meaningful discussions. Such tools have been used successfully by academic programs to enhance peer review at satellite locations (5,7). Web-based applications through which virtual meetings can be conducted also allow increased utilization of the peer-review process.

Another strategy, particularly for physicians working at multiple locations, is "offline" peer review of contours using a central server. Contours would be completed by a physician along with relevant clinical information, and peers would be notified to review the case in the planning system as soon as possible and suggest modifications and/or ask questions. If interconnectivity with planning system is not possible, files with images of target volumes can also be uploaded to a secure server (Figure 15.2) along with relevant clinical information, where other physicians are able to access these files and review contours. By introducing flexibility into the process, this method of peer review of contours allows for more widespread use of a peer-review system, although live interactive sessions are ideal for appropriate discussion and should be the goal whenever possible. Additionally, it allows for peer review early in the process during target delineation, a stage at which in-depth review is needed.

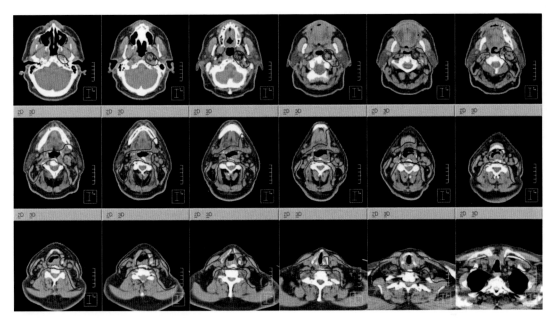

FIGURE 15.2 Sample PDF created from Pinnacle planning system for "offline" peer review of contours.

DECISION TO TREAT

The decision to use radiation therapy as a component of patients' treatment is an important area for peer review, particularly when considering proton beam therapy. This is assigned level 2 importance in the ASTRO recommendations and may be even higher priority for patients being considered for proton therapy. Use of radiation therapy in various clinical settings is guided by published guidelines, but appropriateness of a patient for proton therapy is an individual decision and can benefit significantly from peer review by radiation oncologists with expertise in proton therapy. This is also true because of the complexity and variety of patients treated at proton therapy centers, with relatively more patients getting reirradiation for rare tumors.

One particular strategy is to have daily "intake rounds"—multidisciplinary meetings during which all prospective patients are discussed before the formal consultation with a physician. The available data are reviewed for appropriateness for radiation therapy, particularly proton therapy. The presence of multiple physicians at this meeting, as well as nurses, physicists, dosimetrists, and radiation therapists, can further enhance this process. It also adds to the efficiency of workflow if appropriate patients are identified early and additional data that are required for consultation and treatment can be requested at the earliest time point. It can help the team better prepare for patient consultation by gathering relevant patient data, imaging, prior treatment records, and potential further testing. It also benefits patients who are not appropriate

for treatment and can thus be directed to other appropriate intervention sooner.

REVIEW OF TARGET VOLUMES

As with any conformal treatment, the highest level of importance is on peer review of target volume delineation, ideally, before the initiation of treatment planning. Target volumes (contours) guide all subsequent treatment decisions and are highly variable depending on the patient. Multiple studies have also demonstrated that target definitions may vary significantly between radiation oncologists (8,9), and AAPM Task Group-100 has identified target delineation as the single highest risk point for intensity-modulated radiation therapy (IMRT) treatments. Studies have also shown that contour review leads to meaningful patient-related changes in treatment. Cox et al published their experience with a prospective contouring rounds program and showed 9% rate of target volume modifications. A modification to contours after treatment planning has been completed or after the patient has started treatment leads to duplication of the work for the treatment planning and technical QA team and can be a significant strain on resources. Because of the amount of work involved with making such modifications after treatment has started, there may also be hesitation to suggest changes. Planning for proton therapy is time intensive and complex, and re-planning due to modifications would likely lead to patient treatment delays, inefficiencies, and possibly prohibitive costs. Thus, a comprehensive peer-review program for

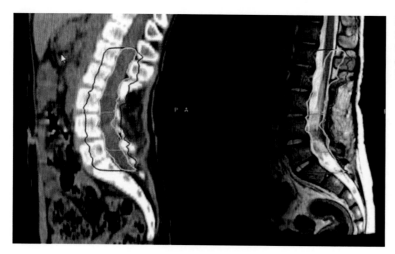

FIGURE 15.3 Detailed peer review of target volume definition with simulation CT and diagnostic imaging viewed side by side.

proton therapy, as well as other conformal therapy, must include prospective review of contours (5).

Oftentimes, we use diagnostic imaging to guide our contours, thus making the review of diagnostic imaging and fusion with simulation CT also very important. This is given a level 2 priority in the ASTRO guidelines. At our biweekly chart rounds, the presentation of contours is done with a split-screen view showing the fused diagnostic imaging (PET/CT, MRI, etc.) alongside simulation CT (Figure 15.3). The presence of radiologists during contour review could also be very valuable, particularly for complex cases, and may be feasible with the "offline" approach described earlier.

PROTON TREATMENT PLANNING AND PEER REVIEW

Proton therapy treatment planning and delivery are associated with unique challenges that have to be considered and addressed during the peer-review process. In proton therapy treatment planning peer review, there should be a particular focus on technical considerations, including immobilization and density changes in the path of the proposed beams. The precision of daily set-up can result in significant alterations in radiographic path length in the beam direction. For instance, patient rotations and variations in patient set-up may cause high-density tissues to move in or out of the beam path, thus resulting in changes in dose distribution. These may be accounted for with the use of appropriate planning target volume (PTV) margins, which may be beam specific, or with the use of range compensator "smearing" to address uncertainties in patient alignment or organ motion. Furthermore, changes in patient and/or tumor anatomy during the course of treatment due to weight loss or tumor growth/shrinkage may have unexpected consequences with respect to potential overdosing of distal normal tissues or underdosing

of target volumes. Tumor motion due to respiration may affect proton delivery as well, and discussion during the peer-review process can be held regarding whether techniques such as 4D-CT and internal target volume (ITV) constructs can adequately address these issues for each individual case. Finally, uncertainties regarding the beam range calculations and increases in relative biological effectiveness (RBE) at the end of the beam range require additional consideration, particularly when choosing beam angles that may be directed toward critical structures.

Thus, robustness of proton treatment planning is highly sensitive to patient- and tumor-specific variables and requires careful assessment at many levels. Peer review of proton treatment planning necessitates the participation of a multidisciplinary group, including physicians, physicists, dosimetrists, and radiation therapists, to identify and address these treatment planning issues, many of which are unique to proton therapy.

AN EXAMPLE PEER-REVIEW PROGRAM

A peer-review program for proton therapy must be comprehensive and so constructed as to most efficiently use resources including treatment planning. We have developed a comprehensive, prospective review process with specific needs of proton therapy treatment delivery in mind.

Since January 2013, we have implemented a policy of a comprehensive peer review. Cases are reviewed for appropriateness for proton therapy at daily intake rounds. Here all prospective patients are discussed before the formal consultation with a physician, and the available data are reviewed for appropriateness for radiation therapy, particularly proton therapy. All patients who are appropriate for radiation undergo simulation and are then presented at our biweekly chart rounds. A web-based application is used for participation from off-site physicians and physicists. All team members are encouraged to attend, and a minimum of two physicians are required to be present at each session; on average, there are four physicians present. The attending physician presents a detailed history and physical exam findings pertinent to the case, along with the planned prescription dose. Gross tumor volumes (GTVs), clinical target volumes (CTVs), and delineation of organs at risk (OARs) are reviewed on each axial slice along with appropriately fused relevant diagnostic imaging. Any suggested modification is documented. Also at this time, there is discussion about treatment planning considerations with selection of beam angles, a decision regarding treatment on fixed-beam versus gantry, passive versus active scanning, length of time needed for treatment planning, and patient start date, as well as specific treatment planning goals regarding target volumes and normal tissues (4).

Once volumes are approved, treatment planning begins. Treatment plans are again reviewed at chart rounds for each patient, with review of beam approach, beam weighting with special attention to end of range, robustness of plan, target coverage, and OAR doses. Isodose lines are reviewed on each axial slice, which provide the spatial information lacking in dose volume histograms. Standardized dose constraints that have been established at the center for each disease site are reviewed. This also provides the opportunity to discuss possible toxicity and management or anticipate the need for replanning during the course of a patient's treatment owing to anatomy changes. Documentation of the chart rounds sessions is done, which includes whether a patient was approved or modifications were suggested.

Over a six-month period from June 2013 to November 2013, 223 new patients were treated, and documentation of peer review at chart rounds was completed for 222 of the 223 patients (99.6%). An average of 9.2 cases were reviewed in each hourly chart rounds session. Modifications were suggested for 13 patients (5.9%) during contour review and for 17 patients (7.7%) during treatment plan review. An average of four physicians were present at each session (4).

Comprehensive prospective peer review is feasible, has led to significant treatment modifications, and provides a template that can be used by academic and community-based practices. In addition, use of web-based remote access to the sessions can increase participation and efficacy for practices with multiple locations.

REFERENCES

1. American College of Radiology. ACR–ASTRO practice parameter for radiation oncology. 2014. http://www.acr.org/~/media/7B19A9CEF68F4 D6D8F0CF25F21155D73.pdf

2. Marks L, Adams R, Pawlicki T, et al. Enhancing the role of case-oriented peer review to improve quality and safety in radiation oncology: executive summary. *Pract Radiat Oncol.* 2013;3:149–156.

3. Lawrence Y, Whiton M, Symon Z, et al. Quality assurance peer review chart rounds in 2011: a survey of academic institutions in the United States. *Int J Radiat Oncol Biol Phys.* 2012;84(3):590–595.

4. Fontanilla H, Cahlon O, Cardinale R, et al. Individual patient based peer-review at a proton center. Abstract presented at: American Society of Therapeutic Radiation Oncology; September 14–17, 2014; San Francisco, CA: American Society of Therapeutic Radiation Oncology.

5. Cox B, Kapur A, Sharma A, et al. Prospective contouring rounds: a novel, high-impact tool for optimizing quality assurance. *Pract Radiat Oncol.* 2015;5:e431–e436.

6. Hamilton S, Hasan H, Parson C, et al. Canadian radiation oncologists' opinions regarding peer review: a national survey. *Pract Radiat Oncol.* 2015;5:120–126.

7. Ballo M, Chronowski G, Schlembach P, et al. Prospective peer review quality assurance for outpatient radiation therapy. *Pract Radiat Oncol.* 2014;4:279–284.

8. Valicenti R, Sweet J, Hauck W, et al. Variation of clinical target volume definition in three-dimensional conformal radiation therapy for prostate cancer. *Int J Radiat Oncol Biol Phys.* 1999;44(4):931–935.

9. Spolestra F, Senan S, Le Péchoux C, et al; Lung Adjuvant Radiotherapy Trial Investigators Group. Variations in target volume definition for postoperative radiotherapy in stage III non-small-cell lung cancer: analysis of an international contouring study. *Int J Radiat Oncol Biol Phys.* 2010;76(4):1106–1113.

16 | Technical Issues of Safety in a Resource-Limited Environment

Mary Coffey and Ola Holmberg

INTRODUCTION

While there is broad agreement among experts that radiotherapy is a safe form of treatment, with more than 5 million treatments delivered annually in the world (1), it is also recognized that safety measures have to be further progressed at several levels for this rapidly developing medical application. Additionally, complex radiotherapeutic technology and procedures are increasingly being introduced into resource-limited countries and regions where they may not previously have been employed, and where safety challenges might be considerable. This chapter explores the issues of quality and safety in radiation oncology that are specific to resource-limited environments.

RADIATION ONCOLOGY IN A GLOBAL CONTEXT

The developing world now accounts for a high number of new cases of cancer globally. In many patients, cancer is diagnosed late and limits the effectiveness of life-saving treatment. Radiotherapy has long been recognized as an effective modality in the treatment of cancer, and it is estimated that more than 50% of patients with cancer would benefit from external beam radiotherapy (2). In many developing countries, there is no access at all to this treatment modality, and in a number of countries where there is some limited access, the availability may be extremely low. Rosenblatt et al (3) highlighted that in nearly 20 low- to middle-income countries, each radiotherapy unit available covers 5 million people, or more, compared with one radiotherapy unit for around 250,000 people in high-income countries. Expanding radiotherapy into countries and areas without current access has the potential to save many lives, but it is mandatory that the expansion be done with safety in mind, considering the complexity of this high-technology treatment modality and the potential for serious consequences when something goes wrong.

The term *resource-limited environment*, in the context of health care, has various definitions. Health care expenditure, or number of hospital beds in a country, are two approaches. The United Nations Scientific Committee on the Effects of Atomic Radiation (UNSCEAR) (1) uses a four-level health care model for the analysis of medical exposures, stratifying countries according to the number of physicians per head of population (Table 16.1). Compared with other models, this model was seen to have better correlation between stratification of country and number of medical radiation procedures overall in the country.

It is estimated (1) that around 50% of the world's population live in countries that are at level II, and that this percentage has been relatively constant for the last 25 years, whereas the world's population increased by 60% between the years 1977 and 2006. The other half of the world's population is roughly equally distributed between level I and level III/IV. It should be remembered, however, that resource-limited environments can also be heterogeneously distributed in a country; for example, a high-income country may have areas with lower resources, or a country may have a single very well-equipped and well-staffed radiotherapy facility but other radiotherapy facilities with much more limited resources. Overall, it has been observed (1) that the medical uses of radiation continue to increase in the majority of countries in the world, irrespective of their levels of health care.

THE SAFETY GAP AND NEEDS

In reviewing safety records in radiotherapy, it has been established that over the last three decades, at least 3,000 patients have been affected by radiotherapy incidents and accidents (4). Radiation accidents from medical uses have accounted for more early acute health effects and deaths

Table 16.1 Four-Level Health Care Model for the Analysis of Medical Exposures Used by UNSCEAR

Level	Number of Physicians per Head of Population
I	At least 1 for every 1,000 people
II	1 for every 1,000–2,999 people
III	1 for every 3,000–10,000 people
IV	Less than 1 for every 10,000 people

Source: From Ref. (1). United Nations Scientific Committee on the Effects of Atomic Radiation. *2008 Report to the General Assembly: Annex A on Medical Radiation Exposures.* New York, NY: United Nations Scientific Committee on the Effects of Atomic Radiation; 2010.

than any other type of radiation accident, including accidents at nuclear facilities (5). These accidents affect not only patients directly (e.g., harm and death), but also their family and friends, and might also undermine the public's confidence in the safety of such treatments. In addition, it has also been established that preventable medical errors, overall, cost billions of dollars each year (6).

Many types of resources are needed in a facility and in a country for the safe and effective performance of radiotherapy. These include a sufficient number of qualified experts who are well educated, specialized, and competent health professionals, such as radiation oncologists, radiation therapists, medical physicists, engineers, and radiation protection officers. There also has to be an appropriate regulatory framework, with competent national authorities (both radiation regulatory authorities and health authorities) establishing requirements and guidelines, authorizing and inspecting facilities and activities, and enforcing legislative and regulatory provisions. Additionally, it is essential to utilize only medical radiological equipment and software that is fully functional, safely designed, and in conformity with applicable standards. However, even when a facility or country has these resources, the safe and effective performance of radiotherapy is not guaranteed. An active and ongoing pursuit of safe practice supported by a positive safety culture is needed. This chapter examines each of these points in turn.

INTERNATIONAL STANDARDS AND REGULATION

The International Basic Safety Standards

Safety requirements covering medical uses of ionizing radiation are defined by national regulations. International harmonization of safety requirements is provided by the International Atomic Energy Agency (IAEA) by means of safety standards. The IAEA safety standards provide a system of Safety Fundamentals, Safety Requirements, and Safety Guides. They reflect an international consensus on what constitutes a high level of safety for protecting people and the environment from the harmful effects of ionizing radiation.

The relevant radiation safety requirements for radiation protection and safety in medicine are the *International Basic Safety Standards for Radiation Protection and Safety of Radiation Sources: International Basic Safety Standards* (BSS) (7) issued in 2014, cosponsored by the Food and Agriculture Organization (FAO), the International Labor Organization (ILO), the Nuclear Energy Agency (NEA), the European Commission (EC), United Nations Environment Program (UNEP), the World Health Organization (WHO), and the Pan American Health Organization (PAHO). The regulation of safety is a national responsibility, and many countries around the world adopt the BSS for use in their national regulations. Its requirements cover all practices, encompassing uses of radiation not only in medicine, but also in agriculture, industry, research and teaching, and intervention in the event of accidents and in chronic exposure situations such as those due to residues from past activities. Recommendations on how to comply with the requirements of the BSS are given within the IAEA Safety Standards Series in Safety Guides. When considering safety in medical uses of ionizing radiation, it is necessary to consider the patients, workers, carers and comforters, and volunteers in biomedical research, as well as the public.

Importance of a regulatory framework

The government is responsible, either through its own actions or through the actions of others, as required by law, to protect the safety of the public and the environment. Having an active regulatory program that performs all pertinent activities (authorization, inspection, and enforcement) is essential for the safe and secure use of radiation in medicine. The government's responsibility is to establish and maintain the legal and regulatory framework; establish regulations and guides; and perform inspections and enforcement actions.

The regulatory program has two main objectives: to protect public health and safety by preventing the availability and use of unsafe practices and equipment, and also to promote safe and effective practices and equipment that will enhance the public health and safety. A regulatory body typically does this by developing regulations, conducting inspections, and enforcement.

The IAEA supports its member states in establishing and strengthening national legal and regulatory frameworks, providing clear safety requirements for workers, patients, and public protection, and for control of radioactive sources from their production or import to their disposal or export, through the development of standards and guidance and the assistance to member states to implement these standards (8).

AVAILABILITY OF QUALIFIED EXPERTS

When developing a new radiotherapy center; expanding or refurbishing an existing center; or introducing new technology, techniques, or procedures, it must be ensured that the personnel delivering the service are competent in their area and that sufficient staff are available in each discipline; "excessive workload and a poor working environment can endanger patient safety" (9). In a resource-limited environment, this can create many difficulties. The number of professionals required in each discipline will be low, and therefore specialist education may not be considered viable locally or nationally. Difficulties with staff recruitment are also a recognized problem in resource-limited environments where salaries and career opportunities are necessarily limited. Often, in these situations, problems are exacerbated by the recruitment of expert staff by wealthier countries experiencing their own shortages, which can offer significantly better pay and conditions.

Primary education issues can be addressed, for example, by integrating with existing programs in related areas or sending identified personnel abroad for specialist education with a contractual requirement for a defined period on return. Continuing education, including preparation for the introduction of new technologies, techniques, or procedures, can be facilitated by industry, through e-learning or fellowships offered by organizations such as the IAEA or European Society for Radiotherapy and Oncology (ESTRO). Education programs at both primary and continuing levels should contain a module on safety and risk management. Education and experience provide the background knowledge and understanding that, although not leading to zero incidents, will enable staff to recognize both incidents that do occur and the potential weaknesses in the system where incidents might occur in the future.

Before initiating a service, it is important to define the roles, responsibilities, and the staffing levels required for safe practice. Recommendations on staffing levels have been devised on the basis of patient numbers by the IAEA (10). It is acknowledged "that staffing levels based on patient numbers are rigid in that they do not take into account variations in techniques, technology and services" and, based on this concept, the IAEA has, more recently, issued a report on the development of an activity-based algorithm (11). This activity-based algorithm gives greater flexibility to managers, allowing them to determine staffing requirements according to the local equipment level and types, workload, procedures, and techniques.

Complex techniques with associated small fields and high doses carry additional safety risks, and when developing the first center in a country or region, techniques such as three-dimensional conformal radiation therapy (3D-CRT) should be the starting point for implementation. Once staff become familiar with these techniques and have gained experience at this level, more advanced techniques can be pursued.

The regulatory body must require that health professionals with responsibilities for medical exposure specialize in the appropriate area and that they meet the requirements for education, training, and competence in the relevant specialty.

EQUIPMENT CONSIDERATIONS

The procurement, acceptance testing, and commissioning of new equipment (especially linear accelerators) is considered in detail in Chapter 7. The issues discussed there are relevant for any environment. The following sections focus on specific considerations for resource-limited environments, including the maintenance of equipment and the use of refurbished equipment.

Procurement

In modern radiotherapy, it is important to ensure that equipment specification is coordinated for the whole treatment chain. Ensuring connectivity between the treatment equipment and the equipment used for patient treatment planning, record-and-verify systems, and quality assurance is important when considering the correct transfer of essential data in the treatment chain. Manufacturers can help by incorporating effective safety design features, supplying easily understood user instructions and interfaces in the appropriate languages, and providing equipment that is compatible between different manufacturers (12). As part of the procurement procedure, accessory devices and quality assurance and radiation protection equipment must be included in the tender. In the decision-making procedure, all safety aspects must be considered. This should include consideration of future developments, new technologies or techniques, and increasing workload, as more referrals will be expected once the service is established. The essential accessory devices that should be included in procurement include laser alignment systems, immobilization devices, and a method of patient observation, preferably camera based. Procurement should also include an agreement for on-site applications training in the specific safety aspects associated with the individual equipment for purchase.

A qualified expert must be available to carry out the safety checks before the commencement of treatments and, ideally, should be involved in the full planning and decision-making process.

Maintenance and servicing considerations

As part of the tendering process, maintenance and servicing considerations must be taken into account. Service agreements must be drawn up to ensure consistency of service and prevent unnecessary downtime and potential equipment failure. The sustainability of service is a key component of effective radiotherapy, and it is vital for facilities in resource-limited environments to consider this aspect carefully.

The equipment maintenance program at a facility should be developed in cooperation with the manufacturer of the equipment. The level of on-site support will often depend on the availability of timely support from the manufacturer and the experience of the local engineer. The approach for unplanned maintenance should also be considered locally and in discussion with the manufacturer. This may be a critical area in resource-limited environments, and should be seriously considered and addressed in any tendering process, if feasible. The person authorized to perform a particular service on a piece of equipment, and the appropriate set of quality control measurements that must be taken by the medical physicist before equipment is returned to clinical use, must be documented and adhered to. Serious safety issues have resulted from lapses in this regard (13).

Refurbished equipment

Refurbished equipment can come in different forms. Equipment that has previously been installed and used in another facility may have been returned to its original operational status, or it may only have been cosmetically refurbished, whereas internal components may not have been replaced or updated. In regard to the acquisition of refurbished equipment, a number of issues merit serious consideration, including the following: (a) older equipment does not necessarily represent the current state of technology and may be less suited to deliver the benefits associated with modern technology; (b) spare parts may be in short supply or totally unavailable to support older equipment, in particular, mechanical parts; (c) older equipment may carry a higher risk of failure or breakdown; (d) training for new users of older equipment may be more difficult to arrange than for newly released equipment; (e) operation and service manuals for older equipment may be difficult to obtain; (f) connectivity with other pieces of equipment in the treatment chain may be more of an issue with older equipment than with newer equipment.

Sustainability of use must be carefully considered when intending to acquire and use refurbished equipment.

Maintenance and service of the refurbished equipment can be difficult with older pieces of equipment, including types of equipment with limited support from manufacturers. Facilities should consider costs of service contracts and extended warranties for the expected remaining life of the equipment and take this into account when refurbished equipment is purchased or donated. It must also comply with international safety standards, which should be documented in writing before purchase.

TECHNICAL CONSIDERATIONS AND SAFETY BARRIERS

Safety barriers at each step in the radiotherapy process

What are safety barriers?

James Reason, a psychologist and internationally recognized leader in the area of medical safety, developed the now famous Swiss cheese model (14) to illustrate the multifactorial nature of incidents. He proposed that most accidents or incidents could be traced to a number of underlying levels of failure. Safety barriers constitute a defense against specific failure points in a system. The introduction of safety barriers at perceived points of weakness limits the potential for incidents or accidents. To identify the points in a system where safety barriers would be most effective, it is first necessary to map the full process and, either through retrospective incident reporting or prospective analysis, or both, to determine potential risks before an incident occurs. Having identified the actual or potential risk, an appropriate safety barrier can be introduced. It is important to consistently review safety barriers as technology, techniques, or procedures evolve or change, and to remove barriers that are no longer effective or necessary as well as introducing new ones.

Overarching these safety barriers is the incident and near incident reporting and learning system, which, among other things, provides information on how well safety barriers are functioning. It should be emphasized that reporting is just one element of a safety culture where the information received is used to learn and improve safety through the introduction of safety barriers at an identified critical point. A recent study, carried out over a two-year period, demonstrated that having a departmental incident learning system resulted in an increased rate of reporting and staff participation with a decline in the severity of the near miss risk index over the same period (15).

A few safety barriers are presented later, in the context of the overall process steps where they may have an impact. There are more extensive lists of these types of barriers in other sources (16).

Patient evaluation. Comprehensive patient evaluation is an important aspect to consider and can affect both outcome and long-term quality of life. The decision to use radiotherapy as part of the overall treatment should be made at a multidisciplinary meeting. The timing of radiotherapy is important in the wider safety context reflected in the technique and dose to be used. Where a multidisciplinary team is not in place, consideration can be given to the use of teleconferencing to seek advice from external experts. This may also be a consideration in more resource-limited environments, where specialized external experts may complement the local experts. Incorrect decisions with respect to the optimum use of radiotherapy can result in higher risk to the patient.

The decision on the radiotherapy prescription should be made within clearly defined departmental protocols. These protocols should be developed by an interdisciplinary radiotherapy team to ensure that all perspectives are included. Protocols should be evidence based and reflect international best practice. Deviations from protocols should be clearly documented and justified. Having a variation in technique based on personal preference or local tradition, rather than evidence, leads to confusion and raises the potential for incidents to occur. Safety barriers at this level include checking that protocols have been adhered to or deviations clearly justified and peer-reviewed.

Peer review has been shown to be an effective safety barrier at several points in the radiotherapy pathway. The Royal Australian and New Zealand College of Radiologists developed a Peer Review Audit Tool for Radiation Oncology (PRAT) in 2006, which, following a review of its effectiveness, was revised in 2013 (17). External peer review can take the form of an external comprehensive clinical audit (18). The issue of peer review is considered further in Chapter 15 (and most of Section III) also with reference to issues that arise in environments with limited resources.

Pretreatment preparation—including image acquisition. The attention to detail with which the pretreatment preparation is carried out will reflect on the accuracy of the subsequent treatment and outcomes.

As in other parts of the radiotherapy treatment chain, ensuring the correct patient identification is crucial in the pretreatment preparation. Although this is not specific to resource-limited environments, there are several ways of addressing this, including the following:

- Patient identification card.

- Photos of the patient. To ensure patient confidentiality when photographs are used, the computer control panel should be positioned so as not to be visible to other patients or visitors.

- Verifying with patients their name and date of birth, to help ensure that the correct patient is being imaged.

- Biometric identification systems. Some centers are also introducing systems such as fingerprint scanners or eye recognition for secure patient identification.

Although some of the measures listed previously rely on high-technology measures that may be difficult to employ in a more resource-limited environment, there is no reason for any health care facility to abstain from using other low-technology safety measures in this regard. These types of safety barriers can act together to form a "defense-in-depth" against a misidentification of a patient at the time of image acquisition, which may affect the whole of the subsequent treatment.

Patient set-up reproducibility starts at the time of image acquisition. To ensure accurate reproducibility wherever possible, the same laser light system should be used throughout the department, both before treatment and at treatment. Centrally mounted and lateral laser lights are recommended for positioning to ensure accuracy in all directions and to avoid any lateral rotation. This may be more difficult in resource-limited environments, where equipment may be shared with, for instance, the diagnostic imaging department, and discussion may be necessary with the imaging department to provide an acceptable laser alignment system. When considering the purchase of a laser alignment system, it is important to select a system with fine laser lines for precision. Wide laser lines can lead to error in situations of patient remarking, and over the course of treatment a significant shift can occur in the skin markings. The laser system should be checked routinely as part of the quality assurance/quality control (QA/QC) program.

Other imaging considerations that manifest themselves in various ways in resource-limited environments include the following: CT bore size (may restrict imaging in the actual treatment position, and must be taken into account); CT slice thickness (for 3DCRT or intensity-modulated radiation therapy [IMRT], a slice thickness of 2–3 mm may be used; 5 mm for some other techniques); scan length (ensure that it is adequate for the planning purposes, and this should be protocol driven); flat tabletop insert (consistent with that of the treatment unit; must be available if the CT scanner is shared with the diagnostic imaging department); and indexing (tabletop inserts should allow for indexing for immobilization devices again to ensure accurate reproducibility (19)). If image fusion with MRI is being carried out, then it is important to ensure, as far as possible, that the patient is in the same position for both scans.

During simulation, it is also advisable that an RTT (radiation therapy technologist, a title recognized by ESTRO and the IAEA) accompanies the patients who are being imaged for radiotherapy to ensure accurate positioning for the purposes of treatment reproducibility, particularly in resource-limited environments, where the availability of the recommended accessory equipment may be limited.

During the image acquisition process, care and attention must be given to the identification of reference points for subsequent isocenter positioning. Shifts from reference marks denoted at the time of image acquisition have been identified as a significant cause of error (19). An example of this type of error is given in the Health Protection Agency Radiotherapy Newsletter (20). Clear and precise documentation of the reference points used is essential.

Treatment planning. Treatment planning is a critical safety step in the implementation of the treatment prescription. Errors introduced at treatment planning are systematic and may have serious consequences for the patient. Incidents reported to the IAEA-developed Safety in Radiation Oncology (SAFRON) reporting and learning system show that 612 of 1,306 event reports (47%) are related to the treatment planning phase (21).

Physicists, dosimetrists, or RTTs, depending on the resources available and the local circumstances, may carry out treatment planning. The critical issue is to ensure that whoever is carrying out the treatment planning is appropriately trained, and an important safety barrier is to have an independent verification of the treatment plan by a different health professional. An example of lapses in independent verification include the accident in Glasgow (22), which might have been prevented if a truly independent calculation check had been used.

Clinical peer review of treatment plans prior to treatment delivery is an additional safety barrier. This allows for independent verification of how well the treatment plan fulfills the prescription, and ensures that protocols are adhered to and deviations from the protocol are discussed and agreed to among peers.

Accurate data transfer is essential in the reproducibility of the treatment prescription. In its publication *Radiotherapy Risk Profile—Technical Manual,* the WHO reported that 38% of reviewed incidents in radiotherapy related to information transfer (4). Electronic transfer of data through a network system is the safest method, but in settings where this is not possible, transfer using a CD-ROM may be an alternative. A record-and-verify system is an important feature of safety, and it has been shown that reduction in the level of manual transfer that is required is directly linked to reduction in systematic error. Wherever possible, all equipment should be networked to the record-and-verify system. All data-transferred information should be double-checked by two independent professionals.

Immobilization devices. Accurate reproducibility is key to successful treatment outcome, particularly in the environment of 3DCRT and IMRT. Having positioned the patient correctly at image acquisition, it is then necessary to, in some way, fix that position for the duration of the treatment process. A wide range of immobilization devices and aids is available, but at a significant cost, and this must be considered in a resource-limited environment where one must make optimum use of the resources that are available. Immobilization devices should be index-linked to the treatment couch.

For some disease sites (e.g., head and neck), individualized immobilization masks are recommended, but in resource-limited environments, the cost of materials may make this policy difficult to implement, and immobilization masks may have to be reused. In this instance, it is essential that used masks be thoroughly cleaned and sterilized before second use. Using immobilization masks more than twice is not recommended, as the rigidity is reduced with each usage.

Immobilization devices should be appropriate to the site being treated and the patient condition. Patients who are comfortable will find it easier to maintain their position for the duration of the treatment delivery. An example of an appropriate immobilization device is use of a five-point fixation mask, which immobilizes the shoulders, when treating tumors in the lower neck region or below. If the patient has a tracheostomy in situ, the mask can be cut out to accommodate this. If this is not possible because of limited resources, an alternative method of shoulder fixation should be used.

Patients immobilized with masks must be carefully monitored throughout treatment as weight changes (loss or gain) resulting from treatment or treatment side effects, variation in nutritional support, or medication will result in an ill-fitting mask and therefore greater inaccuracy. Marking on immobilization masks must be both accurate and clear. Where a boost or additional treatment phase is prescribed the field marking for the additional fields must be clearly differentiated from the first field marking.

Breast boards can also be used for other thoracic treatments and are worth considering even in resource-limited environments. A good workshop can produce useful additional immobilization aids that significantly reduce the costs but can be equally effective; examples include knee rolls and foot stocks, which are very useful in stabilizing patient position for pelvic treatments. "It is often more practical and accurate to have minimal immobilization aids accurately placed by a skilled team of RTTs, than an over complex system" (23).

Treatment delivery and verification. Visual representation of the patient treatment position is a useful safety barrier and minimizes the possibility of treatment of an incorrect patient or site. In some cultures, patient images are unacceptable, so a detailed description of the set-up position must be provided; this description should include a diagrammatic representation.

The purpose of imaging at the initial treatment session is to verify that the treatment position is consistent with the prescription and the treatment plan. A systematic error may be detected at this stage before the commencement of treatment. Systems such as electronic portal imaging (EPI) depend on imaging of the bony anatomy and have limitations with respect to soft tissue motion; where soft tissue motion is likely to occur, 3D volumetric imaging is required. In many centers, the policy is to image on the first 3 days and on review of these images to make adjustments as necessary. The concept behind this approach is that the patients are naturally nervous on the first days of treatment and as they relax, a more accurate image of their position is gained. If there is a very significant difference at the time of the first image, this must be discussed with the clinician and adjustments made if considered appropriate. Imaging may then be carried out with a frequency determined by the resources available and the policy of the center.

In terms of verification of the dose delivered, in vivo dosimetry is one important safety barrier. In vivo dosimetry measures the actual dose delivered to the patient at the time of delivery. It can be used to verify the actual dose delivered to the field or to determine the out-of-field dose to a specific organ at risk (such as the lens of the eye). Correlations can be drawn between the dose measured at the skin surface and the dose delivered to the treatment volume. A wide range of detectors is available, and their use and cost should be assessed as a part of the equipment procurement process. Mijnheer et al (24) describe the range of detectors in their 2013 paper.

It is advisable that audio and visual systems be put in place for observing and communicating with patients during the treatment procedure. One reason for this is that the patient may become distressed, and termination of the treatment may be required to prevent a physical accident.

It is important to be able to speak to patients to reassure and calm them in these circumstances.

Weekly physician review is an important safety check. In addition to monitoring the patient response to treatment and to managing any side effects, during weekly review, dose errors can be detected and managed at an early stage in the process. In some instances, where radiation oncologist numbers are limited, weekly review can also include a suitably trained RTT or nurse or preferably both. Weekly review does not preclude the need for careful attention and daily monitoring of the patient by the treating RTTs.

Follow-up. Follow-up of patients is an important aspect both in respect of patient outcome and also to assess the effectiveness of the treatment approach. Follow-up has also resulted in the identification of unanticipated side effects, particularly in a group of patients that might indicate systematic errors. From the analysis of the Radiation Oncology Safety Information System (ROSIS) data, 23 of 754 errors were detected at follow-up (25). It would be preferable for follow-up to be carried out by a radiation oncologist, who will have a detailed knowledge of anticipated side effects and sites of possible metastatic spread. Where this is not possible, detailed follow-up guidelines should be provided with feedback to the radiation oncologist responsible for the patient.

REFERENCES

1. United Nations Scientific Committee on the Effects of Atomic Radiation. *2008 Report to the General Assembly: Annex A on Medical Radiation Exposures*. New York, NY: United Nations Scientific Committee on the Effects of Atomic Radiation; 2010.

2. Delaney G, Jacob S, Featherstone C, et al. The role of radiotherapy in cancer treatment: estimating optimal utilization from a review of evidence-based clinical guidelines. *Cancer*. 2005;104(6):1129–1137.

3. Rosenblatt E, Acuna O, Abdel-Wahab M. The challenge of global radiation therapy: an IAEA perspective. *Int J Radiat Oncol Biol Phys*. 2015;91(4):687–689.

4. World Health Organization. *Radiotherapy Risk Profile: Technical Manual of the World Health Organization*. Geneva, Switzerland: World Health Organization; 2008.

5. United Nations Scientific Committee on the Effects of Atomic Radiation. *2008 Report to the General Assembly: Annex C on Radiation Exposures in Accidents*. New York, NY: United Nations Scientific Committee on the Effects of Atomic Radiation; 2010.

6. Kohn LT, Corrigan JM, Donaldson MS, eds. *To Err Is Human: Building a Safer Health System*. Washington, DC: National Academy Press; 2000.

7. European Commission, Food and Agriculture Organization of the United Nations, International Atomic Energy Agency, International Labor Organization, OECD Nuclear Energy Agency, Pan American Health Organization, United Nations Environment Program, World Health Organization. *Radiation Protection and Safety of Radiation Sources: International Basic Safety Standards*. Vienna, Austria: International Atomic Energy Agency; 2014. IAEA Safety Series No. GSR Part 3.

8. Abdel-Wahab M, Rosenblatt E, Holmberg O, et al. Safety in radiation oncology: the role of international initiatives by the International Atomic Energy Agency. *J Am Coll Radiol*. 2011;8:789–794.

9. The Royal College of Radiologists. *Toward Safer Radiotherapy*. London, UK: The Royal College of Radiologists; 2008. www.rcr.ac.uk.

10. International Atomic Energy Agency. *Setting Up a Radiotherapy Program: Clinical, Medical Physics, Radiation Protection and Safety Aspects.* Vienna, Austria: International Atomic Energy Agency; 2008.

11. International Atomic Energy Agency. *Staffing in Radiotherapy: An Activity Based Approach.* Vienna, Austria: International Atomic Energy Agency; 2015.

12. Gilley DB, Holmberg O. Addressing patient safety through the use of "criteria of acceptability" for medical radiation equipment. *Radiat Prot Dosimetry.* 2013;153(2):155–157.

13. Spanish Society of Medical Physics. *The Accident of the Linear Accelerator in the "Hospital Clínico de Zaragoza."* Madrid, Spain: Spanish Society of Medical Physics; 1991.

14. Reason J. Human error, models and management. *Brit Med J.* 2000;320(7237):768–770.

15. Nyflott MJ, Zeng J, Kusano AS, et al. Metrics of success: measuring impact of a departmental near-miss incident learning system. *Pract Radiat Oncol.* 2015;5(5):e409–e416.

16. Ford EC, Fong de Los Santos L, Pawlicki T, et al. Consensus recommendations for incident learning database structures in radiation oncology. *Med Phys.* 2012;39(12):7272–7290.

17. Faculty of Radiation Oncology, The Royal Australian and New Zealand College of Radiologists. *Peer Review Audit Tool for Radiation Oncology.* Sydney, Australia: The Royal Australian and New Zealand College of Radiologists; 2013.

18. International Atomic Energy Agency. *Comprehensive Audits of Radiotherapy Practices: A Tool for Quality Improvement.* Vienna, Austria: International Atomic Energy Agency; 2007.

19. Mutic S, Coffey M, Purdy JA, et al. Simulation in the definition and determination of the treatment planning. In: Levitt SH, Purdy JA, eds. *Technical Basis of Radiation Therapy: Practical Clinical Applications.* New York, NY: Springer; 2012.

20. Public Health England. *The Radiotherapy Newsletter of the Health Protection Agency Supplementary Guidance Series: Good Practice in Radiotherapy Error Reporting*—No. 2. London, UK: Public Health England; 2010.

21. International Atomic Energy Agency. 2016. https://rpop.iaea.org/SAFRON.

22. Johnston AM. *Report of an Investigation by the Inspector Appointed by the Scottish Ministers for the Ionizing Radiation (Medical Exposures) Regulations 2000—Unintended Overexposure of Patient Lisa Norris During Radiotherapy Treatment at the Beatson Oncology Center, Glasgow in January 2006.* Edinburgh, UK: Scottish Executive; 2006.

23. International Atomic Energy Agency. *Transition from 2-D Radiotherapy to 3-D Conformal and Intensity Modulated Radiotherapy.* Vienna, Austria: International Atomic Energy Agency; 2008. IAEA-TECDOC-1588.

24. Mijnheer B, Beddar S, Izewska J, et al. In vivo dosimetry in external beam radiotherapy. *Med Phys.* 2013;40(7):070903.

25. Cunningham J, Coffey M, Knoos T, et al. Radiation Oncology Safety Information System (ROSIS)—profiles of participants and the first 1,074 incident reports. *Radiot Oncol.* 2010;97(3):601–607.

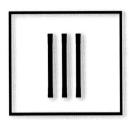

Quality in the Clinical Practice Setting

Adam P. Dicker

17 Creating a Culture of Safety and Empowerment

Dennis R. Delisle and Nicholas A. Thompson

INTRODUCTION

Millions of individuals suffer from the result of unsafe care such as medication errors and hospital-acquired conditions (1,2). The estimated annual cost of such errors, of which nearly 80% are system-derived, is $17 to $29 billion (3,4). These staggering issues were thrust into the public spotlight through the Institute of Medicine (IOM) reports *To Err Is Human* and *Crossing the Quality Chasm* (3,5). Economic and financial pressures have forced the health care industry to face these issues head on (6). The situation is exacerbated by U.S. gross domestic product projections estimating health care expenditures to account for nearly 20% of national spending by 2020 (7).

Health care executives acknowledge patient safety and quality as the number one priority. The close tie to financial reimbursement and the threat posed by safety and quality issues to an organization's fiscal health are also significant (8). In response to the unsustainable financial crises, the federal government continues to drive reform through reimbursement models tied to outcomes. Provider payments are now tied to performance and value. Providers will no longer receive reimbursement for hospital-acquired conditions, readmissions, and other harm-related events (9–11). Pressure from Centers for Medicare and Medicaid

Services (CMS) and other third-party payers has made the monitoring of quality data a critical component in the delivery of care (12).

In 1999, the Agency for Healthcare Research and Quality (AHRQ) was appointed as the federal lead in patient safety. AHRQ was tasked with developing research and partnerships aimed at improving the reliability and safety of health care delivery by: (a) identifying preventable errors; (b) developing effective strategies and approaches to reduce errors and improve safety; and (c) sharing knowledge and best practices across the industry (13). In the complicated health care delivery environment, systems and processes must align with organizational culture. Many errors result from the fragmented systems and processes, as does a culture that neither promotes nor supports transparency and teamwork.

Table 17.1 describes the elements of effective and safe health care delivery as defined by the IOM. Achieving these aims is difficult in the health care setting, which is layered with intricate levels of complexity and variability. Health care providers face challenges with individual patient variability (e.g., comorbidities, socioeconomic status), incomplete or insufficient information (e.g., lack of electronic health records (EHRs) or EHR interoperability),

Table 17.1 IOM Elements of Health Care

Safe	Patients should not be harmed by the care that is intended to help them.
Effective	Care should be based on scientific knowledge and offered to all who could benefit, not to those unlikely to benefit.
Patient-centered	Care should be respectful of and responsive to individual patient preferences, needs, and values.
Timely	Waits and sometimes harmful delays in care should be reduced both for those who receive care and for those who give care.
Efficient	Care should be given without wasting equipment, supplies, ideas, or energy.
Equitable	Care should not vary in quality because of personal characteristics such as gender, ethnicity, geographic location, and socioeconomic status

Source: From Ref. (5). Institute of Medicine. *Crossing the Quality Chasm: A New Health System for the 21st Century*. Washington, DC: National Academy Press; 2001.

rapidly evolving technologies, and financial constraints and regulatory pressures (5,3,14). Improvement efforts, driven by groups such as AHRQ, IOM, and the Institute for Healthcare Improvement (IHI), seek to reduce safety-related errors by addressing the various components (9). Safe, effective care must be balanced with optimal resource consumption and standardization. Accountability and learning can drive improvements in safety, and also yield cost reductions (15). The culture of safety becomes an integral driving force of such change.

CULTURE OF SAFETY

The culture of safety describes the environment within which health care providers work and their perception of and ability to improve and maintain safety. The culture of blaming people for errors is prominent, despite meaningful and significant progress in quality and safety over the years. In a 2012 AHRQ annual patient safety culture survey, results showed, on average, that 65% of respondents worried that mistakes they made were kept in their personnel files, and 50% agreed that staff felt that their mistakes were held against them (16). Traditionally, when errors are made, the approach has been to seek out, blame, and punish the employee at the source of the event. This short-sighted view omits the contributions of system and process gaps that lead to these errors, such as lack of communication and transparency, and poor teamwork (17).

Just Culture

Lucian Leape stated: "The single greatest impediment to error prevention in the medical industry is that we punish people for making mistakes" (18,19). This blame culture generates a fearful environment that results in an unnecessarily high number of medical errors (5,19–21). Consequentially, employees fear punitive measures for their mistakes, which prevents open admittance of errors and shared learning (19,22,23). Kelleher (24) and Marx (22) identified this environment as one of the biggest threats

to a successful organization; instead, they advocate for Just Culture—often referred to as "just safety culture"—which creates a supportive environment of open dialogue to facilitate safer practices (21,25).

Just Culture enables improvements in patient safety by managing human error and leveraging these errors as learning experiences for collective improvement (21,22,25). It includes proactively identifying, reporting, and investigating incidents to take corrective action and avoid reoccurrences (21,22,26). Specifically, Just Culture enables uninhibited reporting and identification of adverse events, thorough evaluations of these events, information sharing of safety issues, organizational learning, staff training and education in patient safety, and teamwork around safety issues (21,26,27). Instead of focusing on who caused the problem, the focus is on what went wrong. However, culture change is challenging, and health care organizations are encountering difficulties in creating and sustaining Just Culture from their current blame-based culture (21).

Table 17.2 describes the way in which behaviors are categorized. *Human error* defines inadvertent actions that deviate from what should have been done. To manage human errors, leaders need to consolidate and reinforce the processes and procedures to ensure increased awareness and understanding. *At-risk behavior* increases the potential for safety issues. The individual may be unaware of these behaviors or mistakenly assume that his or her actions are justified, not risky. At-risk behaviors require immediate coaching and guidance to enhance the individual's situational awareness. Lastly, *reckless behavior* describes a disregard of risks. Such behaviors must be met with the appropriate remedial or punitive responses given the significance and implications of reckless actions. The balance lies in differentiating between the various behaviors and system/process issues (28).

System and process issues mainly drive errors. Error prevention cannot be achieved through individuals working harder in broken systems of care (29). Errors are inevitable, but the goal for providers is to ensure that the error does not reach the patient (30). System and process improvement

Table 17.2 Types of Behaviors

Behavior	Description	Ways to Manage
Human error	Inadvertently doing other than what should have been done; lapse, mistake	Console and reinforce through process and procedure training
At-risk	Behavior that increases risk where risk is not recognized, or is mistakenly believed to be justified	Coach to increase situational awareness Align incentives for positive behavior
Reckless	Behavioral choice to consciously disregard a substantial and unjustifiable risk	Remedial action Punitive action

Source: From Ref. (34). Page A. *Making Just Culture a Reality: One Organization's Approach.* San Francisco, CA: Agency for Healthcare Research and Quality; 2007; Marx D. Patient safety and the just culture. Talk presented at: The Just Culture Community; 2007.

can reduce the risk of future errors and enhance the effectiveness of safety protocols and procedures (31).

Communication is central to fostering a culture of safety. Poor teamwork and communication is the biggest barrier to ensuring a safe environment for patients (8). In the health care setting, communication issues are compounded given the diversity of care providers and settings. Handoffs pose a significant risk of error when patients transition across the care continuum or even between providers (31).

Elements of safety that have to be incorporated into the culture are (32):

- Emphasis on learning—focus on learning from experiences and from others, learning from errors or near misses

- Systems perspective—processes and employees should align toward common goals and be designed to reduce or eliminate the risk or occurrence of errors

- Leadership—clinical and nonclinical support, promoting transparency, accountability, and blame-free environment

The formation of a Just Culture requires a concerted effort, not just isolated training programs and the use of some quality improvement tools (5,20,21,33). The entire organization must place a high value on near-miss and incident reporting. Learning from errors or near misses helps direct attention toward safety (34). Staff begin to shift thinking toward risk assessment, error or near-miss reporting, solution development, and low-risk behavior (28). Patient safety is everyone's responsibility, but it requires the support and diligence of leadership to maintain focus. Cultural change is a slow and deliberate process that requires focus, discipline, and transparency (32). To drive change, health care leaders need to commit to zero patient harm, incorporate safety principles throughout the organization, and deploy best practices and improvement methodologies to drive results (31). In order to identify where to begin, leaders need to assess the cultural environment.

Assessing the culture

Assessing the safety culture enables identification of high-risk areas and processes. Various surveys cover a variety of

depth and breadth, from organizational to unit-specific (35). Many health care organizations annually conduct employee patient safety surveys to assess the culture (i.e., annual) (16,36). Safety can be evaluated on three dimensions: (a) organizational; (b) unit; (c) individual. Table 17.3 outlines the components within each dimension. Organizationally, leaders must have a commitment to and engagement with patient safety activities (e.g., safety huddles, root cause analyses). Leaders need to commit resources to develop, support, and improve safety-related efforts. This financial commitment demonstrates the level of priority leaders place on safety. Transparency in clinical outcomes and dashboard reporting further emphasize the importance of safety within the health care setting. At a local level, units drive safety through policies and procedures as well as recognition and support activities. Individual elements of safety include the perception of shame or blame for errors as well as the viewpoint on learning from mistakes. These dimensions offer a holistic view of an organization.

External pressure to improve safety has led to many organizations taking an introspective view of their culture. Payers, regulators, and accreditors have used safety assessments to inform policy, reimbursement, and other changes (37). AHRQ's Patient Safety Indicators are an example of a methodology employed to assist organizations quantify patient safety events and high-risk areas (16). Additionally, AHRQ developed the Hospital Survey on Patient Safety Culture to assess the culture of safety.

High-reliability organizations

High-reliability organizations (HRO) are defined by their results. Organizations that are highly reliable have predictable and effective operations within a high-risk setting and produce consistent, safe outcomes (38,39). Industries such as air traffic control and nuclear power exemplify HROs. The study and implementation of high-reliability principles has transitioned into health care (31). Organizations that embrace high reliability are said to have a "collective mindfulness" across all employees. Employees are relentlessly looking for and reporting deviations or unsafe conditions before those conditions manifest into a substantial risk or issue (40). In health care, *reliability* can be defined as patients receiving the appropriate tests, medications, and information at the right time (41).

Table 17.3 Evaluating Safety

Organizational	Unit	Individual
Engagement in patient safety activities	Safety policies/procedures	Fear of shame
Commitment of organizational resources	Recognition and support for safety	Fear of blame
Emphasis on safety		Learning

Source: From Ref. (35). Singer S, Meterko M, Baker L, et al. Workforce perceptions of hospital safety culture: development and validation of the patient safety climate in healthcare organizations survey. *Health Serv Res*. 2007;42(5):1999–2021.

HROs embrace safety as everyone's responsibility. Their commitment to the culture of safety has these main principles (42):

- Understanding and appreciation of organization's high-risk nature and need to ensure safe operations

- Blame-free environment, promoting transparency and reporting of errors or near misses

- Collaboration across teams, hierarchy, disciplines to solve problems

- Commitment of organizational resources to address safety concerns

The principles of reliability have been demonstrated in various industries and have direct application in the health care setting. The methods of evaluation and improvement provide a systematic framework to align systems and processes with employees to produce consistent results (43). HROs hardwire the principles into everything they do. The intense, relentless focus on error prevention and risk identification is a hallmark of HROs (31). Not only are employees expected to speak up, they have an obligation to do so, as part of the mission to ensure safety. Table 17.4 describes the safety and high-reliability continuum for organizations. As organizations move from the initial states to approaching zero-harm, trust is ingrained, accountability is self-managed, errors and near misses are transparent and consistently reported, systems are proactively improved, and the safety culture assessment is an integral element of the organization's performance.

Developing a culture of safety

Developing and sustaining a culture of safety requires a significant organizational commitment. Organizational structures, systems, and processes have to align with safety goals, as do individual behaviors, performance assessments, and rewards (15). From senior leaders to frontline staff, employees need to be engaged, trained, and evaluated on their contributions to safety (32,44). Organizationally, groups like AHRQ are dedicated to providing the insight, resources, and best practices to drive health care safety through areas such as (13)

- Information technology

- Performance reporting

- Medication safety

- Simulation and training

- Evidence-based tools and resources

Table 17.4   Safety Culture and High Reliability

Safety Culture	Beginning	Developing	Advancing	Approaching
Trust	Trust is not assessed	Behavioral expectations developed and adopted in some areas	Leaders establish trusting environment through role modeling	High level of trust in all areas; self-management of behaviors
Accountability	Blaming culture, emphasis on individuals, not processes	Disciplinary processes are equitable and aligned with system versus individual error	Equitable and transparent disciplinary procedures aligned with elements of safety culture	All staff recognize and own their personal accountability; transparent disciplinary procedures adopted throughout organization
Identifying unsafe conditions	Limited root cause analyses, near misses are not evaluated	Near-miss reporting begins, some early interventions developed	Staff recognize and report unsafe conditions	Close calls and unsafe conditions routinely reported; early and preventive interventions developed and implemented
System improvement	Limited assessment of system performance and gaps	Begin conducting root cause analyses to assess opportunities for improvement	System issues identified, prioritized, and addressed	Proactive system assessment and improvement throughout organization
Evaluation	No evaluation of culture	Limited assessment and scope of safety culture	Safety culture assessed throughout organization; improvement efforts developed	Safety culture measures reported to board and component of organization's performance scorecard

Source: From Ref. (31). Chassin MR, Loeb JM. High-reliability health care: getting there from here. *Milbank Q.* 2013;91(3):459–490. doi:10.1111/1468-0009.12023.

High reliability and safety are founded on three main concepts: prevention, identification and mitigation, and redesign (43). Prevention emphasizes proactive improvements of potentially high-risk areas, systems, and processes. Identification and mitigation target deviations from standards, confusion in processes/procedures, and workarounds that could lead to errors. Redesign is a result of learning and evolution in processes and structures to reduce or eliminate the likelihood of an error occurring in the future. Each step of this reliability model reduces opportunities for error and enhances individual, unit, and organizational performance and reliability (43).

There is a proven set of improvement methodologies that augment the use of reliability principles. Lean, Six Sigma, and change management have been shown to effectively improve clinical and operational performance as well as enhance employee engagement (45,46). Process improvement and cultural transformation require systematic approaches through a formal framework. This enables direct linkage from individual tasks and responsibilities to organizational results and priorities (47).

IMPROVING THE CULTURE OF SAFETY THROUGH EMPOWERMENT

An empowered workforce is defined by a learning culture—one that recognizes there is always more to learn and strives to continuously improve (48). Organizations like Toyota, Microsoft, Apple, Zappos, and UPS could not have generated high-quality products, maintained service quality at low costs, or achieved high growth rates without such an empowered workforce (48). These high-reliability organizations, among others, hold lessons for the health care industry as it progresses toward enhanced quality and safety.

Improvement strategies

Empowering employees and forming a Just Culture are only the initial steps toward improving quality and patient safety. Improvement strategies, including TeamSTEPPS and Lean Six Sigma as well as nine other strategies drawn from other industries, will lead to enhanced quality and safety.

TeamSTEPPS

TeamSTEPPS—Team Strategies and Tools to Enhance Performance and Patient Safety—was developed by the AHRQ and the Department of Defense to improve quality and safety in health care settings, and combines lessons from more than 25 years of team performance research (49). As a teamwork and communication tool focused on four competencies—leadership, situational awareness, mutual support, and communication—TeamSTEPPS is used to change cultures, develop team cohesion, impact the quality of work environments, and improve employee retention (50–56).

Of the four competencies, leadership is the most important and should be emphasized, especially because most health care professional education does not adequately address it and leadership directly affects the level of success achieved by the other competencies (51,57). *Leadership* in this case is defined as "the process of influencing others to accomplish a mission" (51,58). In contrast, *management* is defined as the "organization and coordination of the activities of an enterprise in accordance with certain policies and in achievement of clearly defined objectives" (51). Situational monitoring includes an awareness of the patient's status, fellow team members, and the surrounding environment as the team pursues its missions or goals (51,52). This awareness enables proactive identification of potential risks and enables another core competency: mutual support. Mutual support entails team members, especially leaders, recognizing when another's workload becomes overwhelming in order to proactively prevent even the risk of errors (49). Communication is the last competency and includes verbal and nonverbal strategies to improve team cohesion and interactions (51,52).

TeamSTEPPS is built on the foundation that teams make better decisions than individuals, and the TeamSTEPPS model is meant to be used by groups that solve unique problems through coordinated action (49). Through TeamSTEPPS, health care professionals are encouraged to use specific tools and strategies. For example, TeamSTEPPS provides various strategies to improve team cohesion and communication, including check-back, Situation Background Assessment Recommendation (SBAR), callout, and I PASS The BATON (51,52). Check-backs validate information communicated between team members through a closed loop, whereas callouts convey critical information during an emergency (51). SBAR is a standardized method used to give patient status updates to physicians, and I PASS The BATON is a mnemonic for patient handovers outlining introduction, patient, assessment, situation, safety, background, actions, training, ownership, and next (51).

Briefings, huddles, and debriefings are also used to promote leadership and support the team. *Briefings* are discussions of the objectives of the work and the roles each team member will play in achieving the expected outcomes (49). A *huddle* is used to discuss critical events or emergencies (49). Lastly, the *debriefing* is used to continuously improve processes and systems through discussion of any near misses and proactive prevention (49).

Successful TeamSTEPPS implementation results in three outcomes: knowledge, attitude, and performance (49). Similar to team unity, the knowledge outcome is a mutual understanding of situations and a consistent alignment of team members toward the same goals (49). Mutual trust is the attitude outcome of TeamSTEPPS that results from teams working through situations together, and can only be built in organizational cultures that focus on accountability rather than blame (i.e., Just Culture) (49). Finally, performance outcomes include the team's ease of adapting to new situations, accuracy of decisions, efficiency, productivity, and overall safety (especially in relation to the patient) (49).

TeamSTEPPS began with crew resource management (CRM) in the 1970s. CRM was first used in a National Aeronautics and Space Administration (NASA) workshop to improve safety and reduce the number of fatal accidents and injuries due to human error (49,59). NASA shifted its attention from errors attributed to mechanical failure and training to team communication and CRM. Today, TeamSTEPPS has been used in hospital operating rooms (ORs), the Veterans Health Administration, and in neonatal intensive care units (NICUs).

The importance of effective communication in the OR cannot be overstated: a patient's life depends on the coordination and functioning of the surgical team. The team must be able to share information quickly and accurately to ensure successful patient outcomes (49). Utilizing briefings and debriefings resulted in an improvement in the appropriate use of prophylactic antibiotics from 85% to 97%, and the number of issues requiring follow-up fell from 44% to 0% (49). In addition, 79% of team members felt that the introduction of briefings and debriefings improved patient safety and team cohesion in the OR (49).

In a different OR, the on-time start rates and operative times of cases performed by urology services were vastly improved through TeamSTEPPS implementation. The OR experienced a reduction of 10% in overall case time, and the on-time first-start rate increased from 49% to 70% (60). With OR time costing approximately $15 per minute, the 10% reduction in overall case time will significantly improve revenues (60,61). Additionally, overall patient safety issues declined from 16% to 6% ($P <.001$) (60).

Texas Health Resources (THR) is a nonprofit health care system of 14 acute care hospitals that implemented TeamSTEPPS with positive results (51,62). THR realized increases in all four competencies at 8 of the 10 hospitals that implemented TeamSTEPPS; inconsistencies in leadership are correlated with the two facilities that did not see improvements (51).

As the nation's largest health care system, the Veterans Health Administration (VHA) is made up of 153 total hospitals throughout the United States (49,63). The VHA used TeamSTEPPS to study the relationship between team training and surgical outcomes. Through a retrospective study, the VHA confirmed that team training reduced surgical mortality. Annual mortality fell by 18% at 74 facilities, whereas 34 facilities that did not have the training experienced a reduction of only 7% (49,63).

Sawyer et al (64) reports that positive teamwork behaviors have been correlated with higher quality of care during neonatal resuscitation. In order to study this correlation, NICU staff completed TeamSTEPPS training courses and were tested in medical simulations (64). The staff completed pre- and posttraining questionnaires about attitudes and knowledge of teamwork, as well as a pre- and posttraining simulation (64). The training resulted in significant improvements in teamwork skills during neonatal resuscitation and an increase in the chances of a nurse speaking up and preventing the incorrect medication dose ordered by the physician (64).

Lean Six Sigma

To increase revenues, reduce costs, and improve quality, health care leaders are adopting creative solutions such as a Lean Six Sigma (65). Lean is a set of concepts, principles, and tools used to create and efficiently deliver the most value from the customer's perspective by utilizing the knowledge and skills of those performing the work (31,66–68). Sigma is a measure of variability (i.e., standard deviation), which means that the higher the sigma level, the higher the performance of the system; for example, 4σ represents 6,210 defects, whereas 6σ represents 3.4 defects per million opportunities (65,69,70). Six Sigma tools focus on improving the outcomes of a process by reducing the frequency of defects; together, Lean and Six Sigma tools produce improved processes that translate into enhanced quality that is implemented and sustained through change management (31,45,46,65). Lean Six Sigma is focused on improving customer satisfaction, reducing cycle time, and decreasing defects (65).

Before Lean Six Sigma was applied for quality improvement in the 1990s, it was used in manufacturing to reduce defects and variation, and eliminate errors (65). It can be applied in health care to enhance patient safety and medical errors, which are the leading cause of death in the United States (65).

Lean Six Sigma can be applied through the DMAIC approach to problem solving. DMAIC—Define, Measure, Analyze, Improve, Control—provides a five-step improvement cycle to improve processes and continuously reduce errors (70). The first step, Define, is defining the project by identifying problems, establishing scope, and defining objectives; the current performance should then be measured and compared with data, often through a value-stream map that shows all of the process steps (70,71). The third step—Analyze—consists of identifying root causes or the source of the problems, as well as understanding best practices (70). The Improve step includes testing solutions, measuring results, and standardizing solutions to fix and prevent problems (70). Finally, continuous improvement is built into the process through controls (70). Lean quality improvement initiatives are often made through kaizen—"change for better"—events (72).

Numerous scenarios exist in health care where Lean Six Sigma can be applied to improve quality, reduce waste, and increase efficiency. For example, rearranging work areas, standardizing workflows, and improving labeling in storage closets are all potential opportunities for the application of Lean Six Sigma (73). Other examples include reducing the number of transfers, improving ED flow and reducing waiting time, improving scheduling of appointments, and reducing turnaround time for patient tests (65,74). The examples that follow outline applications of Lean Six Sigma, including improved surgical quality, medication-related patient safety events, and resident team response to a hospital-based cardiopulmonary arrest.

Although surgical quality depends on numerous factors, the quality of instrument delivery is imperative (72). Errors in processing may lead to wasted time, increased costs, and decreased quality, including surgical infections and perioperative morbidity (72). Improvements were made in surgical instrument processing through a series of 1- to 5-day kaizen events that were further improved through team huddles (72). These kaizens generated greater efficiency through process redesign and standardization, along with physical rearrangement of the space to create better flow (72). The new process included successive checks to prevent errors, better definition of each operator's role, and communication back to the team through the recording and posting of identified errors (72). After the process was implemented, there were only 44 errors out of 4,594 surgical procedures, which represented a 69.3% improvement in the rate of errors for the same time frame (72).

Headwaters Health Care Center is an 87-bed hospital in Ontario, Canada, that experienced 1.3 serious medication-related patient safety events per 10,000 orders (71). Through value stream mapping, opportunities were identified to eliminate waste, improve flow, and standardize the process from a physician writing a medication order to the receipt of medicine by the patient (71). The hospital made a public commitment to reducing medication-related patient safety events by half within a one-year period and involved patients in the initiative; the improvement was inexpensive to implement and resulted in a significant impact: a reduction from 1.3 to 0.07 events per 10,000 orders within 10 months (71).

Residents are often excluded from quality improvement training and initiatives, but present an opportunity to improve patient care and expand the reach of process improvement initiatives (67). Residents were trained in Lean thinking, and one team piloted a Lean thinking approach to evaluate the response to an in-hospital cardiopulmonary arrest (67). The team created a current and future state value stream map with frontline staff and other stakeholders to optimize the process (67). The team successfully addressed a safety issue while engaging in a learning experience to improve the future delivery of patient care (67).

Other strategies

User-centered designs utilize visibility, affordance, constraint, and forcing functions. Visibility could include a written set of instructions to use on a piece of equipment or labels that denote where a piece of equipment should be stored. Affordance shows how an activity should be performed; this may include marking the correct arm before surgery to eliminate the chance of wrong-side surgery. A constraint makes it difficult to do the wrong thing, and a forcing function makes the wrong thing impossible to do (27).

Making processes similar by eliminating waste and standardizing them decreases the memory burden associated with them. Protocols and checklists remind staff of the processes to follow and minimize problem solving. For example, auto-populating the usual dose of a medication into an electronic order system is just one way to simplify and standardize processes (27).

Interruptions, distractions, long hours, and staffing can all affect patient safety. The burden of these can be reduced through teamwork, the reduction of distractions from the workspace such as cell phones or food, and the creation of "safe zones" to reduce distractions and interruptions.

It is unreasonable to expect staff to remain vigilant without aids for 10- to 12-hour shifts. Breaks, rotating staff, alarms, and checklists can all maintain staff vigilance for longer periods (27). For example, having different alarms for more serious situations than those for less serious situations decreases reliance on staff vigilance (27).

As showcased through TeamSTEPPs, teamwork and collaboration are both extremely important to promote effective communication and generate a culture of safety (27). Effective teamwork and communication are especially important during patient handoffs and in time-sensitive situations, such as during surgery (27). Importantly, many health professionals lack formal training in teamwork, which leads to deficits when teams are mobilized in the workplace (51,52).

Patients are the customers of health care. Similar to the way Lean Six Sigma places an emphasis on the customer, patients and their families should be at the center of the health care delivery process, especially when making decisions about medications or treatments and creating discharge plans (27). Putting patients and families at the center gives them some control, enables a better understanding of the care they are receiving, and allows them to correct any misinformation (27). The "voice of the customer" is essential to generating the highest quality care outcomes for patients as well as optimizing processes that directly affect them (31).

Utilizing frontline staff when creating new processes and pilot-testing these processes when implementing them helps overcome many pitfalls and obstacles before widespread implementation begins (27). For example, piloting a new electronic incident reporting system in a few practices would be more successful than undertaking a larger implementation, because a smaller rollout would be easier to change if any problems occur.

Even the best plans and designs may be subject to errors, but proactive planning for recovery will allow easier and faster resolution of errors. Simulations and drills to practice events such as infant abductions or fires enable smoother, less stressful recoveries in real-life situations (75). Additionally, even the most reliable process is subject to potential issues; high-reliability organizations are consistently preoccupied with failures and are always able to correct processes if problems arise (31). "The hallmark of a high reliability organization is not that it is error-free, but that errors don't disable it" (31,40).

Information to make informed decisions must be available when care is being delivered (75). This just-in-time information may include drug formularies, patient records, or laboratory results, which are often provided through electronic or mobile programs (75).

REFERENCES

1. Institute of Medicine. *Preventing Medication Errors: Quality Chasm Series*. Washington, DC: National Academies Press; 2007.

2. Klevens RM, Edwards JR, Richards CL Jr, et al. Estimating health care-associated infections and deaths in U.S. hospitals, 2002. *Public Health Rep.* 2007;122(2):160–166.

3. Kohn LT, Corrigan JM, Donaldson MS & Committee on Quality of Health Care in America,Institute of Medicine. (1999). *To err is human: Building a safer health system.* The National Academies Press.

4. Leonard M, Frankel A, Simmonds T, et al. *Achieving Safe and Reliable Healthcare: Strategies and Solutions.* Chicago, IL: Health Administration Press; 2004.

5. Institute of Medicine. *Crossing the Quality Chasm: A New Health System for the 21st Century.* Washington, DC: National Academy Press; 2001.

6. Lee TH. Turning doctors into leaders. *Harv Bus Rev.* 2010;88(4):50–58.

7. Office of the Actuary, National Health Statistics Group. 2012. www.cms.gov/research-statistics-data-and-systems/statistics-trends-and-reports/nationalhealthexpenddata/nationalhealth acountsprojected.html.

8. Makary M. *Patient Safety; Hospital Risk— Perspectives of Hospital C-Suite and Risk Managers.* New York, NY: American International Group; 2013.

9. DesHarnais SI, Nash DB. Reforming way medical students and physicians are taught about quality and safety. *Mt Sinai J Med.* 2011;78(6):834–841. doi:10.1002/msj.20302; 10.1002/msj.20302.

10. Normand SL, Wolf RE, Ayanian JZ, et al. Assessing the accuracy of hospital clinical performance measures. *Med Decis Making.* 2007;27(1):9–20. doi:10.1177/0272989X06298028.

11. Wachter RM. Patient safety at ten: unmistakable progress, troubling gaps. *Health Aff.* 2010;29(1):165–173. doi:10.1377/hlthaff.2009.0785.

12. Gould BE, Gray MR, Huntington CG, et al. Improving patient care outcomes by teaching quality improvement to medical students in community-based practices. *Acad Med.* 2002;77(10):1011–1018.

13. Agency for Healthcare Research and Quality. *A Decade of Evidence, Design, and Implementation.* Rockville, MD: Agency for Healthcare Research and Quality; 2012.

14. Schulman PR. General attributes of safe organisations. *Qual Saf Health Care.* 2004;13(Suppl 2):ii39–ii44. doi:10.1136/qshc.2003.009613.

15. Carroll JS, Rudolph JW. Design of high reliability organizations in health care. *Qual Saf Health Care.* 2006;15(Suppl 1):i4–i9. doi:10.1136/qshc.2005.015867.

16. Agency for Healthcare Research and Quality. *Hospital Survey on Patient Safety Culture: 2012 User Comparative Database Report.* Rockville, MD: Agency for Healthcare Research and Quality; 2012.

17. Institute for Healthcare Improvement. (2009). Overview of the IHI 5 million lives campaign. Retrieved from http://www.ihi.org/offerings/Initiatives/PastStrategicInitiatives/5MillionLivesCampaign/Pages/default.aspx.

18. Leape LL. *Testimony, United States Congress.* Washington, DC: House Committee on Veterans' Affairs; 1997 (October 12).

19. Abujudeh H, Bruno M. *Quality and Safety in Radiology.* New York, NY: Oxford University Press; 2012.

20. Cook HH, Guttmannova K, Joyner JC. An error by any other name. *Am J Nurs.* 2004;104(6):32–43.

21. Khatri N, Brown GD, Hicks LL. From a blame culture to a Just Culture in health care. *Health Care Manage Rev.* 2009;34(4):312–322. doi:10.1097/HMR.0b013e3181a3b709.

22. Marx D. *Patient Safety and the "Just Culture": A Primer for Health Care Executives.* New York, NY: Agency for Healthcare Research and Quality; 2001.

23. Tucker AL, Nembhard IM, Edmondson AC. Implementing new practices: an empirical study of organizational learning in hospital intensive care units. *Manag Sci.* 2007;53(6):894–907. doi:10.1287/mnsc.1060.0692.

24. Kelleher, B. Engaged employees = high-performing organizations. *Financial Executive.* 2011;27(3):51-53.

25. Scott-Cawiezell J, Vogelsmeier A, McKenney C, et al. Moving from a culture of blame to a Just Culture in the nursing home setting. *Nurs Forum.* 2006;41(3):133–140.

26. Kirk S, Parker D, Claridge T, et al. Patient safety culture in primary care: developing a theoretical framework for practical use. *Qual Saf Health Care.* 2007;16:313–320. doi:10.1136/qshc.2006.018366.

27. Barnsteiner J. Teaching the culture of safety. *Online J Issues Nurs.* 2011;16(3):1–14. doi:10.3912/OJIN.Vol16No03Man05.

28. Marx D. Patient safety and the Just Culture. New York, NY: Talk presented at: The Just Culture Community; 2007.

29. Gibson R, Singh J. *Wall of Silence: The Untold Story of the Medical Mistakes That Kill and Injure Millions of Americans.* Washington, DC: LifeLine Press; 2003.

30. Gawanda A. *Complications: A Surgeon's Notes on an Imperfect Science.* New York, NY: Henry Holt; 2002.

31. Chassin MR, Loeb JM. High-reliability health care: getting there from here. *Milbank Q.* 2013; 91(3):459–490. doi:10.1111/1468-0009.12023.

32. Singer S. *What We've Learned About Leveraging Leadership and Culture to Affect Change and Improve Patient Safety.* San Francisco, CA: Agency for Healthcare Research and Quality; 2013.

33. Pronovost PJ, Weast B, Holzmueller CG, et al. Evaluation of the culture of safety: survey of clinicians and managers in an academic medical center. *Qual Saf Health Care.* 2003;12(6):405–410.

34. Page A. *Making Just Culture a Reality: One Organization's Approach.* San Francisco, CA: Agency for Healthcare Research and Quality; 2007.

35. Singer S, Meterko M, Baker L, et al. Workforce perceptions of hospital safety culture: development and validation of the patient safety climate in healthcare organizations survey. *Health Serv Res.* 2007;42(5):1999–2021.

36. Sexton JB, Helmreich RL, Neilands TB, et al. The safety attitudes questionnaire: psychometric properties, benchmarking data, and emerging research. *BMC Health Serv Res.* 2006;6:44. doi:10.1186/1472-6963-6-44.

37. Carroll J, Hatakenaka S. Driving organizational change in the midst of crisis. *Sloan Manag Rev.* 2001;(42):70–79.

38. Weick K, Sutcliffe K, Obstfeld D. Organizing for high reliability: processes of collective mindfulness. In: *Research in Organizational Behavior.* 1st ed. Stamford, CT: JAI Press; 1999:81–123.

39. Roberts K. Some characteristics of one type of high reliability organization. *Org Sci.* 1990;1:160–176.

40. Weick K, Sutcliffe K. Managing the unexpected: resilient performance in an age of uncertainty. San Francisco, CA: Jossey-Bass; 2007.

41. Nolan T, Resar R, Haraden C, et al. Improving the reliability of health care. IHI Innovation Series White Paper. Boston, MA: Institute for Healthcare Improvement; 2004.

42. Agency for Healthcare Research and Quality. Patient safety primers. 2014. https://psnet.ahrq.gov/search?Site2Search=PSNet&q=Patient+safety+primers&f_resource_typeID=220.

43. Institute for Healthcare Improvement. (2009). Overview of the IHI 5 million lives campaign. Retrieved from http://www.ihi.org/offerings/Initiatives/PastStrategicInitiatives/5MillionLivesCampaign/Pages/default.aspx.

44. Pronovost PJ, Berenholtz SM, Goeschel CA, et al. Creating high reliability in health care organizations. *Health Serv Res.* 2006;41(4, pt 2):1599–1617.

45. Delli-Fraine JL, Langabeer JR, Nembhard IM. Assessing the evidence of Six Sigma and Lean in the health care industry. *Qual Manag Health Care.* 2010;19(3):211–225. doi:10.1097/QMH.0b013e3181eb140e.

46. DuPree E, Martin L, Anderson R, et al. Improving patient satisfaction with pain management using Six Sigma tools. *Jt Comm J Qual Patient Saf.* 2009;35(7):343–350.

47. McAlearney A, Song P, Garman A, et al. Promoting safety and quality through human resource practices. Chicago, IL: Agency for Healthcare Research and Quality; 2011. Contract Final Report No. 290-06-0022-5X.

48. Hirsh S. Learning is the "secret sauce" for any high-performing organization. *J Staff Dev.* 2014;35(1):76.

49. Plonien C, Williams M. Stepping up teamwork via TeamSTEPPS. *AORN J.* 2015;101(4):465–470. http://dx.doi.org/10.1016/j.aorn.2015.01.006.

50. Clapper TC. Next steps in TeamSTEPPS®: creating a just culture with observation and simulation. *Simulation & Gaming.* 2014;45(3):306–317. doi:10.1177/1046878114543638.

51. Clapper TC, Kong M. TeamSTEPPS®: the patient safety tool that needs to be implemented. *Clin Simulat Nurs.* 2012;8(8):e367–e373. doi:10.1016/j.ecns.2011.03.002.

52. Agency for Healthcare Research and Quality. TeamSTEPPS fundamentals course: Module 4. In: *Situation Monitoring: Instructor's Guide.* Rockville, MD: Agency for Healthcare Research and Quality; 2006. http://www.ahrq.gov/professionals/education/curriculum-tools/teamstepps/index.html.

53. Harvey EM, Wright A, Taylor D, et al. TeamSTEPPS® simulation-based training: an evidence-based strategy to improve trauma team performance. *J Cont Educ Nurs.* 2013;44(10):484–485. doi:10.3928/0022012420131025-92.

54. Howe EE. Empowering certified nurse's aides to improve quality of work life through a team communication program. *Geriatr Nurs.* 2014;35(2):132–136. doi:10.1016/j.gerinurse.2013.11.004.

55. Liaw SY, Lau TC, Siau C, et al. An interprofessional communication training using simulation to enhance safe care for a deteriorating patient. *Nurse Educ Today.* 2014;34(2):259–264. doi:10.1016/j.nedt.2013.02.019.

56. Meier AH, Boehler ML, McDowell CM, et al. A surgical simulation curriculum for senior medical students based on TeamSTEPPS®. *Arch Surg.* 2012;147(8):761–766. doi:10.1001/archsurg.2012.1340.

57. Hicks CM, Bandiera GW, Denny CJ. Building a simulation-based crisis resource management course for emergency medicine, phase 1: results from an interdisciplinary needs assessment survey. *Acad Emerg Med.* 2008;15(11):1136–1143. doi:10.1111/j.1553e 2712.2008.00185.x.

58. United States Army Cadet Command. *Citizenship in Action and Leadership: Theory and Application.* Boston, MA: Pearson; 2005.

59. Marshall D. *The History of Crew Resource Management: From Patient Safety to High Reliability.* Centennial, CO: Safer Healthcare; 2010.

60. Weld L, Stringer M, Ebertowski J, et al. TeamSTEPPS improves operating room efficiency and patient safety [published online ahead of print on April 17, 2015]. *Am J Med Qual.* doi:10.1177/1062860615583671.

61. Bacchetta MD, Girardi LN, Southard EJ, et al. Comparison of open versus bed-side percutaneous dilatational tracheostomy in the cardiothoracic surgical patient: outcomes and financial analysis. *Ann Thorac Surg.* 2005;79(6):1879–1885.

62. Sheppard F, Williams M, Klein VR. TeamSTEPPS and patient safety in healthcare. *J Health Care Risk Manag.* 2013;32(3):5–10. doi:10.1002/jhrm.21099.

63. Neily J, Mills PD, Young-Xu Y, et al. Association between implementation of a medical team training program and surgical mortality. *JAMA.* 2010;304(15):1693–1700.

64. Sawyer T, Laubach VA, Hudak J, et al. Improvements in teamwork during neonatal resuscitation after interprofessional TeamSTEPPS training. *Neonatal Netw.* 2013;32(1):27–33. doi:10.1891/0730-0832.32.1.26.

65. Turney J. Six Sigma and Lean Six Sigma. *Radiol Technol.* 2007;79(2):191–192.

66. Lean Enterprise Institute. What is Lean? 2015. www.lean.org/WhatsLean.

67. Kim KS, Lukela MP, Parekh VI, et al. Teaching internal medicine residents quality improvement and patient safety: a Lean thinking approach. *Am J Med Qual.* 2010;25(3):211–217. doi:10.1177/1062860609357466.

68. Womack JP, Jones DT. *Lean Thinking, Banish Waste and Create Wealth in Your Corporation.* 2nd ed. New York, NY: Free Press; 2003.

69. Pande P, Holpp L. *What Is Six Sigma?* New York, NY: McGraw-Hill; 2003.

70. Taner MT, Sezen B, Antony J. Overview of Six Sigma applications in healthcare industry. *Int J Health Care.* 2007;20(4):329–340. doi:10.1108/09526860710754398.

71. Critchley S. Improving medication administration safety in a community hospital setting using Lean methodology. *J Nurs Care Qual.* 2015;30(4):1–7. doi:10.1097/NCQ.0000000000000112.

72. Blackmore CC, Bishop R, Luker S, et al. Applying Lean methods to improve quality and safety in surgical sterile instrument processing. *Jt Comm J Qual Patient Saf.* 2013;39(3):99–106.

73. Norris B. Human factors and safe patient care. *J Nurs Manag.* 2009;17(2), 203–211. doi:10.1111/j.1365-2834.2009.00975.x.

74. Pexton C. One piece of the patient safety puzzle: advantages of the Six Sigma approach. 2005. www.psqh.com/janfeb05/sixsigma.html.

75. Barnsteiner, J. Teaching the culture of safety. *The Online Journal of Issues in Nursing.* 2011;16(3): 1-14. doi:10.3912/OJIN.Vol16No03Man05.

18 Clinical Testing of Quality and Safety Measures

Kevin L. Moore and Arno J. Mundt

WHY TEST FOR QUALITY AND SAFETY?

As the motivations for improving quality and safety in radiation oncology have been extensively discussed in the preceding chapters, in this contribution we consider how to establish whether a particular initiative did in fact result in improved quality and safety. This may strike the reader as a strange question, or perhaps one that should be rephrased to consider instead *whether* a quality and safety initiative should require testing at all. We can begin here and advance the argument that any new initiative that alters previous practice of any kind deserves at least the consideration of validation testing, although the exact nature of that testing will depend on the intervention and a cost-benefit analysis of administering any systematic investigation.

To frame the discussion of clinical testing of quality and safety, consider an analogy to therapeutic drug administration. If a new drug purports to offer higher quality therapy than an existing standard-of-care pharmaceutical, it must undergo the well-known (and incredibly expensive) battery of clinical trial testing, culminating in a phase III randomized controlled trial (RCT). However, some ancillary systems in drug administration, for example, an infusion pump, will be implemented without undergoing anything like a RCT. Needless to say, all of the systems involved in drug delivery have undergone testing of some kind or another, although the precise nature of the validation study will depend strongly on the degree to which the intervention separates itself from existing processes. A new infusion pump with a purportedly more accurate administration of intravenous pharmaceuticals need demonstrate little more than safe medical operation before clinical implementation; an expensive double-blind trial comparing old and new infusion pumps would be laughably inappropriate.

For quality and safety interventions in radiation oncology, a similar spectrum clearly exists between low-impact, low-cost changes up to high-impact, high-cost changes, with the degree of validation testing required scaling up in proportion to the expected impact of the new intervention and the amount to which the new system departs from established past experience. A clinician's responsibility is, first and foremost, to the well-being of the patients, but this responsibility must extend to the demonstration of what effect new interventions have on existing processes. We would argue that early adopters of a new technology have an added responsibility to demonstrate, at least to themselves, what benefit (if any) is offered by the incorporation of a new process to the patients under their care. The responsibility to the larger medical community is perhaps less direct, yet, thankfully, the incentives of academicians are generally coaligned with the sharing of an institution's experience so that these studies can inform the decision-making process of the wider community. Quantifying the magnitude of any quality improvements and their implementation costs allows others to have requisite information for a cost-benefit analysis of whether to adopt new technologies or not. This does not let late adopters off the hook, of course, as their fiduciary duty to their patients would compel them to at least verify to some degree the benefits claimed by early adopters, even if this verification can be of a much smaller scale than earlier foundational studies.

To this point we have spoken of these clinical tests of quality and safety measures either in analogy or in the abstract. For the sake of this discussion, we identify a *quality intervention* as one involving the use of a tool or system to improve some known or suspected continuous variable associated with a radiotherapy treatment (e.g., reduced normal tissue complication risk from improved treatment planning, or better concordance between planned and delivered dose distributions from the use of on-treatment imaging). By way of contrast, we identify a *safety intervention* as the use of a tool or system to prevent some discrete negative action from occurring (e.g., a retina scanning system designed to disallow treatment unless the correct patient is properly identified prior to treatment). The reader is encouraged not to take this distinction as a strict one; obviously, if a particular continuous quality variable deviates by a very large amount, this could represent a safety concern. However, this functional distinction will, we hope, help clarify the differences in the testing of new safety interlocks from quality improvement measures such as knowledge-based treatment plan quality assessment.

The remainder of this chapter focuses on examples and designs of clinical tests of quality and safety measures in radiation oncology. The full spectrum of quality and safety interventions in radiation oncology spans a much wider set of examples than could possibly be covered here, but we hope that this chapter can help the reader identify what test is most appropriate for the particular quality or safety intervention under consideration.

RETROSPECTIVE QUALITY AND SAFETY INVESTIGATIONS

A retrospective study is perhaps the most widely used clinical investigation method, owing to the relatively low cost of conducting such studies and the minimal regulatory oversight required; that is, a waiver of patient consent is readily obtained from an institutional review board (IRB) in the context of a research investigation. As a tool to identify the need for a quality and safety intervention, retrospective studies are invaluable and irreplaceable. Multipatient chart reviews can identify systematic weaknesses and patterns of care in clinical practice, multipatient treatment plan quality surveys can identify exactly how existing systems are performing with respect to known clinical quality criteria (1), and data mining of incident reporting systems can yield insight into the frequency and root causes of errors and/or near misses (2–7).

As a tool for clinically testing the value of new quality and safety measures, however, retrospective studies suffer from an obvious failing: the results of these studies are obtained only after a particular intervention has been in use for some significant portion of time, meaning that any quantification of the value of the intervention will likely come long after the system is entrenched in the clinic in question. In the case of some interventions, particularly those of the discrete safety variety, waiting a sufficient amount of time to develop a statistically significant number of observations to ascertain effectiveness may be unavoidable. For this we only advocate that a clinical testing effort should begin with forethought as part of a more prospective data collection endeavor, as opposed to an afterthought roughly akin to "Hey, why don't we see what happened after we implemented X into the clinic . . . maybe a project for a resident?" Although not without value, such studies rarely elevate the testing of the new system to the priority it deserves and almost certainly delay the ability to share the experience of the investigating institution with the wider community.

For some quality interventions, it can be stated categorically that a mere retrospective study would be inappropriate as compared with alternative study designs discussed subsequently. As we argue in the following sections, the contention that retrospective quality studies are always of lower cost/effort does not hold water when sufficient planning for real-time data collection and analysis is implemented with adequate forethought.

COMPARATIVE PRECLINICAL QUALITY TESTING AND BENCHMARKING

A companion investigation to a retrospective quality and safety study is that of a preclinical test on retrospective data. Like a retrospective data-mining endeavor, preclinical testing performed on prior data is an invaluable tool when properly employed, but, in its ideal form, should be coupled with a plan for a complementary postclinical study.

Preclinical testing of a new quality system is most readily accomplished by collecting a representative sample of prior clinical data, applying the new technique, then comparing known quality metrics between the new and the old techniques. These *in silico* studies are replete in the treatment planning literature, for example, comparing 3D conformal radiotherapy (3D-CRT) with intensity-modulated radiation therapy (IMRT) (8–13), IMRT with protons (14–16), IMRT with volumetric modulated arc therapy (VMAT) (17–21), multicriterial optimized IMRT with unconstrained IMRT optimization (22–24), and knowledge-based IMRT with manual IMRT (25–31). Similar *in silico* studies in auto-contouring (32–35), image alignment (36–38), and dose calculation algorithms (39–43) are not difficult to find in the literature. If human judgment is involved in making superiority assessments (for example, evaluating the quality of human contouring versus autosegmentation), "blinding" the preclinical evaluators can inoculate the study against any bias toward a new system.

Preclinical testing of a new safety system is typically more difficult than a quality comparison, as in many instances, the incidents that the safety system is attempting to prevent cannot be repeated. However, sometimes it is possible to apply new safety systems to a plurality of previous clinical data to detect previously observed errors and, potentially, discover errors that had gone unnoticed previously. As such errors are usually infrequent, a large survey of prior data is typically required to estimate error rates and their detection probabilities. It is also possible to introduce cases with known problems, which could help establish detection probabilities, although it does not advance any understanding of the underlying probabilities of these errors in clinical practice.

It must be flatly stated that preclinical quality studies, although necessary, are not sufficient to establish the performance of a particular quality and safety system without follow-up after clinical implementation. Critiques of preclinical studies as the exclusive means by which to establish the validity of a new system are that the test itself is too removed from normal clinical processes and, if not controlled properly, open to bias on the part of the investigators (e.g., plan quality comparisons that do not fairly represent the best possible result with one or more of the comparison techniques). One can roughly generalize the features of a strong preclinical quality study by tallying how many of the following elements are present in the investigation:

- Retrospective data pulled from a relevant clinical sample
- Quality controls on techniques under comparison to ensure fair comparisons
- Multiple institutions contributing to retrospective data pool
- Blinded test subjects making quality assessments
- Includes plan for postclinical follow-up to confirm quality improvements against same quality criteria used in original study
- Multiple institutions involved in postclinical testing

A similar scoring list can be generated for testing clinical safety systems:

- Retrospective events pulled from relevant clinical sample
- Conditions precisely repeated in testing of safety intervention
- Multiple institutions' experiences contributing to the data pool
- Sufficient statistics on prior events to make predictions about the error detection performance (e.g., receiver operator characteristic curve) after implementation
- Includes plan for postclinical confirmation of error detection performance with new safety system
- Multiple institutions involved in postclinical testing

Not all studies can or must satisfy all criteria, but this list could help consumers of these studies assess the likely generalizability of any individual intervention to another clinic.

One example of a quality study that satisfies most of these criteria (save the multi-institutional components) would be the published experience of Princess Margaret Hospital in the implementation of automated breast planning (44,45). This included a sizeable sample of prior data with quality comparisons in the initial publication, with a subsequent publication years later documenting the true performance of the system in clinical practice on a tenfold larger dataset (158 patients in the preclinical study (44) vs. 1,661 in the long-term follow-up study (45)).

An example of preclinical testing of a safety system that boasts several of these criteria is Kalet et al (46), wherein the authors describe the design and testing of a Bayesian network designed to detect errors in radiotherapy treatment plans (e.g., prescription errors, laterality transposition, inappropriate treatment techniques). The study utilized 4,990 previous clinical cases to train and analyze the performance of the system. As the errors the system was designed to detect were rare, the investigators introduced known errors into the previous cases to establish the error detection performance of the system, ultimately quantifying the receiver operating characteristic (ROC) curve for the system with ample statistics to compare against the reference system (human physicists, in this case). Finally, as the system was implemented in a commercial oncology informatics system (OIS), it natively has the ability to incorporate the system into clinical use and expand to multiple institutions with the same OIS, both endeavors reportedly under way.

PROSPECTIVE TESTING OF QUALITY AND SAFETY INTERVENTIONS

All too frequently, new quality and safety measures are clinically implemented without a robust plan for prospective evaluation of their effectiveness. Although this may be a result of the presumed expense and effort of running a prospective trial, depending on the design of the prospective evaluation, the resources required to implement this level of testing need not exceed that of a retrospective investigation beyond effort of forethought.

Pre–post testing (quasi-experiments)

The natural complement to the preclinical testing discussed in the previous section is a plan for collecting some equivalent postintervention data to compare the "before" and "after" groups. Such pre–post tests have the somewhat disparaging moniker of "quasi-experiments" as they lack the element of random assignment (47), although in many ways a properly designed prospective before-intervention versus after-intervention may strike the best balance for most quality and safety initiatives that necessarily replace existing processes; few quality and safety measures represent a degree of intervention that would warrant the expense of a fully randomized prospective trial. Perhaps the most emblematic case of a quality and safety intervention that would trigger a pre–post study would be the replacement or upgrade of one system to another, for example, a new linear accelerator system or a major software upgrade that displaces an existing installation. In this instance, the investigating institution has no choice but to divide the study into "before" and "after" periods.

A few principles can guide these pre–post studies to make them as robust and as free of bias as possible:

1. Use preclinical survey to identify the quantity (or quantities) that the quality and safety measure is hypothesized to improve.

2. Strike a balance of gaining statistical significance against a tight temporal correlation in pre- and postintervention. Intuitively, the longer the duration of the study, the higher the likelihood that some other time-dependent element could be confounding the result (for example, rotating personnel, refined procedures, other new systems implemented in the same time frame, etc.).

3. Whenever feasible, incorporate ongoing data collection and plan for a long-term follow-up study to confirm that any postintervention was not due to low statistical power in the initial pre–poststudy.

Adding in a long-term follow-up component clearly represents a significant resource in time, effort, and data collection. Again, the magnitude of the intervention and the stage of implementation of the system (early vs. late adoption) can guide whether a long-term follow-up effort is warranted or whether that effort would be better apportioned elsewhere. The same logic would apply to the incorporation of a multi-institutional evaluation, which obviously expands the statistics and generalizability of the final results but proportionally scales up the resources required to conduct such a large-scale endeavor.

Concurrent quality comparisons

For quality and safety measures that will ultimately replace existing processes, it can be highly desirable to prospectively conduct a "real-time" concurrent study that sets the new system against the process it is intended to supplant. Comparison studies closely resemble the design of the pre–post studies (see Figure 18.1(A) and (B)), but should enjoy a slight preference in that the safety profile of maintaining existing processes while quantitatively establishing the effect of new processes is clearly superior to pre–post studies. Stated another way, if it is possible to operate the old system while implementing a new system, then a concurrent study should be preferred over a pre-post study.

Like a pre-post study, the quality metric(s) of interest are stated up front, and the old and new systems are compared in their ability to achieve quality metric X or detect error Y in real clinical practice. Secondary components such as efficiency can also be tracked in this time period. When possible, some element of blinding can help remove any bias in favor of the new system. One excellent example of this in the literature is the study by Wu et al (48), wherein an automated head-and-neck planning tool is hypothesized to be superior to the existing human-driven planning process. With specified quality parameters and plan-effect size determining the accrual to support the primary hypothesis that the automated plans were superior in clinical practice, treatment plans were generated using both the standard manual planning process and automated systems in the same treatment planning system. Either plan was capable of being delivered to the patient; that is, all existing safeguards regarding dose calculation, treatment planning system quality assurance (QA), and so on were in place. The candidate plans were then blinded to reviewing physicians, who simply selected the better of the two plans presented. This last step largely inoculates the study against charges that the authors were biased in favor of the technology they developed, especially as the quality metric comparisons were presented alongside the blinded physician's plan selections that represented the primary results.

Randomized controlled trials

Little need be said regarding the well-known structure of a RCT (49) (Figure 18.1(C)); the question for quality and safety initiatives is primarily whether such an endeavor is (a) ethical, (b) practical, or (c) warranted given the scale of the intervention. As for (a), one can nearly exclude all safety initiatives from contention for a RCT, as an equipoise condition is nearly impossible to satisfy because safety initiatives are almost never an either-or proposition. If one is implementing a new safety system with the hypothesis that this safety system will outperform existing safeguards, a RCT would be ethical only if it necessarily excludes the possibility of combining the new system with the existing system. As new safety interventions almost always *add* to existing safeguards, incorporating any safety system into use can only hold fixed or lower the probability of events. In the rare cases where a new safety system does fully supplant an existing safeguard, such as the introduction of a computer automated pretreatment check replacing a review previously done by a human, a RCT could perhaps be considered; however, as it is almost always possible to run a concurrent study on the intervention instead of a RCT, this is unlikely to be appropriate.

A RCT regarding a quality intervention is easier to envision, and we can look to the history of implementing IMRT over 3D-CRT as an instructive case study that, as should hopefully be obvious to the reader, did represent a new intervention in the name of improved quality. IMRT represented a dramatic shift in the manner in which we treat our patients and manage quality assurance in our clinics, purporting to offer substantial clinical benefits but also introducing new risks to patients that, in at least one well-publicized instance, were implicated in a fatal radiotherapy delivery mishap (50). A change of this magnitude in the name of improved quality of treatment would seem to demand RCT evidence before becoming

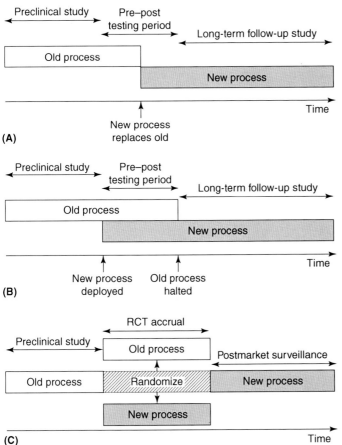

FIGURE 18.1 Options for prospective testing of a new clinical quality and safety measure. In all cases, a preclinical study should precede the new intervention to establish baseline performance of the quality metric of interest. (A) In the case of a pre–post study, the new process replaces the existing process at a particular moment in time. The comparison duration is kept brief to eliminate any other time dependencies influencing the quality element of interest. When feasible, long-term follow-up can strengthen the evidence for the effect of the new process, especially when there were low statistics in the pre–post evaluation period. (B) A concurrent study closely resembles a pre–post study, yet is preferred when the new process does not exclude the preceding process. (C) Finally, in the case of new quality interventions with unproven clinical effects (i.e., a sufficiently large departure from previous experience) that necessarily replace previous systems, a RCT could be considered. Assuming statistically significant results supporting the primary hypothesis that the new process is superior to the old, the new process is adopted and enters the postmarket surveillance phase.

the new standard of care, and yet even 20 years after IMRT began to be clinically implemented, there is only one RCT that directly compared IMRT with its predecessor technology (51).

First, as to the question of whether a RCT for comparing IMRT versus 3D-CRT is warranted, it easily passed the "is it warranted" criterion, as it clearly represented a huge departure from previous standard-of-care treatments. As regards whether a RCT for IMRT versus 3D-CRT would be ethical, the issue was perhaps less clear. If it is possible to deliver a plan that spares a patient's parotid glands from a 3D-CRT treatment that would guarantee permanent xerostomia, is it ethical to deny that patient the presumably better plan? Now perhaps this question can clearly be answered in the negative; however, in the years when IMRT was initially being adopted, there was not yet evidence that the parotid sparing IMRT offered was not offset by a loss of, say, clinical target coverage and/or compromised dose delivery that affected other aspects of an patient's treatment. The PARSPORT trial (51) went through the effort of a RCT in IMRT versus 3D-CRT, providing the evidence that had been lacking behind the clinical intuition that IMRT is always superior, although

there is some evidence for the improved outcomes of IMRT in secondary endpoints of large-scale clinical trials (52–54).

As for the issue of practicality for RCTs for a quality initiative, one quality intervention that would easily fail this criterion is deep inspiration breath hold (DIBH) breast irradiation (55). As this technique is primarily designed to reduce long-term radiation-induced cardiac morbidity, the timescale for evaluating the primary endpoint of any DIBH RCT would be far too long to be practical. Thus, DIBH techniques were tested using dosimetric comparison studies that fall short of a RCT, yet closely resemble some of the other studies described in this chapter (55–59).

Thus, we can say that, whether for ethical or practical reasons, the majority of quality and safety interventions do not warrant a full RCT to establish their effectiveness. This still leaves a substantial menu of options for demonstrating the efficacy of new quality and safety systems, which, given the obvious constraints in implementing clinical testing of any magnitude, need not be disparaged against this gold standard unless an argument can be made that a RCT is the only way to fully establish the efficacy of a practice-changing technique.

A NOTE ON THE PUBLICATION OF QUALITY AND SAFETY STUDIES WITH PROSPECTIVE DATA COLLECTION

As identified in a recent editorial (60), the prospective collection of clinical data can easily become complicated by human research regulations. As stated in §46.111(a)(4) of the U.S. Code of Federal Regulations (C.F.R.) (61), "Informed consent will be sought from each prospective subject." Unfortunately, in the context of considering the challenges to prospective investigations of clinical interventions, the following statement must be made: managing informed consent presents a nearly insurmountable logistic (and financial) barrier on large-scale data collection investigations, and there is a well-known phenomenon of institutional IRBs erroneously categorizing quality and safety studies as research.

Faden (62,63), Kass (64), and colleagues have argued for the ethical framework of a learning health care system in which, owing to the burdensome impediments associated with its adherence, informed consent should *not* always be required. The experience of the National Neurosurgery Quality and Outcomes Database (N²QOD) is also an instructive one, wherein Asher et al (65) describe the N²QOD effort to set up a large-scale multi-institutional clinical registry while avoiding unnecessary administrative burdens associated with quality improvement efforts. The bias toward classifying clinical registries as human subjects research was evident at 5 of 23 N²QOD sites, where local IRBs concluded that the identical project description was human subjects research and insisted on full oversight and informed consent of all patients. The N²QOD effort sought clarification directly from the US Department of Health and Human Services regarding the interpretation of federal regulations, ultimately receiving official confirmation on the following points relevant for regulatory compliance of investigations into clinical registries:

- Human Subjects Research regulations ("The Common Rule," 45 C.F.R. 46) do not apply to practice sites submitting data as part of normal clinical care, irrespective of funding status of the project.

- The Common Rule does not apply to Registry Institution unless federal funds are used to support the project; then a "waiver of consent" will be required.

- Privacy Rules do apply; that is, business associate agreements must be in place, and all data must be handled in a Health Insurance Portability and Accountability Act (HIPAA)–compliant fashion.

- If protected health information (PHI) is used for research, a waiver of HIPAA authorization from a single/central IRB is required.

- Neither the Privacy nor Common Rules apply to the analysis and/or transfer of de-identified data sets; therefore, secondary analysis of de-identified data does not constitute "human subjects research." IRB review and patient consent/authorization are not required.

For the purposes of implementing new clinical quality and safety systems, even in a multi-institutional context, this ultimately means that as long as PHI protections are robust, these prospective quality studies may become part of a published research investigation without incurring the extremely high costs of managing informed consent on all patients. The one exception to this must be the case of a RCT, on the hypothesis that the new quality intervention is superior to the existing "standard-of-care" process; informed patient consent *must* be a component of such an experimental design.

CONCLUSIONS

So what is the ideal clinical test of quality and safety measures? As should be clear from the foregoing, there is no one answer to that question, although we would argue that the ideal *framework* for designing a test of a particular clinical intervention does exhibit some common features: an initial retrospective data-mining effort into the quality/safety feature of interest, preclinical testing (if available) of the intervention, a plan for ongoing data collection, and a final analysis that directly compares the "after-intervention" period with either the "before-intervention" period or externally sourced benchmarks (if they exist).

REFERENCES

1. Moore KL, Brame RS, Low DA, et al. Quantitative metrics for assessing plan quality. *Semin Radiat Oncol.* 2012;22:62–69.

2. Klein EE, Drzymala RE, Purdy JA, et al. Errors in radiation oncology: a study in pathways and dosimetric impact. *J Appl Clin Med Phys.* 2005;6(3):81–94.

3. Terezakis SA, Harris KM, Ford E, et al. An evaluation of departmental radiation oncology incident

reports: anticipating a national reporting system. *Int J Radiat Oncol Biol Phys.* 2013;85(4):919–923.

4. Mutic S, Brame RS, Oddiraju S, et al. Event (error and near-miss) reporting and learning system for process improvement in radiation oncology. *Med Phys.* 2010;37:5027–5036.

5. Ford EC, Fong de los Santos L, Pawlicki T, et al. The structure of incident learning systems for radiation oncology. *Int J Radiat Oncol Biol Phys.* 2013;86:11.

6. Ford EC, Fong de los Santos L, Pawlicki T, et al. Consensus recommendations for incident learning database structures in radiation oncology. *Med Phys.* 2012;39:7272–7290.

7. Ford EC, Terezakis S, Souranis A, et al. Quality control quantification (QCQ): a tool to measure the value of quality control checks in radiation oncology. *Int J Radiat Oncol Biol Phys.* 2012;84(3):e263–e269.

8. Kam MK, Chau RM, Suen J, et al. Intensity-modulated radiotherapy in nasopharyngeal carcinoma: dosimetric advantage over conventional plans and feasibility of dose escalation. *Int J Radiat Oncol Biol Phys.* 2003;56:145–157.

9. Arbea L, Ramos LI, Martínez-Monge R, et al. Intensity-modulated radiation therapy (IMRT) versus 3D conformal radiotherapy (3DCRT) in locally advanced rectal cancer (LARC): dosimetric comparison and clinical implications. *Radiat Oncol.* 2010;5:17.

10. MacDonald SM, Ahmad S, Kachris S, et al. Intensity modulated radiation therapy (IMRT) versus three dimensional conformal radiation therapy (3DCRT) for the treatment of high grade glioma: a dosimetric comparison. *J Appl Clin Med Phys.* 2007;8(2):47–60.

11. Ashman JB, Zelefsky MJ, Hunt MS, et al. Whole pelvic radiotherapy for prostate cancer using 3d conformal and intensity-modulated radiotherapy. *Int J Radiat Oncol Biol Phys.* 2005;63:765–771.

12. Cheng JC-H, Wu J-K, Huang C-M, et al. Dosimetric analysis and comparison of three-dimensional conformal radiotherapy and intensity-modulated radiation therapy for patients with hepatocellular carcinoma and radiation-induced liver disease. *Int J Radiat Oncol Biol Phys.* 2003;56:229–234.

13. Piroth MD, Pinkawa M, Holy R, et al. Integrated-boost IMRT or 3-D-CRT using FET-PET based auto-contoured target volume delineation for glioblastoma multiforme: a dosimetric comparison. *Radiat Oncol.* 2009;4:57.

14. Trofimov A, Song L, Wala JA, et al. Evaluation of the utility of parametrized expectation values of dose-volume metrics for quality control in IMRT and proton therapy planning for prostate carcinoma. *Int J Radiat Oncol Biol Phys.* 2011;81(2):S822–S823.

15. Trofimov A, Nguyen PL, Coen JJ, et al. Radiotherapy treatment of early-stage prostate cancer with IMRT and protons: a treatment planning comparison. *Int J Radiat Oncol Biol Phys.* 2007;69:444–453.

16. Weber DC, Trofimov AV, Delaney TF, et al. A treatment planning comparison of intensity modulated photon and proton therapy for paraspinal sarcomas. *Int J Radiat Oncol Biol Phys.* 2004;58:1596–1606.

17. Verbakel WF, Cuijpers JP, Hoffmans D, et al. Volumetric intensity-modulated arc therapy versus conventional IMRT in head-and-neck cancer: a comparative planning and dosimetric study. *Int J Radiat Oncol Biol Phys.* 2009;74:252–259.

18. Palma D, Vollans E, James K, et al. Volumetric modulated arc therapy for delivery of prostate radiotherapy: comparison with intensity-modulated radiotherapy and three-dimensional conformal radiotherapy. *Int J Radiat Oncol Biol Phys.* 2008;72:996–1001.

19. Popescu CC, Olivotto IA, Beckham WA, et al. Volumetric modulated arc therapy improves dosimetry and reduces treatment time compared to conventional intensity-modulated radiotherapy for locoregional radiotherapy of left-sided breast cancer and internal mammary nodes. *Int J Radiat Oncol Biol Phys.* 2010;76:287–295.

20. Lee T-F, Chao P-J, Ting H-M, et al. Comparative analysis of smartarc-based dual arc volumetric-modulated arc radiotherapy (VMAT) versus intensity-modulated radiotherapy (IMRT) for nasopharyngeal carcinoma. *J Appl Clin Med Phys.* 2011;12(4):3587.

21. Cozzi L, Dinshaw KA, Shrivastava SK, et al. A treatment planning study comparing volumetric arc modulation with rapidarc and fixed field IMRT for cervix uteri radiotherapy. *Radiot Oncol.* 2008;89:180–191.

22. Craft D. Calculating and controlling the error of discrete representations of pareto surfaces in convex multi-criteria optimization. *Phys Med.* 2009;26(4):184–191.

23. Monz M, Kufer KH, Bortfeld TR, et al. Pareto navigation: algorithmic foundation of interactive multi-criteria IMRT planning. *Phys Med Biol.* 2008;53:985–998.

24. Hong TS, Craft DL, Carlsson F, et al. Multicriteria optimization in intensity-modulated radiation therapy treatment planning for locally advanced cancer of the pancreatic head. *Int J Radiat Oncol Biol Phys.* 2008;72:1208–1214.

25. Tol JP, Delaney AR, Dahele M, et al. Evaluation of a knowledge-based planning solution for head and neck cancer. *Int J Radiat Oncol Biol Phys.* 2015;91:612–620.

26. Li N, Carmona R, Sirak I, et al. Validation of a knowledge based automated planning system in cervical cancer as a clinical trial quality system. *Int J Radiat Oncol Biol Phys.* 2015;93(3):S40.

27. Moore KL, Schmidt R, Moiseenko V, et al. Quantifying unnecessary normal tissue complication

risks due to suboptimal planning: a secondary study of RTOG 0126. *Int J Radiat Oncol Biol Phys.* 2015;92:228–235.

28. Shiraishi S, Tan J, Olsen LA, et al. Knowledge-based prediction of plan quality metrics in intracranial stereotactic radiosurgery. *Med Phys.* 2015;42:908–917.

29. Shiraishi S, Moore K. Knowledge-based prediction of three-dimensional dose distributions for external beam radiotherapy. *Med Phys.* 2016;43(1):378–387.

30. Appenzoller LM, Michalski JM, Thorstad WL, et al. Predicting dose-volume histograms for organs-at-risk in IMRT planning. *Med Phys.* 2012;39:7446.

31. Moore KL, Brame RS, Low DA, et al. Experience-based quality control of clinical intensity-modulated radiotherapy planning. *Int J Radiat Oncol Biol Phys.* 2011;81:545–551.

32. Chao KC, Bhide S, Chen H, et al. Reduce in variation and improve efficiency of target volume delineation by a computer-assisted system using a deformable image registration approach. *Int J Radiat Oncol Biol Phys.* 2007;68:1512–1521.

33. Rodrigues G, Louie A, Videtic G, et al. Categorizing segmentation quality using a quantitative quality assurance algorithm. *J Med Imaging Radiat Oncol.* 2012;56:668–678.

34. Han X, Hibbard LS, O'Connell NP, et al. Automatic segmentation of parotids in head and neck CT images using multi-atlas fusion. *Med Image Anal Clin Grand Chall.* 2010:297–304.

35. Castadot P, Lee JA, Parraga A, et al. Comparison of 12 deformable registration strategies in adaptive radiation therapy for the treatment of head and neck tumors. *Radiot Oncol.* 2008;89:1–12.

36. Robar JL, Clark BG, Schella JW, et al. Analysis of patient repositioning accuracy in precision radiation therapy using automated image fusion. *J Appl Clin Med Phys.* 2005;6.

37. Kessler ML. Image registration and data fusion in radiation therapy. *Br J Radiol.* 2014;79(1):S99–S108.

38. Khamene A, Bloch P, Wein W, et al. Automatic registration of portal images and volumetric CT for patient positioning in radiation therapy. *Med Image Anal.* 2006;10:96–112.

39. Vanderstraeten B, Reynaert N, Paelinck L, et al. Accuracy of patient dose calculation for lung IMRT: A comparison of Monte Carlo, convolution/superposition, and pencil beam computations. *Med Phys.* 2006;33:3149–3158.

40. Aarup LR, Nahum AE, Zacharatou C, et al. The effect of different lung densities on the accuracy of various radiotherapy dose calculation methods: implications for tumor coverage. *Radiat Oncol.* 2009;91:405–414.

41. Mihaylov IB, Siebers JV. Evaluation of dose prediction errors and optimization convergence errors of deliverable-based head-and-neck IMRT plans computed with a superposition/convolution dose algorithm. *Med Phys.* 2008;35:3722–3727.

42. Siebers JV, Kawrakow I, Ramakrishnan V. Performance of a hybrid MC dose algorithm for IMRT optimization dose evaluation. *Med Phys.* 2007;34:2853–2863.

43. Dogan N, Siebers JV, Keall PJ, et al. Improving IMRT dose accuracy via deliverable Monte Carlo optimization for the treatment of head and neck cancer patients. *Med Phys.* 2006;33:4033–4043.

44. Purdie TG, Dinniwell RE, Letourneau D, et al. Automated planning of tangential breast intensity-modulated radiotherapy using heuristic optimization. *Int J Radiat Oncol Biol Phys.* 2011;81:575–583.

45. Purdie TG, Dinniwell RE, Fyles A, et al. Automation and intensity modulated radiation therapy for individualized high-quality tangent breast treatment plans. *Int J Radiat Oncol Biol Phys.* 2014;90:688–695.

46. Kalet AM, Gennari JH, Ford EC, et al. Bayesian network models for error detection in radiotherapy plans. *Phys Med Biol.* 2015;60:2735.

47. Shadish WR, Cook TD, Campbell DT. *Experimental and Quasi-Experimental Designs for Generalized Causal Inference.* Boston, MA: Wadsworth Cengage Learning; 2002.

48. Wu B, McNutt T, Zahurak M, et al. Fully automated simultaneous integrated boosted–intensity modulated radiation therapy treatment planning is feasible for head-and-neck cancer: a prospective clinical study. *Int J Radiat Oncol Biol Phys.* 2012;84(5):e647–e653.

49. Piantadosi S. Clinical trials: a methodologic perspective. New York, NY: John Wiley & Sons; 2013.

50. Bogdanich W. Radiation offers new cures, and ways to do harm. *New York Times.* January 23, 2010.

51. Nutting CM, Morden JP, Harrington KJ, et al. Parotid-sparing intensity modulated versus conventional radiotherapy in head and neck cancer (parsport): a phase 3 multicentre randomized controlled trial. *Lancet Oncol.* 2011;12:127–136.

52. Michalski JM, Yan Y, Watkins-Bruner D, et al. Preliminary toxicity analysis of 3-dimensional conformal radiation therapy versus intensity modulated radiation therapy on the high-dose arm of the radiation therapy oncology group 0126

prostate cancer trial. *Int J Radiat Oncol Biol Phys.* 2013;87:932–938.

53. Lin C, Donaldson SS, Meza JL, et al. Effect of radiotherapy techniques (IMRT vs. 3D-CRT) on outcome in patients with intermediate-risk rhabdomyosarcoma enrolled in COG d9803—a report from the children's oncology group. *Int J Radiat Oncol Biol Phys.* 2012;82:1764–1770.

54. Vikström J, Hjelstuen MH, Mjaaland I, et al. Cardiac and pulmonary dose reduction for tangentially irradiated breast cancer, utilizing deep inspiration breath-hold with audiovisual guidance, without compromising target coverage. *Acta Oncol.* 2011;50:42–50.

55. Korreman SS, Pedersen AN, Nøttrup TJ, et al. Breathing adapted radiotherapy for breast cancer: comparison of free breathing gating with the breath-hold technique. *Radiot Oncol.* 2005;76:311–318.

56. Remouchamps VM, Letts N, Vicini FA, et al. Initial clinical experience with moderate deep-inspiration breath hold using an active breathing control device in the treatment of patients with left-sided breast cancer using external beam radiation therapy. *Int J Radiat Oncol Biol Phys.* 2003;56:704–715.

57. Mageras GS, Yorke E. Deep inspiration breath hold and respiratory gating strategies for reducing organ motion in radiation treatment. *Semin Radiat Oncol.* 2004;14(1):65–75.

58. Pedersen AN, Korreman S, Nyström H, et al. Breathing adapted radiotherapy of breast cancer: reduction of cardiac and pulmonary doses using voluntary inspiration breath-hold. *Radiot Oncol.* 2004;72:53–60.

59. Borst GR, Sonke J-J, den Hollander S, et al. Clinical results of image-guided deep inspiration breath hold breast irradiation. *Int J Radiat Oncol Biol Phys.* 2010;78:1345–1351.

60. McNutt TR, Moore K, Quon H. Needs and challenges for big data in radiation oncology. *Int J Radiat Oncol Biol Phys.* 2016;95(3):909-915. doi:10.1016/j.ijrobp.2015.11.032.

61. Code of Federal Regulations: Title 45 Public Welfare. In: *Part 46: Protection of Human Subjects.* Washington, DC: Department of Health and Human Services; 2009. www.hhs.gov/ohrp/human-subjects/guidance/45cfr46.html.

62. Faden RR, Beauchamp TL, Kass NE. Informed consent, comparative effectiveness, and learning health care. *N Engl J Med.* 2014;370:766–768.

63. Faden RR, Kass NE, Goodman SN, et al. An ethics framework for a learning health care system: a departure from traditional research ethics and clinical ethics. *Hastings Cent Rep.* 2013;43:S16–S27.

64. Kass NE, Faden RR, Goodman SN, et al. The research-treatment distinction: a problematic approach for determining which activities should have ethical oversight. *Hastings Cent Rep.* 2013;43:S4–S15.

65. Asher AL, McGirt MJ, Glassman SD, et al. Regulatory considerations for prospective patient care registries: lessons learned from the national neurosurgery quality and outcomes database. *Neurosurg Focus.* 2013;34:E5.

19 | Quality and Safety Training in Graduate Medical Education

Erin F. Gillespie, Derek Brown, and Arno J. Mundt

ESTABLISHING QUALITY IMPROVEMENT EDUCATION IN RESIDENCY

The Accreditation Council for Graduate Medical Education (ACGME) is a nongovernmental organization responsible for the accreditation of United States residency training programs. It was established in 1981 as the first independent accrediting body, in response to increasing demand for better consistency across residency programs as well as formalization of subspecialty training (1). ACGME's mission is to promote high-quality resident education in an environment that fosters trainee professionalism and well-being. In 1999, the ACGME, in collaboration with the American Board of Medical Specialties, introduced the following six domains of clinical competency to the medical profession (2):

1. Patient Care and Procedural Skills

2. Medical Knowledge

3. Practice-Based Learning and Improvement

4. Interpersonal and Communication Skills

5. Professionalism

6. Systems-Based Practice

At the same time, the Institute of Medicine (IOM) was conducting a multiyear investigation of health care quality in the United States. The landmark 1999 report, *To Err Is Human: Building a Safer Health System,* extrapolated that as many as 98,000 deaths occurred from preventable disease in the United States each year (3). Serious concerns regarding variability in patterns of care and quality were further outlined in *Crossing the Quality Chasm: A New Health System for the 21st Century* (3,4). Then, in a follow-up 2003 report, an interprofessional panel convened by the IOM recommended that health professional education (both medical schools and residency training programs) become the center of focus for improvement, with the hope that training future leaders in patient-centered care, systems-based practice, interdisciplinary teamwork, quality improvement, and information technology would instigate generational change in the health care system (5). Because these skills must be learned and practiced in the clinical setting, much of the burden has fallen to residency training programs (6).

With this alignment of the ACGME's and IOM's vision for the future of health care, the Advisory Committee on Educational Outcome Assessment undertook a significant effort, called the ACGME Outcome Project, to identify high-quality assessment methods for residency programs to use in order to assign tangible outcome measures to the aforementioned competencies. Their 14-month work period ended in September 2008 with the publication of a formal report, which included an outline for implementation of the Next Accreditation System (NAS). The overarching goal of the NAS is to train physicians no longer as independent actors, but as team players and leaders in a collaborative care delivery model that serves the public by being sensitive to cost-effectiveness and incorporating health information technology into the improvement of care for individuals and populations (7). In this new system, each specialty was tasked with developing educational Milestones (separated into five levels) for each of the six competencies, to facilitate the assessment of resident progress. One of the most revolutionary components of the NAS was the creation of the Clinical Learning Environment Review (CLER) program, which addresses the following six focus areas (8):

1. Patient Safety

2. Health Care Quality

3. Care Transitions

4. Supervision

5. Duty Hours and Fatigue Management and Mitigation

6. Professionalism

The program involves routine CLER site visits, which are built to model continuous quality improvement (CQI) by evaluating benchmarks and providing encouragement and promotion of the clinical learning environment at each institution. This feedback is intended to help the clinical sites better train residents to provide safe, high-quality patient care. To facilitate institution and resident engagement, the ACGME created CLER *Pathways to Excellence*, which provides a framework with actionable items, expanding the six focus areas to include 34 pathways and 89 properties that represent specific outcome measures (9).

PRACTICAL IMPLEMENTATION OF QUALITY IMPROVEMENT EDUCATION

As is often the case, practical implementation of such guidelines can prove challenging, with many approaches available, but each with its own set of barriers (10). A systematic review of the literature was undertaken in 2014 by the American College of Surgeons to investigate the availability of QI curricula (11). Among 50 relevant references identified, 31 publications outlined curricula, the majority of which were in primary care residencies (52%), followed by general surgery (19%), generic to all GME programs (16%), radiology (7%), critical care (3%), and emergency medicine (3%). Plan, Do, Study, Act was the most common QI content presented (39%), followed by root cause analysis (16%), Lean thinking (7%), and Six Sigma (3%). Most of the QI instruction was delivered in a lecture or didactic setting (84%), although various other methods were also incorporated, including small groups (19%), web-based modules (19%), QI projects (19%), and experiential/bedside teaching (16%). About one-fourth of curricula used validated assessment tool kits (QIKAT, QIPAT), whereas most (54%) involved simply direct observation with feedback (12). The most comprehensive curricula were designed as an elective (nonmandatory) experience, such that a minority of residents were recipients of the educational experience.

In 2015, a survey of otolaryngology program directors was performed to assess the status of QI education in otolaryngology training (13). With a 39% response rate, 90% of program directors considered QI education to be important or very important, yet only 23% of programs contained an educational curriculum in QI, and only 33% monitored residents' individual outcome measures. The most common barriers were inadequacy of faculty with expertise in QI (75%), and competing resident educational demands (90%). Every otolaryngology program director considered morbidity and mortality conferences to be an integral component of in QI education. Notably, many programs are looking to utilize these already established conferences to teach ACGME core competencies, with the content including primarily root cause analysis (14–16).

Another common approach is to require residents to complete a QI project. Although this design inherently places the burden on the resident, whose time is already stretched incredibly thin between patient care and educational activities, these activities can foster a culture of collaboration that is central to successful CQI (17). One such project undertaken at the University of Washington is worth discussing (18). During the CLER visit, the administration recognized that patient problem lists were not being routinely used or updated, and noted that this issue was most influenced by residents caring for patients on the hospital wards. Residents were invited to engage in brainstorming and implementation of a possible solution, and with the creation of an electronic problem list manager, they showed a twofold increase in the number of problems entered daily. Alignment of house staff and institutional administration goals is critical to the success of QI (10). More generally, an institution-wide environment of QI and patient safety includes attending physicians playing an active role in mentoring and supporting residents and their projects, as well as collaboration from professionals in other disciplines (17).

One approach being adopted by GME at the University of California at San Diego (UCSD) is to produce and mandate 16 10-minute, online learning modules that provide baseline training in quality and safety in health care. These modules are paired with a list of possible QI projects as well as specific qualified QI champions to serve as resident mentors, from which residents can choose for their QI project. Although this model aims to provide an easily accessible curriculum to all residents in the UC San Diego Health System, and engage residents in their choice of projects and mentors with appropriate expertise, the challenge will be to incorporate this into the resident's clinical workflow and educational experience.

THE APPROACH TO QUALITY AND SAFETY EDUCATION IN RADIATION ONCOLOGY

The field of radiation oncology has long emphasized the importance of quality assurance and patient safety in clinical practice in view of the significant potential for harm in adverse events caused by errors in the delivery of radiotherapy. In 2010, the *New York Times* published multiple articles documenting fatal incidents in radiation oncology, which moved the discussion further to the forefront and included action items that would affect education and training for both radiation oncology and medical physics residents (19–21).

There was a congressional hearing on the topic in February of 2010 (22), which was quickly followed by statements from the major professional organizations for the field of radiation oncology, namely, the American Association of Physics in Medicine (AAPM) and the American Society for Radiation Oncology (ASTRO).

The AAPM established the following set of key points that "could substantially improve safety and quality in the medical use of radiation" (23):

1. Qualifications

2. Accreditation

3. National reporting/tracking

4. Manufacturers and U.S. Food and Drug Administration (FDA) process

5. Improving safety

6. Our responsibility

Meanwhile, ASTRO proposed a Target Safely six-point plan that described the design and deployment of a quality and safety mini-course for radiation oncology and medical physics residents (24). The course content includes lectures on human factors, incident learning systems (ASTRO/ AAPM RO-ILS), process maps and failure modes effects analysis (FMEA), and root cause analysis (RCA), as well as specific medically related topics such as morbidity and mortality, peer review, and CQI. Then in 2012, ASTRO released another body of work, *Safety Is No Accident* (25), which was "designed to address the specific requirements of a contemporary radiation oncology facility in terms of structure, personnel and technical process in order to ensure a safe environment for the delivery of radiation therapy." Although plenty of valuable information is contained in the document, formal education in quality and safety is only mentioned once—as a challenge for medical physicists.

Most recently, the ACGME incorporated direct instructions for quality and safety training into residency programs, with the following requirements for radiation oncology residents:

1. The program must ensure that there are intradepartmental clinical oncology conferences that cover the following topics: new patient management, patient safety, and continuous quality improvement.

2. The program director must ensure that residents are integrated and actively participate in interdisciplinary clinical quality improvement and patient safety programs.

3. Residents are expected to systematically analyze practice using quality improvement methods, and implement changes with the goal of practice improvement.

4. Residents are expected to work in interprofessional teams to enhance patient safety and improve the quality of patient care.

These responses from both professional organizations and the accrediting body for medical residency programs attempt to address a deficit in quality and safety in radiation oncology and propose an actionable plan for curricular development, but so far have resulted in fragmented implementation strategies. The AAPM and ASTRO have both held workshops focused on quality and safety, but these are isolated events instead of sustainable trainings that can be integrated into residency programs on an ongoing basis (26). In 2010, TreatSafely, a nonprofit organization, began providing practical training workshops on the use of quality and safety tools specifically designed for radiation oncology professionals (27). In 2014, UCSD and University of California at San Francisco (UCSF) collaborated to implement the one-day course for 18 radiation oncology and 5 medical physics residents from their institutions. Resident feedback from pre- and posttests was positive, including an increase from 22% to 72% of residents agreeing with the statement "I have adequate education in quality improvement for my current role," and, more specifically, an increase from 9% to 78% in regard to the statement "I have adequate skills and knowledge to head a root cause analysis" (28). Most recently, radiation oncologists at the University of Florida outlined a framework for educational curricula to help guide programs in a radiation oncology–specific approach (29). Our colleagues in diagnostic radiology appear to be more unified in their approach to education, with the American Board of Radiology publishing a Core Quality and Safety Study Guide for residents preparing for board exams that incorporate QI methods (30). A similar document designed for radiation oncology residents would be extremely useful.

With most institutions left to their own devices to develop and deploy curricula to guide QI education, radiation oncology is not unlike the rest of GME in its approach to quality and safety education. For programs with attendings and residents who have a specific interest in quality and safety, such as UCSF, UCSD, and University of Florida, this may be an adequate approach. In fact, one positive result of the fervor around QI process and implementation in training programs has been the development of a new career pathway in Patient Safety and QI (31). However, for the majority of programs that do not have individual champions of quality and safety, education during residency continues to be limited, with many programs mandating a QI project requirement without providing educational guidance, which, as stated earlier, is suboptimal. Recently, the University of Washington conducted a survey of radiation oncology and medical physics residents in collaboration with ASTRO's resident committee, the Association for Residents in Radiation Oncology (ARRO). Preliminary data show that only one-third of residents feel that formal teaching for principles of patient safety and quality management is adequate, and two-thirds agree that radiation oncology training would benefit from more education in safety. The resources requested by residents as being most useful included practical workshops in specific skills (66%), followed by incorporation of principles into morbidity and mortality conferences (55%), QI project development workshops (43%), and online modules (40%) (32).

There is clearly room for expanded, standardized quality and safety training programs within the field of radiation oncology, and it is the authors' opinion that this effort should be undertaken collaboratively by ASTRO and AAPM. A curriculum that provides baseline knowledge of key quality and safety concepts and tools, coupled with suggested QI projects, would go a long way toward improving understanding, and changing culture, in radiation oncology departments.

REFERENCES

1. Federated Council for Internal Medicine. Enhancing standards of excellence in internal medicine training. *Ann Intern Med.* 1987;107(5):775–778.

2. Swing SR. Assessing the ACGME general competencies: general considerations and assessment methods. *Acad Emerg Med.* 2002;9(11):1278–1288.

3. Kohn LT, Corrigan JM, Donaldson MS; Committee on Quality of Health Care in America, Institute of Medicine. *To Err Is Human: Building a Safer Health System.* Washington, DC: National Academies Press; 2000.

4. Committee on Quality of Health Care in America, Institute of Medicine. *Crossing the Quality Chasm: A New Health System for the 21st Century.* Washington, DC: National Academies Press; 2001.

5. Greiner AC, Knebel E; Committee on the Health Professions Education Summit, Board of Health Care Services, Institute of Medicine. *Health Professions Education: A Bridge to Quality.* Washington, DC: National Academies Press; 2003.

6. Armstrong G, Headrick L, Madigosky W, et al. Designing education to improve care. *Jt Comm J Qual Patient Saf.* 2012;38(1):5–14.

7. Nasca TJ, Philibert I, Brigham T, et al. The next GME accreditation system—rationale and benefits. *N Engl J Med.* 2012;366(11):1051–1056.

8. Accreditation Council for Graduate Medical Education. *Clinical Learning Environment Review (CLER) Program.* Chicago, IL: Accreditation Council for Graduate Medical Education; 2012. www.acgme.org/acgmeweb/tabid/436/ProgramandInstitutionalAccreditation/NextAccreditationSystem/ClinicalLearningEnvironmentReviewProgram.aspx.

9. Accreditation Council for Graduate Medical Education. *Clinical Learning Environment Review (CLER) Pathways to Excellence: Expectations for an Optimal Clinical Learning Environment to Achieve Safe and High Quality Patient Care.* Chicago, IL: Accreditation Council for Graduate Medical Education; 2014. www.acgme.org/acgmeweb/Portals/0/PDFs/CLER/CLER_Brochure.pdf.

10. Liao JM, Co JP, Kachalia A. Providing educational content and context for training the next generation of physicians in quality improvement. *Acad Med.* 2015;90(9):1241–1245.

11. Medbery RL, Sellers MM, Ko CY, et al. The unmet need for a national surgical quality improvement curriculum: a systematic review. *J Surg Educ.* 2014;71(4):613–631.

12. Leenstra JL, Beckman TJ, Reed DA, et al. Validation of a method for assessing resident physicians' quality improvement proposals. *J Gen Intern Med.* 2007;22(9):1330–1334.

13. Bowe SN. Quality improvement in otolaryngology residency: survey of program directors. *Otolaryngol Head Neck Surg.* 2016;154(2):349–354.

14. Kravet SJ, Howell E, Wright SM. Morbidity and mortality conference, grand rounds, and the ACGME's core competencies. *J Gen Intern Med.* 2006;21(11):1192–1194.

15. Rosenfeld JC. Using the morbidity and mortality conference to teach and assess the ACGME general competencies. *Curr Surg.* 2005;62(6):664–669.

16. Kauffmann RM, Landman MP, Shelton J, et al. The use of a multidisciplinary morbidity and mortality conference to incorporate ACGME general competencies. *J Surg Educ.* 2011;68(4):303–308.

17. Myers JS, Nash DB. Graduate medical education's new focus on resident engagement in quality and safety: will it transform the culture of teaching hospitals? *Acad Med.* 2014;89(10):1328–1330.

18. Flanagan MR, Foster CC, Schleyer A, et al. Aligning institutional priorities: engaging house staff in a quality improvement and safety initiative to fulfill clinical learning environment review objectives and electronic medical record meaningful use requirements. *Am J Surg.* 2016;211(2):390–397.

19. Bogdanich W, Rebelo K. A pinpoint beam strays invisibly, harming instead of healing. *New York Times.* December 29, 2010.

20. Bogdanich W, Ruiz RR. Radiation errors reported in Missouri. *New York Times.* February 25, 2010.

21. Bogdanich W. Radiation offers new cures, and ways to do harm. *New York Times.* January 23, 2010.

22. *Medical Radiation: An Overview of the Issues—Hearing Before the Subcommittee on Health of the Committee on Energy and Commerce House of*

Representatives. Washington, DC: U.S. Government Printing Office; 2010.

23. Herman MG. Patient safety and errors in the application of medical radiation: our responsibility. *J Appl Clin Med Phys.* 2010;11(2):3329.

24. ASTRO. Target safely. 2010. www.astro.org/Target-Safely.aspx.

25. ASTRO. Safety is no accident: a framework for quality radiation oncology and care. 2012. www.astro.org/uploadedFiles/Main_Site/Clinical_Practice/Patient_Safety/Blue_Book/SafetyisnoAccident.pdf.

26. Thomadsen BR, Dunscombe P, Ford E, et al. *Quality and Safety in Radiotherapy: Learning the New Approaches in Task Group 100 and Beyond.* Madison, WI: Medical Physics; 2013.

27. Pawlicki T, Brown D, Dunscombe P, et al. i.Treatsafely.org: an open access tool for peer-to-peer training and education in radiotherapy. *Med Phys Int J.* 2014;2(2):4077–4409.

28. Fogh S, Pawlicki T. A report on quality and safety education for radiation oncology residents. *Int J Radiat Oncol Biol Phys.* 2014;90(5):988–989.

29. Yeung A, Greenwalt J. A framework for quality improvement and patient safety education in radiation oncology residency programs. *Pract Radiat Oncol.* 2015;5(6):423–426.

30. American Board of Radiology. Diagnostic radiology: core quality and safety study guide. 2015. www.theabr.org/sites/all/themes/abr-media/pdf/Core_Exam_Quality_and_Safety_Syllabus_1st_ed_FINAL.pdf.

31. Nagler A, Chudgar SM, Rudd M, et al. GME Concentrations: a collaborative interdisciplinary approach to learner-driven education. *J Grad Med Educ.* 2015;7(3):422–429.

32. Spraker M et al. "A Survey of Radiation Oncology Residents' Training and Preparedness to Lead Patient Safety Programs in Clinics" in *American Association of Physicists in Medicine Annual Meeting.* 2016. Washington, DC. http://www.aapm.org/meetings/2016AM/PRAbs.asp?mid=115&aid=33826.

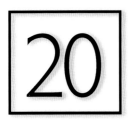

Training: How to Teach Quality and Safety

Laura A. Doyle, Amy S. Harrison, and Yan Yu

INTRODUCTION

You have made it to Chapter 20, which means you are interested in improving your health care system, radiation oncology department, or peers by educating others about quality and safety. A number of high-profile publications have called attention to the need to focus on quality improvement in health care; however, less attention has been devoted to discussing how to fill this educational gap. Sheps and Cardiff (1) describe the long and arduous battle of decreasing the number of patient-related medical errors, owing to the complex nature of the health system and nature of teaching safety events versus concepts of safety science. Teaching quality and safety to health care professionals is one essential component in improving the quality of health care delivery and reducing medical errors (2).

Before embarking on the journey of educating health care providers on the subject of quality, it is important to identify your target audience, subject goals, and method of delivery. The following sections are framed to walk through the steps of implementing an educational program related to quality and safety in health care. The mechanism and goals for teaching quality may vary depending on the particular setting and audience.

Defining your goals

The six key quality aims defined by the Institute of Medicine (IOM) report *Crossing the Quality Chasm* are embedded in almost every aspect of health care (3). Physicians are trained in techniques that have proven *effectiveness* in treating particular ailments; nurses perform tasks to ensure that patients are managed *safely*; administrators design facilities and schedules to increase patient *access* to care and *timeliness* of receiving care. Even without having formal training and education in quality and safety, most clinical personnel have knowledge and experience related to multiple aspects of quality in health care. However, focusing on specific quality improvement tools and methodology can help strengthen a provider's knowledge and practice of quality in the health care system and drive cultural and technical quality improvement efforts.

First determine whether your goal is to solve a specific problem related to health care; if so, your goal might be to gather a team of health care professionals and teach this team one quality improvement tool, such as Six Sigma. The goal of the education program would be to train the team in the basic methodology of the tool, guide them through a practical example, and ultimately improve a real-life problem. If your goal is not specific to an isolated problem, an appropriate goal might be to educate a specific audience in basic safety science concepts.

By setting a goal for your target audience, you can better develop an outcome-centered course design (4). This method encourages the teacher to work backward in the process of course design, first determining the final outcome desired from the students (e.g., remember three different quality improvement tools to use in practice). From the outcome, the teacher can then determine objectives as intermediate steps for achieving the final course outcome. Outcomes should be measurable and detailed. While there are a number of methodologies related to education and transfer of knowledge, perhaps the most widely known taxonomy related to cognition is Bloom's taxonomy. Figure 20.1 lists the six cognitive states of Bloom's framework.

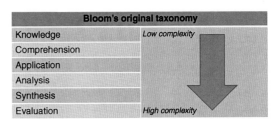

FIGURE 20.1 Six cognitive states of Bloom's framework.

Knowing your audience

Most of the published literature related to teaching quality improvement focuses on the setting of medical students or medical residents (5,6). This population of individuals is an essential focus of teaching quality improvement to ensure that future generations of providers have basic knowledge and understanding of the importance of quality in health care; however, they are not the only audience that benefits from formal education and training about quality-related subject matter. For students and residents who are already immersed in an existing curriculum, quality improvement and safety can be topics integrated into the existing structure, whereas other audiences can be reached by developing an appropriate curriculum and platform for teaching.

When evaluating your audience, consider age and educational levels as well as the needs and learning motivations in selecting the subject matter, rigor, and teaching style. The target audience plays an important role in determining the method for transferring knowledge; a few unique techniques are described in a later section of this chapter, as are the scope of the material, length of the program, and frequency/timing of education.

At the institutional level, perhaps administration is interested in creating a 1-hour educational module to introduce all staff to basic quality and safety terms and definitions. Other programs might be targeted at designated "quality leaders" and focus on more methodology in quality improvement. Prior education of the audience plays a role in defining the starting point, level of depth of covered material, and evaluation criteria. A small group may be provided with background materials, such as journal articles or a basic quality text (7,8), to set the framework for the topic to be discussed in the formal course.

Another concept related to defining your audience is determining their motivating factors. Using extrinsic and intrinsic motivators to engage learners on the topic of quality and safety is a useful part of teaching quality. Most health care professionals have some level of intrinsic motivation related to quality in health care, but framing your lecture with the importance of your objectives in relating quality back to the patient will only strengthen the intrinsic motivation for learners to embrace your teaching experience (9). Extrinsic motivators, while sometimes out of the control of the teacher, might be relevant in some cases. Some examples of extrinsic motivators include availability of discipline-specific continuing medical education credits (often referred to as CMEs) or compensation tied to quality metrics following a program related to implementation of a new quality improvement tool (10).

Major quality topics and theories

This chapter focuses on teaching the concepts of "quality" in health care. For those without a predefined topic or a general interest in expanding the knowledge of peers or employees, where does one begin? Other chapters in this textbook provide appropriate content for teaching the specific topics of quality improvement to the health care professional. Whether it is defining the basics of quality assurance versus quality control or teaching a specific skill, such as how to conduct a root cause analysis (RCA), first identify your audience, define your goals, and select your teaching method. Decide how to evaluate the participants and communicate all aspects of the proposed curriculum before diving into the material. Certain topics may lend themselves to a particular teaching technique, although all may be affected by the other characteristics such as audience, goals, and logistics. A general guide for teaching some of the common topics in quality is outlined in this section.

Lean/Six Sigma

If the goal is to improve efficiency, reduce waste, and identify areas for improvement, the concepts of Lean and Six Sigma can be used independently or in tandem (11,12). A number of publications describe the use of Lean and Six Sigma in practical applications in the health care system, discussing the application of the theory, implementation of the methods, and results of the quality improvement project. Formal coursework exists for training in these methodologies, but application can be customized in the individual setting to optimize efficient deployment of these skills into practice. Often, a small number of employees within a department are trained in full methodology (ranked by "belts") and implement quality improvement projects by educating small groups on the basic philosophy to fulfill a Lean or Six Sigma project.

TeamSTEPPS®

Goals focused on improving patient safety with a "team" as an audience would benefit from the Team Strategies and Tools to Enhance Performance and Patient Safety (TeamSTEPPS) curriculum (13). This methodology is rooted in teamwork to improve specific safety concerns in health care. The Agency for Healthcare Research and Quality has developed a number of tools and materials for implementing this technique. These tools can be used for a variety of applications in radiation oncology and other health care settings. Accessibility and breadth of material make it possible to implement this content more easily in a quality improvement curriculum with an appropriate facilitator for framing and delivering the information.

Root cause analysis

The increasing attention to tracking medical events and near misses, especially through the establishment of patient safety organizations and other national repositories, has increased the use of tools to analyze the factors leading to a mistake or potential mistake (14). Educating staff members on tools such as RCA can help to train individuals to learn to identify potential hazards within the care process, increase reporting of errors, and foster a "no-blame" safety culture.

Failure mode effect analysis

Beyond event investigation, a tool such as failure mode effect analysis (FMEA) can be useful to identify potential safety hazards, prioritize quality improvement projects, and train staff to recognize key factors of risk and severity. When developing a program to teach RCA or FMEA, one might select a representative from each discipline in radiation oncology (therapy, dosimetry, physics, nursing, etc.) to improve the comprehensive evaluation of the health care delivery system.

How to deliver knowledge to your audience

There are a number of forums in which to educate health care professionals. The most commonly published technique includes a formal curriculum, usually as part of a postgraduate education program (5). Additionally, some research focuses on the use of simulation labs as a means of educating health care professionals (15). Beyond these common techniques, literature on this topic is sparse. However, there are several methods to spread knowledge about a particular topic to staff in the health care field.

The technique may depend on the goal of the educational session, the type of material to be presented, and the audience. A variety of tools for teaching arereviewed in this section. There are many ways to categorize teaching techniques. Some of the more traditional or structured teaching methods involve lecturing. Almost every teaching session involves some sort of teacher or facilitator directing learners through the discussion of facts about a particular topic, but the traditional lecture is usually limited to a one-sided presentation of facts for the duration of the educational session, and relies on more passive transfer of information. This teaching style may be achieved in person, or electronically (live or prerecorded) through a range of technological tools. The electronically delivered lecture style also falls into more of a directed lecture style, since the learner is in control of a number of factors, including pace, frequency, and repetition of lectured topics.

Modified lecture teaching styles may include more interactive lecturing, which relies on student participation to drive the direction of the topic incorporating teaching tools, such as group work and presentation of projects, student participation through question and answer, role play, and the like. Case studies and other problem-solving exercises are great teaching tools, especially for the topic of teaching quality. A lot of research in health care has focused on the interactive teaching tool of simulation and its impact on patient safety (16). When feasible, the use of more interactive teaching tools may enhance learner engagement (Figure 20.2).

eLearning: a platform for "quality" learning

The roles of a teacher and student have evolved with technology. Very few courses are driven in person with a single reference or textbook. Electronic access to resources has expanded the ability to use a variety of sources in print and digital media. The electronic media have enabled the use of "eLearning" (electronic educational technology) through a variety of software and web-based applications. From apps to websites, the "classroom" can take on many different roles. eLearning has been defined by three characteristics that make it different from traditional in-person class styles: "asynchronicity, decentralization and electronically mediated interaction and communication" (17).

Teaching through electronic means has a number of advantages and disadvantages. Some of the advantages of teaching through technological tools, often referred to as "distance learning," include the fact that students do not have to be physically present in a classroom, can often view the course material when it is convenient for their schedule, and have access to course material from almost anywhere they can obtain an Internet connection. These advantages are significant to "adult learners" as working professionals. The eLearning platform helps to alleviate some of the logistical hurdles of teaching quality to health care professionals. eLearning can also cater to a large audience and accommodate any length or frequency of educational sessions. Learners are also able to work

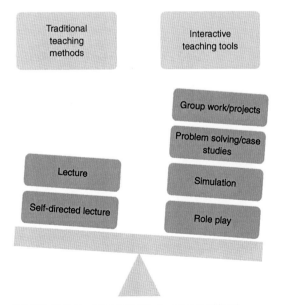

FIGURE 20.2 Teaching techniques, using traditional and interactive teaching methods.

at their own pace and have the ability to repeat concepts that may be important or difficult to master.

eLearning resources are abundant, covering a range of options from open source to commercial applications and platforms. Products are available for large or small populations, and come with a variety of tools to facilitate live versus prerecorded lectures, facilitate communication between teacher and student and among students, and evaluate users through electronic tests and other deliverables. Some highly utilized vendors include Adobe, Apple, Google, and Blackboard. Adobe products such as Captivate and Connect allow presentation of prerecorded lecture material that includes sound and visuals as well as live presentations. Both products are useful for demonstrating quality improvement tools, such as checklists integrated in an electronic medical record, or use of a patient safety organization for recording medical errors. Captivate can integrate screen captures into video lectures to supplement traditional lectures using programs such as Microsoft PowerPoint. Apple applications such as FaceTime and iCloud sharing, and Google applications such as Google Docs and Hangout are more informal applications that support sharing of information and virtual conferencing. Other general applications, such as YouTube® and Skype®, are useful tools for sharing digital educational material or facilitating communication between the mentor and the students. Finally, there are many applications designed specifically for eLearning. They include Blackboard, Canvas, Coursera, edX, ePals, Moodle, Schoology, and Sakai. Each specific application has advantages and disadvantages. The choice of an application should be based on characteristics previously discussed in this chapter, in addition to factors such as convenience, cost, access, ease of use, connectivity, and additional tools.

Disadvantages of the eLearning platform include limitations on activities, group work, and physical interaction. Some learners have challenges accessing information electronically and thrive on real-time discussions. eLearning may also place the additional burden on the facilitator of having to be available to students in addition to creating the material electronically (17). Although students are able to access material on their own time, the amount of time spent accessing electronic classrooms and completing assignments may exceed that spent in a physical classroom to cover the same material.

When possible, a combination of teaching strategies using eLearning followed by periodic on-site meetings can be deployed to enhance the learning experience. This hybrid technique has been praised by teachers and students as offering the advantage of both styles of education and improving student outcomes (18).

Deliverables and evaluation

The final step in crafting an educational offering related to the topic of quality for health care workers is to evaluate the competency of participants who have completed the educational coursework. Evaluation does not have to consist of a formal grading system, but could well be a short survey, or a presentation from participants of practical implementation of skills learned in the curriculum.

A course focusing on the Six Sigma principles might culminate in a project completed by small groups or all participants. The project may be participant directed, but submitted to the facilitator for feedback. An annual educational session on quality might end with a short 10-question, multiple-choice quiz on the topics covered. Participant evaluation is a great way to document that each learner was not only in attendance, but also grasped the material covered. This formal evaluation is very useful in distance learning courses where participants are not physically present for educational sessions. The evaluation may also be delivered through a distance learning platform, and the results of the evaluation communicated back to the participant in similar fashion.

SUMMARY

Taking the time to prepare, defining your audience and goals, designing a curriculum, and selecting an appropriate teaching style and evaluation method are important factors in teaching health care professionals about the topic of quality. Time is a valuable resource, and you want to make the most out of your investment. Employees throughout the health care system can benefit from learning about a variety of topics related to quality. Even the concepts that appear obvious are of considerable value in translating the methodology of quality into practical use of quality concepts. We wish you the best of luck in teaching your team members about quality in health care.

REFERENCES

1. Sheps SB, Cardiff K. Patient safety: a wake-up call. *Clin Govern Int J.* 2011;16(2):148–158.

2. Batalden P, Davidoff F. Teaching quality improvement: the devil is in the details. *JAMA.* 2007;298(9):1059–1061.

3. Institute of Medicine. *Crossing the Quality Chasm: A New Health System for the 21st Century.* Washington, DC: National Academy Press; 2001.

4. Nilson L. *Teaching at Its Best: A Research-Based Resource for College Instructors.* 3rd ed. San Francisco, CA: Jossey-Bass; 2010.

5. Weeks W, Robinson J, Brooks B, et al. Using early clinical experiences to integrate

quality-improvement learning into medical education. *Acad Med.* 2000;75:81–84.

6. Vinci L, Oyler J, Johnson J, et al. Effect of quality improvement curriculum on resident knowledge and skills in improvement. *Qual Saf Health Care.* 2010;19:351–354.

7. Wachter R. *Understanding Patient Safety.* New York, NY: McGraw Medical; 2008.

8. Nance J. *Why Hospitals Should Fly: The Ultimate Flight Plan for Patient Safety and Quality Care.* Bozeman, MT: Second River Healthcare Press; 2011.

9. Marshall M, Harrison S. It's about more than money: financial incentives and internal motivation. *Qual Saf Health Care.* 2005;14:4–5.

10. Anderson LW, Krathwohl DR. *A Taxonomy for Learning, Teaching, and Assessing.* Boston, MA: Allyn & Bacon; 2001.

11. Koning H, Verver J, van den Heuvel J, et al. Lean Six Sigma in healthcare. *J Healthc Qual.* 2006;28(2):4–11.

12. Black J. *The Toyota Way to Healthcare Excellence: Increase Efficiency and Improve Quality With Lean.* Chicago, IL: Health Administration Press; 2008.

13. Agency for Healthcare Research and Quality. TeamSTEPPS: national implementation. 2015. http://teamstepps.ahrq.gov.

14. Thomadsen B, ed. *Quality and Safety in Radiotherapy: Learning the New Approaches in Task Group 100 and Beyond.* Madison, WI: Medical Physics; 2013.

15. Gaba D. The future vision of simulation in health care. *Qual Saf Health Care.* 2004;13(Suppl 1):i2–i10.

16. Aggarwal R, Mytton O, Derbrew M, et al. Training and simulation for patient safety. *Qual Saf Health Care.* 2010;19(Suppl 2):i34–i43.

17. Koch L. The nursing educator's role in e-learning: a literature review. *Nurse Educ Today.* 2014;34(11):1382–1387.

18. Veneri D, Gannotti M. A comparison of student outcomes in a physical therapy neurologic rehabilitation course based on delivery mode: hybrid versus traditional. *J Allied Health.* 2014;43(4):e75–e81.

21 Making Metrics Matter

Amy S. Harrison, Laura A. Doyle, and Yan Yu

INTRODUCTION

The Institute of Medicine's (IOM's) (1) six aims for closing the quality chasm included safe, timely, effective, efficient, patient-centered, and equitable care. These six goals represent ideals for health care improvement through continuous quality improvement. In order to improve health care quality, *quality of care* had to be defined. Avedis Donabedian (2) created a framework for assessing the quality of health care through analysis of performance of the providers, the institutions, the technical quality, best practice standards, interpersonal communication or the art of health care, patient participation, and community care. Each level of assessment has both value and costs, which must be addressed by society, the provider, the patient, and the payer. This nearly 30-year-old paper clearly outlined what could be assessed to define quality and provided an approach to this assessment in the form of three classifications: structure (material resources, human resources, and organization), process (patient and provider activities, from seeking care to treatment implementation), and outcome (clinical effects of care as well as patient satisfaction) (Figure 21.1).

These classifications lend themselves to the creation of metrics and measures within each category. The terminology of metrics and measures is frequently crossed, and caution should be used to understand the context of use when employing these phrases. By technical definition, according to the National Institute of Standards and Technology, a *metric* is a data unit that can be directly measured or collected, whereas a *measure* is a value derived or interpreted from one or more metrics (3). However, in health care, definitions broaden from this basic concept. For example, the American College of Cardiology/American Heart Association Task Force on Performance Measures (4) define *performance measures* as developed with an association methodology, in collaboration with multiple organizations, and include the public process of review and comment, whereas *quality metrics* are internal metrics created to assess performance at a provider, hospital, or health care system level. In practice, many other terms are used,

including quality or improvement measures. McGlynn (5) writes, "Measures may also include thresholds, standards or other benchmarks of performance." Benchmarks may be internal or departmental goals, defined institutionally, regionally, or nationally. The prefixes of "quality" or "performance" are used interchangeably; some may say performance is more for process indicators. For this chapter, the term *metrics* will represent the simple data unit that can be directly measured or collected; the term *measure* will be the value derived from analysis and assessment of one or more metrics.

Measures should incorporate scientifically sound evidence of quality on the basis of best practice and using defined parameters (numerator and denominators) from reproducible data. Data must be available for collection, analysis, and reporting through a reasonable process, and all measures have to be relevant to the stakeholders, the system being measured, and third parties such as accrediting bodies or payers (6). More importantly, measures have to have meaning to the end user as well as the stakeholders

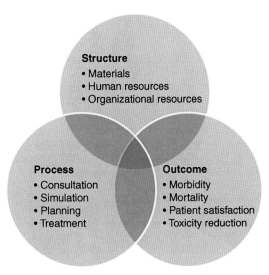

FIGURE 21.1 Donabedian quality framework for health care.

and providers creating the measures. Collected data have to be framed for the context of use not just by the end goal (benchmarking on a standard, comparison of care to competitors, or continuous quality improvement), but also by the presentation of data. How does the measure or metric work, and is it effective?

FRAMING THE DATA

Many metrics are intrinsically locked into place by common practice standards and simple definitions. For example, if you work at a nationally designated cancer institute, your institution will have already delivered structure metrics to the National Cancer Institute that include research protocol participation levels, research infrastructure, documentation of shared resources, and quantification of department leadership. If a hospital has accreditation from the American College of Radiology (ACR), structure metrics on existing equipment, staffing levels, and process metrics such as quality practices will have been delivered to the ACR for review. The Joint Commission has a set of core measurements, which a hospital must meet to establish or maintain accreditation; much of these data are collected through vendors with limited hospital employee effort. Payers such as insurance companies and Medicare require specific measures to be reported to define pay rates or reimbursement levels for work; this concept of "pay for performance" is supported through quality measures. In fact, Medicare.gov (7) provides the opportunity to compare hospitals on the basis of these

metrics through its "Compare Hospitals" web page (Figure 21.2).

This comparison of Hospitals A and B includes structure items such as the type of hospital and whether emergency services are provided, and patient satisfaction scores (Figure 21.3), as well as process (use of imaging equipment, timeliness, and value) and outcomes measures (complications, readmissions, and deaths). Comparisons include regional and national averages for items where numerical values are assessed. From this government database, one can compare hospitals on multiple measures. Figure 21.3 shows patient satisfaction scores for physician communication, nursing communication, staff helpfulness, pain management, understanding medicines, cleanliness, quiet, discharge orders, whether patients gave an overall score of 90%, and whether patients would recommend this hospital. Patient satisfaction scores represent a significant measure at all levels of care, as patients are the consumers of health care services and their satisfaction drives utilization and care preferences in their peer groups. Most institutions survey patients through national satisfaction surveys; these data should be presented and shared with staff.

Most existing core metrics are for ambulatory care or specialty services such as cardiology or surgery. There are limited existing cancer care– or radiation oncology–specific metrics. Most of these measures are process measures, owing to the inherent difficulties of quantifying patient clinical outcomes. With a goal of cancer care to improve survival, metrics such as a 5-year survival have significant

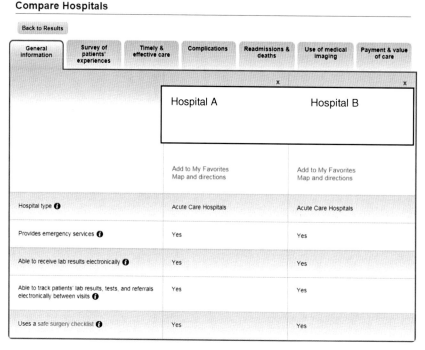

Compare Hospitals

| Back to Results |

General information	Survey of patients' experiences	Timely & effective care	Complications	Readmissions & deaths	Use of medical imaging	Payment & value of care

	Hospital A	Hospital B
	Add to My Favorites Map and directions	Add to My Favorites Map and directions
Hospital type ⓘ	Acute Care Hospitals	Acute Care Hospitals
Provides emergency services ⓘ	Yes	Yes
Able to receive lab results electronically ⓘ	Yes	Yes
Able to track patients' lab results, tests, and referrals electronically between visits ⓘ	Yes	Yes
Uses a safe surgery checklist ⓘ	Yes	Yes

FIGURE 21.2 Hospital structure comparison from Medicare.gov website.

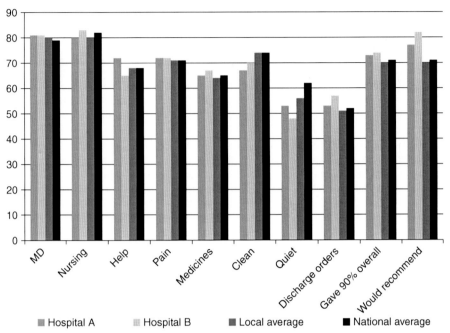

FIGURE 21.3 Hospital-compared patient satisfaction data for two hospitals with the local average scores and national averages.

delay for evaluating current state of care. Hayman (8) stated that radiation oncology outcomes measures are "problematic" owing to a multitude of factors, including: (a) length and patterns of care make connections between intervention and results unclear and not singularly attributable, (b) case-mix/risk adjustments are difficult and costly, and (c) statistical significance from benchmarks is difficult to establish owing to limited case events and the size of patient populations. According to Shekelle et al (9), the validity of 50% of all clinical practice guidelines has a 5.8-year shelf life, with 10% or more requiring modifications after 3.6 years. Compounding the problem of maintaining the shelf-life validity of practice guidelines are the rapid changes in radiation delivery technology and practice patterns, so it comes as no surprise that outcome benchmarks can become quite variable and complicated in nature.

Efforts from the National Initiative on Cancer Care Quality (NICCQ), the National Quality Forum (NQF) part of an American Society of Clinical Oncology (ASCO) study, and the ASCO Quality Oncology Practice Initiative; professional societies; patient advocates; and researchers all contributed to the establishment of quality measures for breast and colon cancer. These NICCQ measures were investigated in 2006 by Malin et al (10) by extracting the patient lists from the American College of Surgeons (ACS)–approved cancer registry for five metropolitan areas. To gather these metrics, patients were contacted via surveys for record release, and post-patient consent medical records from cancer providers and primary care

physicians were reviewed by trained nurses. From these data, 86% of breast patients and 78% of colorectal cancer patients received recommended care. A care provider might view these rates and perceive them as reasonable for this level of care and this type of disease; however, patients could interpret these data to mean they have a 1 in 5 chance of being treated outside of the recommendations of care.

In 2006, the National Comprehensive Cancer Network (NCCN) and ASCO collaborated to generate quality measures for breast and colon cancer that could be easily implemented into a clinical care workflow and used for accountability and pay for performance (11). During the same time period, the National Quality Forum, a multi stakeholder (payer, provider, consumer, and researcher) organization, assembled to establish quality measures for breast and colon cancer as well as symptom management and end-of-life/palliative care. The NQF measures were adopted by the Centers for Medicare and Medicaid Services (CMS). Ultimately, both the NCCN-ASCO and NQF measures were harmonized. These standards were presented with details on measuring the population (denominator) and expected intervention (numerator) with exclusions and explanations. Reporting the measures to CMS created accountability in utilization of care, but widespread implementation of data collection remains difficult. The simplest extraction point is from billing codes, but these lack clinical data needed to define the subset of patients. Data such as tumor size or estrogen receptor status remain in the medical record, but must be extracted by knowledgeable staff unless electronic medical records are fully engaged with mineable data fields as opposed to free text data entry (12). The National Cancer Institute's Surveillance, Epidemiology, and End Results (SEER) program combined with Medicare billing claims can provide much of the data needed, but is generally not up to date; also, Medicare data exclude patients 65 or younger. Hospital-based registry data provide a useful data-mining tool, but many times lack information related to all specialty care such as chemotherapy and radiation. Additionally, there is little incentive to invest in this labor-intensive data mining, beyond academic investigations. In creating these measures, considerations were made to allow physician exclusions when recommendations were not followed, but these exclusions were denied owing to fear of data biasing; however, certain measures were adjusted by age such that frail patients or those with comorbidities would be excluded from the metric entirely.

Nolan and Berwick (13) defined three types of measurements in health care: item-by-item, composite measures and all-or-none measurements. "Item-by-item measurement" separates each care item as a rate or per-centage. The NQF-endorsed ASTRO measurement for bony metastasis uses item-by-item measures where the numerator is all patients with painful bony metastases and no prior radiation to the same anatomic site who receive "30 Gy/10 fxns, 24 Gy in 6 fxns, 20 Gy/5 fxns, or 8 Gy/1 fxn." The denominator is all patients with painful bony metastases and no previous radiation who receive external beam therapy. "Composite measures" compute percentages across a range of measures such that the rate represents all care that was given divided by all care that should have been given. This measure gives partial credit for completing some of the measures. Last, the "all-or-none measurement" gives no partial credit across a group of composite measures and thereby shows whether a patient received all the care he or she should have received. This measure has all the patients who received all the care in the numerator. This all-or-nothing measurement is most in line with patient desires for measures, as patients perceive all measures as equally important to their outcomes, and this score is tied directly to the individual patient receiving all required quality care. Candidate measures for all or none should be "indisputable" basics of good care for a condition. However, presenting the data in this "all-or-nothing" format amplifies errors, as one poor score degrades the entire measurement. The Joint Commission on Accreditation of Health Care Organizations uses this type of measurement. When used, Nolan and Berwick concluded, "all-or-none" measures drive quality improvements because they require investigation into the entire chain of care.

Quality measures, benchmark data, and performance indicators are all tools for communication of data; the purpose of these data can be for end users to select care providers, which indirectly leads to improvement; or for direct improvement by using these values to track improvements from changes in processes (14), the latter

being the basis of continuous quality improvement and leading health care to statistical process control in health care. Any population of hospitals, physicians, or health care plans, when generating and providing data, publicly creates the opportunity for patients or payers to choose/ select them as a provider on the basis of these data. Berwick et al (14) state that problems with using these public guidelines as selection tools include the limited scope of guidelines, lack of understanding of the values by the general public, and local constraints of benchmarks. From the data used for selection, process, and therefore quality, improvements can be implemented and become the measures used for statistical process control (SPC) within the health care environment (15).

SPC was developed in the 1920s by physicist Walter Shewhart to improve industrial manufacturing processes by allowing the visualization of change in outcomes over time through the analysis of run charts/control charts using statistically derived decision rules. These charts are fre-quently used in Six Sigma methodology to remove process defects and minimize variability. Detailed explanation and practice of SPC exceeds the scope of this chapter; the reader is referred to the chapter on statistics. In health care, continuous quality analysis looks toward the work of W. Edwards Deming and the principles of plan–do–study–act, which allow the effect of implemented changes to be tracked using quality measures. Maintaining measures allows the user to verify that implemented changes are sustained over time (16). Thor et al (15) reviewed the application of SPC in health care through a systematic literature review and reported that SPC has been applied in health care over a large range of settings and specialties and that it is used not only by departments and providers but also by patients in managing their own care, showing that this means of data observation, analysis, and performance adjustment is a versatile tool to improve health care.

DATA COLLECTION AND ANALYSIS

As mentioned earlier, data can be collected from na-tional databases such as SEER or CMS, institutional databases, and electronic medical records (institution or departments), or extracted from paper charts/records. The easiest method for data collection is from a fully implemented electronic medical record (EMR) where data entry is in the form of mineable inputs extracted through the software. Even with a fully functional EMR, problems and errors are easily propagated in metric generation. Creating a useful metric may take much iteration without national, local, or societal standards in place. In creating departmental metrics, it is the detail that adds depth and meaning to the performance mea-sures in radiation oncology. Even when an appropriate measure is established, care must be taken to validate metrics, as EMR upgrades or changes in billing codes may invalidate a custom metric output report. Metrics have a life cycle defined by goals, data collection, accuracy, meaningfulness, efficiency and ease of collection/maintenance, presentation of data, needs of the stakeholders, and improvements or changes in the system over time. The metric life cycle is complex and ever evolving (Figure 21.4). As the diagram suggests, most of the processes in the metric life cycle can bring the metric back to the point of conception to have the metric or measure core definition updated in order to strengthen the data collected or add more meaning and significance to the measure. Metrics should be continuously reviewed and reassessed with respect to changes in care, delivery of care, outcomes, and data.

Complexity in creating a valid measure and maintaining it can be shown with the simple metric of patient turnaround time (TAT) from simulation to treatment. In all radiation oncology EMR systems, patient schedules are readily available, and a department may decide to track its patient TAT to seek improvements in the IOM goal of timeliness. Although it is simple to extract the time and date of simulation and time and date of treatment, details are important when trying to create meaning from these two numbers (e.g., should you lump palliative and curative cases together, or simple plans with complex plans; should data be reviewed by treatment machine or physician; and how does the EMR manage weekends and treatment times?). To solve these questions, it is best to clarify the question being asked; still, multiple iterations of the metric may be necessary to focus on the goals of the metric and understand the output in a useable way. Although there is no baseline for TAT in radiation oncology, having a present-state knowledge of performance for a measure is necessary to understand the impact of departmental changes and influences on workflow.

Even when a metric is well defined for measurement, extraction of data may be clouded by lapses in how data are entered (provider/clinical support team), how the EMR stores and retrieves the data, and time needed to validate data and system usability. The American Society for Radiation Oncology generated a measure called External Beam Radiotherapy for Bone Metastases, which is currently incorporated into the Choose Wisely campaign and endorsed by the National Quality Forum. This measure is based on the following clinical guideline recommendation:

Although various fractionation schemes can provide good rates of palliation, numerous prospective randomized trials have shown that 30 Gy in 10 fractions, 24 Gy in 6 fractions, 20 Gy in 5 fractions, or 8 Gy in a single fraction can provide excellent pain control and minimal side effects. The longer course has the advantage of lower incidence of repeat treatment to the same site, and the single fraction has proved more convenient for patients and care givers. (17)

The numerator, denominator, and data exclusion rules are listed, including the billing and diagnosis codes to be used for data collection. The expectation of this metric is an all-or-nothing process measure where 100% is the goal. During the feasibility testing for the measure, payer data from three states and 245 physicians were reviewed. Paper records were randomly sampled: 1,635 cases were treated and 155 patient records were sampled. The percentage rate of cases meeting the quality metric, also called the *performance rate*, was 79.6% after 2% of the cases were excluded as acceptable exclusions from the metric. The billing, diagnosis codes, prescriptions, and fractionation can be extracted from an EMR database; thereafter, only cases that do not meet the prescription rules must have chart documentation reviewed by clinical staff to see if they are allowed exceptions. Problems with this electronic version of the data extraction include physicians not creating a new diagnosis for patients returning with a bony metastasis, and if the correct diagnosis code is not entered per treatment session the patient data will be omitted. Additionally, two of the four exceptions—"patients with femoral axis cortical involvement greater than 3 cm in length" and "patients who have undergone a surgical stabilization procedure"—require two things: (a) the physician must record this information during the patient's history; and (b) there must be a review of patient history data, which remains a free-text portion of the EMR. The need to individually review charts and documentation for exclusions increases the time needed to collect data and overuses department resources, making the metric less appealing to the clinical staff that needs to validate the data or the physician team that must learn or improve on documentation processes.

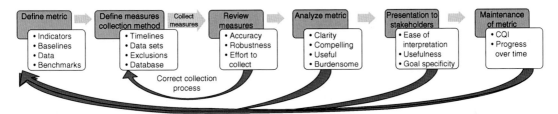

FIGURE 21.4 The metric life cycle.

In addition to workflow problems in the process of extracting data, changes in system structures also create challenges to effective measures collection and metric analysis. System structures include software upgrades, changes in staffing, and procedures or ICD codes, all of which may invalidate an automated data-extraction process and create data corruption that may not be easily discoverable. This is especially true of measures with extended time periods for data collection, such as annually collected metrics. In regard to daily, weekly, or monthly metric data, different complications may arise; for example, data may be unrepresentative if data collection is based on EMR billing codes, or variable if billing codes are not captured and verified in real time. If the billing codes or diagnosis are incorrect and this is not discovered until final billing verification at the end of a 6- to 8-week treatment course, the metric results might be skewed for the months when measures were reported.

If data collected are going to be compared with external benchmarks, standard guidelines and a universal understanding of the data must be created. Benchmarking represents an agreed-upon gold standard for performance. NQF-endorsed measures could be appropriate guidelines for benchmarking quality, as they were formed, assessed, and validated for reliability by experts from various departments relying on published evidence-based data. Benchmarking is frequently disputed owing to case mix (diversity of comparison populations by disease severity and local variations in patient socioeconomic status), which affects baseline health levels and patient engagement in health care. Certain benchmarks provide for risk adjustment on the basis of measurement to normalize comparisons across populations and regions. Risk assessment, however, adds cost and time to data collection and the formation of benchmarks.

Variation in practice can also account for variation in metrics from national benchmarks. For incident learning in radiation oncology, the definition of medical reportable event (MRE) is set by state and/or federal regulatory agencies and is common radiation oncology taxonomy, but incident reporting for nonreportable events is not nationally standardized. One institution may report every variation that occurs in the patient care process or violations in internal procedures such as physicians not drawing volumes in a timely manner or partial treatments, whereas another institution may only report MREs. This variation in practice would equate to one institution having thousands of variations from intended treatment/process and the other institution reporting only a handful. The magnitude of uncertainty in measurement or the reporting process is even vaguer in near-miss reporting, as there is no universally accepted definition of a near miss. The common meaning of a *near miss* is an error in the treatment process that is discovered and corrected before it has an impact on patient care. Physicists routinely discover errors in plans or prescriptions during pretreatment plan checks; each of these discovered "errors" or events could be considered a near miss worthy of reporting. Voluntary national incident learning systems such as the ASTRO/AAPM-supported Radiation Oncology Incident Learning System (RO-ILS) will give all participating departments a glimpse at other practices' event reporting and benchmarking values for treatment event reporting. Although these incident learning systems were never intended to be a benchmarking tool, they could serve as continuous quality improvement (CQI) tools if all institutions were using the same reporting protocol and participating in this database.

Analysis of a metric starts at the point of creation and may require many data extraction validations and presentation formats to both establish meaning and validate the metric (Figure 21.4). *Data extraction validation* is the process of reviewing the raw data points extracted from either the EMR or the patient database to ensure that the numbers used in generating the measure are the correct information in the correct format. The metric should be collected over a relevant time period in order to generate a baseline. From this point, variations over time can be assessed, as well as outcomes from continuous quality improvement practice changes, which might knowingly or unknowingly impact a metric. It is important to note that the raw data should be reviewed for reasonableness, outliers, and exclusions. For TAT using EMR scheduling as a collected data point, if a patient is not canceled from a simulation schedule for not showing up, the TAT data extraction might calculate from an erroneous scheduling point such as a completed appointment time from a prior treatment course, thereby creating a TAT of years instead of days. Reliance and delays in patient start times due to coordinating appointments with medical oncology, surgery, or dental appointments may extend patient TAT and skew data if not explored before the data are presented (Figure 21.5). These outliers in data spotlight system or metric weaknesses. If a patient is on hold from simulation to start of treatment, waiting for an appointment with medical oncology, and this lag is due to medical oncology national meetings or summer vacation schedules, interventions or changes in process or interdepartmental communication can reduce these gaps. The spike in September/October 2014 on the left in Figure 21.5 was a true peak in times owing to the absence of head-and-neck expert physician in both radiation oncology and medical oncology; this spike was addressed by changes in physician cross-coverage in both departments. All decisions regarding metrics should be made by staff members who understand the data, how the data are collected, and department policy. Department leadership in conjunction with the quality committee should address how any data singularities or exceptions should be reported or corrected. Excluding data eliminates an improvement opportunity, whereas keeping the outlier skews overall trends in data resulting from near-random variations that can be clearly explained.

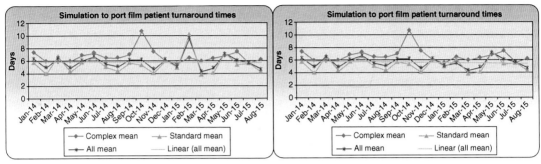

FIGURE 21.5 Simulation to port film patient turnaround time; left image is preanalysis by metric owner; right image has adjustment for February 2015, where an error in the queueing process yielded one data point of >300 days.

In their book, *The Quality Solution*, Nash and Goldfarb (18) provide guidelines for special cause variations in control charts as eight consecutive points above or below the mean; any point in the upper or lower control limit; eight consecutive points that all change in the same direction; nonrandom patterns, including cycles, trends, clusters, and sawtooth data; two consecutive points beyond two sigma from the mean; and four consecutive points beyond one sigma from the mean. Definition of not only the metric but also the investigation level and the level where change must occur should be done at the start of assessing a measure.

PRESENTATION

Presentation of data should be palatable to and efficient for the people receiving the data. Figure 21.5 represents the graph used in a department staff meeting attended by physicians, nursing, administration, radiation therapists, dosimetrists, and physicists. The goal of this visual representation is to show quickly the data and trending of TAT to the entire department. These data are reviewed by a physicist prior to presentation, and during this review the Six Sigma analysis on standard deviations and fluctuations is explored. If data show unacceptable variations, all data are presented to the quality committee to establish if a quality improvement project should be implemented.

As with art, the saying "beauty is in the eye of the beholder" holds true for quality metrics, control charts, and data presentation. Differences in preferences and perspectives will affect how presented data are digested by the audience. The same TAT graph, showing reduced TAT, at a staff meeting might elicit praise from the physician team, whereas administration may ask if this is an opportunity to increase referrals or decrease staffing levels.

Edward Tufte (19), a pioneer in the field of visual data representation, has authored multiple books on how to visually represent quantitative information. In his book *The Visual Display of Quantitative Information*, Tufte

teaches that the basic principle of graphical excellence is the visual communication of complex ideas with clarity, precision, and accuracy. Graphical data displays allow the viewer the quickest consumption of data in the smallest space, wherein multivariate data are usually combined in one graph that displays the truth of data. Tufte's graphical excellence is a "matter of substance, statistics, and design."

These principles are applicable in health care in many formats for radiation oncology. For example, during implementation and ramping up of a stereotactic body radiotherapy program for lung cancer, an institution might decide to track adherence to an NRC/RTOG protocol's guidelines. Figure 21.6 shows the V20 values for all patients treated, as well as the guidelines for deviations from the published protocol. This immediately shows that one case was a major deviation for this dose constraint and that four had minor variations; improvements to this graph could be made by modifying the bullet sizes to be representative of target volume or tumor location, as these items dramatically impact achievement of this dose constraint.

Care should be taken to present data in a meaningful and efficient manner.

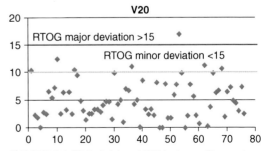

FIGURE 21.6 Clinical data set V20 (volume of lung getting more than 20 Gy) plotted per 76 SBRT plans; the light gray line represents a minor deviation per RTOG 0813 dosimetric guidelines and the dark gray (top) line represents a major deviation.

CONTINUOUS QUALITY IMPROVEMENTS

Without a starting point or baseline measurement, the effects of changes in process, equipment, techniques, personnel, or procedures cannot be tracked for improvement. The principles of CQI rely on creating appropriate measures with clear definitions, knowing one's starting point, and working to improve the outcomes. Quality improvement may be structural (moving to more advanced treatment delivery modes), process related (improved TAT), or outcome related (improved outcomes or lowered toxicities). One must have an understanding of the starting point and continuously track measures to know that (a) there are improvements and (b) these improvements are sustained.

CQI might not even be formalized in an institution in order to track improvements; for example, when the Joint Commission first required standardized indicators for hospital performance, after 2 years they were able to report "consistent improvements in measures reflecting the process of care for acute myocardial infarction, heart failure, and pneumonia" (20). This improvement from external auditing might have been from the Hawthorne effect, where behaviors and following recommended guidelines are improved owing to the effect of being observed, while some improvement would have been from structured interventions. For certain metrics such as handwashing, the Joint Commission measures are collected and reported by their auditors during on-site observation and data collection. The institution may have in place preparations or educational session in order to achieve accreditation, but in this example the external audits create an informal CQI process.

Recommendations for any focused implementation that might improve process should include knowing the base operating level, a concept iterated in all quality improvement methodology. In *The Checklist Agenda*, Atul Gwande (21) discusses multiple interventions in processes where checklists are added to the workflow and documents process measure improvements over time with the addition of a checklist. Fong de los Santos et al (22) recently published medical physics practice guidelines for safety checklists and noted that "gathering, measuring, and providing feedback on clearly defined outcomes" is necessary.

Although quality metrics and measurements may not be driving patient decisions as of yet, they are becoming a factor for purchasers, health plans, regulators, clinicians, and accountable care organizations (ACOs). The trend to show value in radiation oncology is becoming a driving force in competitive markets locations and a useful tool in finding care partners for ACOs. There are certainly barriers to CQI, such as time commitments to collect and analyze data, and political or power struggles when presenting the concept of measuring and trending performance, but having the ability to show current performance levels as well as a commitment to continuous change is only possible through measurement (14). Radiation oncology is slowly generating standards and understanding of practice variations through participation in the Choosing Wisely campaign, data collection through RO-ILS, and structure and process as part of accreditation through APEX. These standards will encourage CPI at a widespread level and improve overall patient care in radiation oncology. The field of radiation oncology uses rapidly changing, advancing technology, and the constant change in this field allows an easy pathway for continuous quality improvement.

REFERENCES

1. Institute of Medicine. *Crossing the Quality Chasm: A New Health System for the 21st Century*. Washington, DC: National Academy Press; 2001.

2. Donabedian A. The quality of care: how can it be assessed? *JAMA*. 1998;260(12):1743–1748.

3. NIST, EWG/ICV Evaluation Working Group, DARPA Intelligent Collaboration and Visualization Program, Chapter 5. http://zing.ncsl.nist.gov/nist-icv/documents/section5.htm.

4. Bonow RO, Masoudi FA, Rumsfeld JS, et al. ACC/AHA classification of care metrics: performance measures and quality metrics. A report of the ACA/AHA Task Force on Performance Measures. *JACC*. 2008;52(24):2113–2117.

5. McGlynn E. Selecting common measures of quality and system performance. *Med Care*. 2003;41(1):I39–I47.

6. Lighter DE. Medical informatics and information resources for quality improvement. In: Lighter DE, ed. *Advanced Performance in Health Care*. Sudbury, MA: Jones and Bartlett; 2011:109–139.

7. Centers for Medicare & Medicaid Services. (2016). Medicare Hospital Compare. Retrieved from https://www.medicare.gov/hospitalcompare/search.html.

8. Hayman JA. Measuring the quality of care in radiation oncology. *Semin Radiat Oncol*. 2008;18:201–206.

9. Shekelle PG, Ortiz E, Rhodes S, et al. Validity of the Agency for Healthcare Research and Quality clinical practice guidelines. *JAMA*. 2001;286(12):1461–1467.

10. Malin JL, Schneider EC, Epstein AM, et al. Results of the National Initiative for Cancer Care Quality: how can we improve the quality of

cancer care in the United State? *J Clin Oncol.* 2006;24:626–634.

11. Desch CE, McNiff KK, Schneider EC, et al. American Society of Clinical Oncology/National Comprehensive Cancer Network quality measures. *J Clin Oncol.* 2008;26:3631–3637.

12. DeMartino JK. Measuring quality in oncology: challenges and opportunities. NCCN Policy Report. *J Natl Compr Canc Netw.* 2013;11(12):1482–1491.

13. Nolan T, Berwick DM. All or none measurement raises the bar on performance. *JAMA.* 2006;295(10):1168–1170.

14. Berwick DM, James B, Coye MJ. Connections between quality measurements and improvement. *Med Care.* 2003;41(1):I30–I38.

15. Thor J, Lundberg J, Ask J, et al. Application of statistical process control in healthcare improvement: systematic review. *Qual Saf Health Care.* 2007;16:387–399. doi:10.1136/qshc.2006.022194.

16. Lighter DE. Essentials of statistical thinking and analysis. In: Lighter DE, ed. *Advanced Performance in Health Care.* Sudbury, MA: Jones and Bartlett; 2011:173–229.

17. 1822 External Beam Radiotherapy for Bone Metastases. National Quality Forum. www.qualityforum.org/QPS/QPSTool.aspx.

18. Nash DB, Goldfarb NI. Analyzing quality data. In: Nash DB, Goldfarb NI, eds. *The Quality Solution: The Stakeholder's Guide to Improving Health Care.* Sudbury, MA: Jones and Bartlett; 2006:73–91.

19. Tufte ER. Graphical excellence. In: Tufte ER, ed. *The Visual Display of Quantitative Information.* Cheshire, UK: Graphics Press, 2001.

20. Williams SC, Schmaltz SP, Morton DJ, et al. Quality of care in U.S. hospitals as reflected by standardized measures, 2002–2004. *N Engl J Med.* 2005;353(3):255–264.

21. Gawande A. *The Checklist Manifesto: How to Get Things Right.* New York, NY: Metropolital Books; 2010.

22. Fong de los Santos LE, Evans S, Ford EC, et al. Medical physics practice guideline 4.a.: development, implementation, use and maintenance of safety checklists. *J Appl Clin Med Phys.* 2015;16(3):5431. www.jacmp.org/index.php/jacmp/article/view/5431. doi:10.1120/jacmp.v16i3.5431.

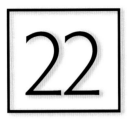

22 | The Patient Perspective on Quality and the Role of the Patient in Safety

Suzanne B. Evans and Sharon Rogers

INTRODUCTION

Much has been made in recent years about providing quality care in medicine. This has been defined in a myriad of ways. However, the Institute of Medicine defined six dimensions of quality as critical targets: that health care is to be safe, effective, patient centered, timely, efficient, and equitable (1). The notion of patient-centered care has been relatively new in the delivery of modern medicine. Measurement of patient satisfaction has been undertaken through a number of different instruments (2,3), which despite variations have been found to be reliable (4). This chapter explores what patients expect from their care providers, how quality is perceived, and ways in which patients can be engaged in safety.

HOW DO CAREGIVERS' AND PATIENTS' EXPECTATIONS OF QUALITY DIFFER?

No piece of data illustrates the chasm between patient and provider perceptions more clearly than the study by Fenton et al (5), which demonstrated higher mortality and costlier care in patients who were more satisfied. Despite this study, there is no doubt that patient satisfaction is a worthy goal. Patient satisfaction is correlated with provider technical competence (6,7), improved compliance with medical recommendations (7), and less litigation (8,9). Additionally, the Centers for Medicare and Medicaid Services, the largest payer of the U.S. health care system, has developed performance-based reimbursement, and patient satisfaction is part of this performance (10).

Providers believe that good care is compliant with the processes that are defined as quality processes, and they place much less emphasis on outcomes (11). For the provider, it is understood that outcomes—particularly in cancer care—are often partially out of their control, and even the best processes can result in suboptimal outcomes. The adage in medicine, "If you aren't seeing any complications, you aren't doing enough procedures," is a prime example of this philosophy. For patients, however, the quality of their care is inextricably linked, at least in part, to their outcome.

Patient Expectations of Medical Care

As with any customer service experience, patient satisfaction is achieved when expectations and experience align. Patients come with expectations about how the health care system works and what the interactions will be like with health care providers. Sometimes these expectations are informed by the stories they read in the newspaper or magazines, by television programs and commercials, or by the experiences of friends and relatives. Sometimes patients have a "sense" of how things work on the basis of their own imagination of the system. Often these expectations are not in line with the way things actually work, and then there is disappointment and distress, and the experience is judged to be negative in some way.

THE DOMAINS OF QUALITY CARE FROM THE INSTITUTE OF MEDICINE: SAFE, EFFECTIVE, PATIENT CENTERED, TIMELY, EFFICIENT, AND EQUITABLE

Safety

Generally speaking, most patients and family members believe that the care they will receive, even if not entirely successful, will be safe, provided efficiently, and monitored by some sort of quality assurance program/set of metrics. Overall, patients and families believe that they will not be harmed by the treatment they are to receive as a result of unsafe practices and procedures. There can be very important exceptions to this rule along cultural, racial, and socioeconomic lines to which clinicians should be sensitive (12–15). Unfortunately, these expectations are not always realized, and the patient/family experience disappointment, anger, distress, and anxiety when something untoward occurs.

Patients and families also come with the expectation that health care facilities will be clean, modern, and almost sterile in appearance and a place where their creature comforts and emotional needs will be addressed. Although these are not specifically safety issues, patients often use these metrics as a facsimile measure of the quality of the organization and the safety of the care that will be provided. This is a sort of halo effect (16) for institutions: Those that appear beautiful are perceived as being "better." Should a patient find an environment or physical layout that is messy, dirty, disorganized, and inefficient, he or she becomes suspicious about the safety controls in place. Interestingly, there are data that the highest quartile hospitals for cleanliness as measured in Hospital Consumer Assessment of Healthcare Providers and Systems (HCAHPS) had fewer iatrogenic infections (17), so this perception may not be wrong. In a sense, the order and professionalism of a clinic or treatment room or the professional appearance and manner of a health care provider can either undermine or enhance the perception of quality and safety for some individuals.

Effectiveness

Patients typically also believe that the health care providers who will attend them are fully competent and qualified. Patients believe that the facility they have chosen can provide the highest level of skill and professionalism in health care providers, with the latest equipment and the most sophisticated technology available. They believe that the staff will all be able to use all of the equipment. Patients expect that every provider is fully trained in and aware of the latest technical advances or the most current research in the specific area that affects the patient. Interestingly, although most of the literature surrounding the "provider" of health care points to the physician as the one who is most correlated to satisfaction (18,19), there are data within radiation therapy that the radiation therapist holds a particularly high standing as a determinant of satisfaction (20) within radiation medicine. Thus, it is essential that the therapist be perceived as skilled, compassionate, and trustworthy.

Patients and family also believe that all systems and resources needed for their care are fully functional and present. There is an expectation that computers are working, supplies are present and at hand, and they are in a well-run, efficient and organized, technical setting. Patients do not really think about "how" this is all measured or guaranteed; they just take for granted that "it is."

Most patients come with the expectation that although trainees may be present and observing, those personnel will not be assigned to "do anything to them" in important

aspects of care (21). Similarly, the notion that temporary workers—who have limited knowledge of the equipment or system—may be assigned to care for them is a surprise to most patients.

Patients believe not only that the equipment and staff will be adequate, but also that the treatments offered by these entities will be effective. They must believe this. Otherwise, they would not subject themselves to the pain and discomfort of the actual procedure; the comorbidities of the treatment; the time taken away from their lives; the time, effort, and money it takes to get to treatment; and the hope one needs to continue on the journey of treatment. When physicians quote success rates of treatment, there is substantial variation on how this is perceived, owing in part to the manner in which it is presented (22). Most patients will focus on the successes and not give much thought to the risks, and the challenge of confronting therapeutic failure is formidable (23). For many patients, a 5% risk factor means that it is 95% of a sure "thing"; however, they do not imagine that if they are in the 5% category, then it is 100% ineffective for them. This is a shock for most patients and family members.

Patient-centered care: cultural issues, issues of dignity, privacy, shared decision making, and quality of life

Patient-centered care is a very old concept (24). Although classically this focuses on the physician–patient relationship, within radiation medicine it is prudent to use the term *provider*. Not only the physician, but also nursing and therapy, would do well to adhere to several of these guiding principles. The components of patient-centered care include (Figure 22.1) (25) the provider exploration of the patient's disease and the illness experience, the provider's understanding of the whole person, the patient and provider finding common ground regarding management, education regarding the prevention of side effects and promotion of health, and the enhancement of the patient–provider relationship over time. To progress in a truly patient-centered manner, it is worth exploring issues of culture, dignity, privacy, shared decision making, and independence/quality of life.

Culture

The concept of cultural issues has become increasingly more complex and sophisticated and many have struggled with it in the past few years. In the Past, cultural issues focused on language difficulties for people who come from different countries and cultures. Now language is only part of the question (26), and people are thinking broadly and deeply about the notion of cultural diversity (27,28)—concepts such as the meaning of health and illness, cultural variation in beliefs about death and dying, the role of family in caring for the sick (29), or

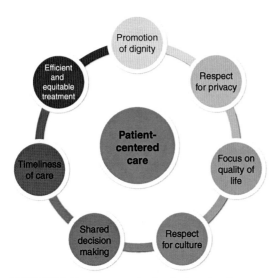

FIGURE 22.1 The components of patient-centered care.

the rituals for care of the patient after death. Challenging questions arise around "What is the current definition of family?" and "How does the health care system response to issues of sexual preference or sexual transition?" Inadequate responses to any of these questions prompt patient dissatisfaction.

Dignity

Donna Hicks, in her 2011 book entitled *Dignity* (30), says that "dignity is an internal state of peace that comes with the recognition and acceptance of the value and vulnerability of all living things." In other words, the patient has an inherent and internal sense of his or her own dignity as a valued and sentient being. The patient comes with the expectation, hope, fear, and wish that his or her own dignity—his or her innate sense of worth and value—will be recognized, acknowledged, and treated well; in essence, the patient hopes that he or she will be treated with respect. The specific domains of dignity within palliative cancer care are symptom distress, existential distress, dependency, piece of mind, and social support (31). When health care providers give patient short shrift in this particular aspect, then patients will judge themselves to have not been treated properly or respectfully.

Privacy

The notion of privacy has also evolved over time. In the past, privacy might have meant maintaining confidentiality about a particular patient's clinical history or personal identity in casual conversation, or the drawing of drapes in an examination room. Today, with the prevalence of and reliance on computers and the innate risks to breaches of patient confidential and personal health information

has resulted in the notion of privacy becoming a more complicated matter that requires complicated protection strategies (32). However, for patients the essence of the issue is the same; although they retain for themselves the right to share information about themselves however they please, they expect that the health care facility and health care providers will not breach their confidentiality in any way.

Shared decision making

The notion that the patient and the health care provider are in an equal relationship where each party has equal power and authority in the decision-making process is false in health care. There is a knowledge imbalance that results in a power imbalance, and "sharing" on the basis of equality will not be possible. However, the patient must be able to give informed consent, and in order to do that, he or she must understand the issue to the best of his or her ability. This means that the health care provider must be precise and understandable in all communications, but particularly in conversations surrounding decision making. With better understanding, the patient will be better able to share in the decision making and will be better able to live with the consequences of his or her decisions, and also will feel more satisfied with the care, with less anxiety (33).

Quality of life

The notion of "quality of life" has been growing in importance over the last two decades, and there is much struggle in the understanding of the definition of the term. It is getting a lot of attention, particularly since patient-reported quality of life has been linked with improved outcomes (34–38). Perhaps, like the notion that "beauty lies in the eye of the beholder," quality of life is determined by the person who must live it. Health care providers must strive for the ideal or the best cure that can be achieved through available technologies and interventions. Patients, in contrast, may be prepared to accept a lesser state. Frank discussion with each patient will help to define exactly what "quality of life" means for that person and what can reasonably be expected for a given disease status.

Timeliness of care

We live in a time of "instantaneous" everything, and expectations are growing around the timeliness of all sorts of services. It is therefore natural for this expectation to be applied to health care services. Certainly, when a patient hears that he or she has cancer, the orientation (after the shock has worn off) is to start treatment immediately to stop the invisible growth of the cancer. But as those who work in health care know, there are many processes and systems that take time to reveal themselves. For example, pathology results cannot be accessed immediately; it takes time to obtain the proper staging studies or procedures; review and consultation take time before unequivocal facts can be established, and not everyone needs immediate treatment.

Most patients understand that health care services will take time to organize and are prepared to wait a reasonable amount of time. Most patients also recognize that some patients are sicker and must be triaged to receive care first. There are some patients, however, whose own fear or own narcissism prevails, and they will honestly say that they are unwilling or unable to wait for services and demand immediate attention. All of the previously noted scenarios require discussion, with the key effective elements in all of these discussions being factual disclosure, forthright explanation, reassurance, and setting out of a plan that is known and understood.

Efficiency

When a patient hears the diagnosis of cancer, the immediate reaction, after the shock and fear have passed, is "When can we start treatment?" Of course, most people realize that there must be some planning to prepare the actual treatment, but generally speaking the amount of time that it takes to complete diagnostics, and staging, and create treatment plans, is much longer than patients imagine. Radiation oncology departments should seek to be proactive about managing start times, understanding how long the treatment-planning process takes, and understand the downstream effects of any upstream delays to allow prompt notification of the patient. Current Six Sigma–type strategies allow for this sort of proactive management (39–41). Once a patient is "in the system," and going through the treatment, the focus and anxiety of "time" recede and the attention is refocused on comorbidities and seeing if the treatment is working.

Equitable care

Unfortunately, despite growing awareness of the existence of health care disparities, they persist (42–45). These inequities, which can be based along racial, cultural, socioeconomic, sexual, or sexual-orientation lines, can inhibit access to care (46). Patients perceive quality care to be free of such inequalities.

THE PATIENT EXPERIENCE OF ERROR

Many organized groups in medicine, particularly in the last two decades, have focused on developing definitions of *patient safety* and *quality of care*. These two concepts are intimately related to one another, and there is quite a bit of research on these topics. These definitions have led to the development of many different types of measureable indicators and standards that are believed to be,

directly or indirectly, an indication of both patient safety and quality of health care. Because organized medicine can only act on those things that can be measured and controlled, the focus has tended to be on the measurement of errors, the prevention of errors, the appropriate use of medical therapies, the timing of various functions (response time), or the efficacy of specific interventions, to name a few.

For many patients, although they recognize that these matters (and many not mentioned) are important, they take such things as a "given." For patients and family members, the most impactful measures of safety are expressed in the following question: "Did I get the right care, done properly, and did I get better?" "Were the people caring/compassionate to me?" "Did they answer my questions and do I understand what happened and what is going to happen to me?"

When a mishap occurs (such as an equipment malfunction in the midst of the procedure, a miscalculation in a setting, or some other event that would be described as an "incident"), the patient is shocked and asks questions such as "How could this have happened?" "How can you let a novice work on me?" "Don't you have systems in place to check on these things regularly?" This is followed almost immediately by self-concern, "What does this mean for me?" "What is going to happen to me?"

In responding to these patient questions, there are often limitations and unknowns that result in less-than-comprehensive responses that, in turn, prompt further anxiety, fear, anger, and suspicion about safety. An example might be helpful here. Take the scenario in which radiation has been set up for a particular patient, and despite double or triple checks, a miscalculation in the radiation dosage is found, and the only explanation is "human error." Patient have a difficult time believing that human error is still possible in a world/circumstance/hospital where science and technology are expected to be sophisticated and standardized and where safety monitoring measures prevail. With respect to the patient's concern as to what will be the consequences or long-term sequelae of a safety error, this is not always known, and this uncertainty amplifies the already existing anxiety and distress on the part of the patient. The reader is directed to Chapter 24 for a more thorough discussion of this topic.

THE ROLE OF THE PATIENT IN SAFETY

Although there is much reluctance on the part of health care providers to bring up the subject of medical error with patients, it is by no means unknown to those receiving health care. Public opinion surveys show that 75% of those surveyed view health care as "moderately safe" and would have concerned about error if hospitalized (47–48). Some patients may not wish to have any involvement in this, which doubtless varies on the basis of demographic factors (49–51) as well as their

Table 22.1 Example Letter (54): Engaging the Patient in Safety

Letter from the Medical Physics Team

Radiation therapy is an extremely effective method for treating cancer, using radiation to kill cancer cells while maintaining normal body functions.

For the radiation therapy to be effective, it must be delivered accurately, to the right locations and in the correct amounts. The processes for making sure that the proper radiation treatment is delivered accurately and safely is termed *quality assurance*. Our entire radiation oncology team is dedicated to making sure that your treatment is delivered in a safe and accurate manner.

The radiation oncology team members responsible for setting up and running our treatment-related quality assurance procedures are UCLA faculty of medical physicists. We are formally trained in physics and medical physics with MS or PhD degrees and have significant additional advanced clinical training following our degrees. All of our senior medical physicists have been certified by the American Board of Radiology in therapeutic medical physics, which serves as an independent certification of our clinical competence. Our responsibilities include making sure that the computer systems that help the radiation oncology team to design the optimal treatment plan for you and the linear accelerators and other machines that deliver the treatments are operating within nationally and internationally accepted specification for accuracy and safety.

Your safety is our primary concern in the design of your treatment plan and in design of our quality assurance program. Our team members include experts in the design of such programs. Whenever available, we also utilize national and international standards in quality assurance, where many members have been involved in the writing of those standards. As part of our routine processes, we continuously review and enhance our quality assurance program on an ongoing basis. As part of our research mission, we seek to develop and test new quality control and quality assurance techniques, comparing them to existing programs in an effort to further enhance the safe delivery of radiation treatment for our patients. During your treatment, you may see some of these processes being evaluated from time to time. Feel free to ask any of the team members about them.

Finally, safe delivery of treatment does not happen by chance, but results from a collaborative effort between the medical professionals of our treatment team with you, the patient. So, we ask you to play an active role as well. Please, always feel comfortable to ask questions at any time about our quality assurance and safety programs as well as about your treatment.

Sincerely,
Nzhde Agazaryan, PhD
Professor and Chief of Clinical Medical Physics
Daniel Low, PhD
Professor and Vice Chair for Medical Physics

Source: Medical Physics: Letter from the Medical Physics Team: Radiation Oncology UCLA, last accessed September 11, 2015. http://radonc.ucla.edu/body.cfm?id=301, with permission.

overall health and disease status (52–53). Patients should be informed about safety checks that they will notice during their care (time-out procedures, wrist banding) so they understand what should take place on a daily basis. They should be invited to question anything that does not make sense to them or seems unusual. However, the desire and inclination of the patient to be actively involved in patient safety will be very individual. The invitation should be extended to the patient in question (see Table 22.1); however, safety remains the responsibility of the treatment team (55).

SUMMARY AND FUTURE DIRECTIONS

Quality cancer care is marked by respect for dignity, the concerns of patients from within their cultural context, and the delivery of safe and effective care. This is a complex process, which requires a well-organized team with empathetic communication skills. Although patients may have varying levels of desire to be integrated into the patient safety process, patients should feel comfortable asking questions about their care and should understand the safeguards that are part of their daily routine.

REFERENCES

1. Institute of Medicine. *Crossing the Quality Chasm: A New Health System for the 21st Century*. Washington, DC: National Academy Press; 2001.

2. Ware J, Snyder M, Wright WR, et al. Defining and measuring patient satisfaction with medical care. *Eval Program Plan*. 1983;6(3/4):247–263.

3. Rubin HR, Gandek B, Rogers WH, et al. Patients' ratings of outpatient visits in different practice settings: results from the medical outcomes study. *JAMA*. 1993;270(7):835–840.

4. Kirsner RS, Federman DG. Patient satisfaction: quality of care from the patients' perspective. *Arch Dermatol*. 1997;133(11):1427–1431.

5. Fenton JJ, Jerant AF, Bertakis KD, et al. The cost of satisfaction: a national study of patient satisfaction, health care utilization, expenditures, and mortality. *Arch Intern Med.* 2012;172(5):405–411.

6. Liptak GS, Hulka BS, Cassel JC. Effectiveness of physician-mother interactions during infancy. *Pediatrics.* 1977;60(2):186–192.

7. Linn BS. Burn patients' evaluation of emergency department care. *Ann Emerg Med.* 1982;11(5):255–259.

8. Hickson GB, Clayton EW, Entman SS, et al. Obstetricians' prior malpractice experience and patients' satisfaction with care. *JAMA.* 1994;272(20):1583–1587.

9. Hickson GB, Clayton EW, Githens PB, et al. Factors that prompted families to file medical malpractice claims following perinatal injuries. *JAMA.* 1992;267(10):1359–1363.

10. Brook RH, McGlynn EA, Cleary PD. Quality of health care: Part 2: measuring quality of care. *N Engl J Med.* 1996;335(13):966–970.

11. Stanowski AC, Simpson K, White A. Pay for performance: are hospitals becoming more efficient in improving their patient experience? *J Healthcare Manage.* 2015;60(4):268–285.

12. Boulware LE, Cooper LA, Ratner LE, et al. Race and trust in the health care system. *Public Health Rep.* 2003;118(4):358–365.

13. Casagrande SS, Gary TL, LaVeist TA, et al. Perceived discrimination and adherence to medical care in a racially integrated community. *J Gen Intern Med.* 2007;22(3):389–395.

14. LaVeist TA, Nickerson KJ, Bowie JV. Attitudes about racism, medical mistrust, and satisfaction with care among African American and White cardiac patients. *Med Care Res Rev.* 2000;57(Suppl 1):146–161.

15. Guadagnolo BA, Cina K, Helbig P, et al. Medical mistrust and less satisfaction with health care among native Americans presenting for cancer treatment. *J Health Care Poor Underserved.* 2009;20(1):210–226.

16. Zebrowitz LA, Franklin RG Jr. The attractiveness halo effect and the babyface stereotype in older and younger adults: similarities, own-age accentuation, and older adult positivity effects. *Exp Aging Res.* 2014;40(3):375–393.

17. Sorra J, Khanna K, Dyer N, et al. Exploring relationships between patient safety culture and patients' assessments of hospital care. *J Patient Saf.* 2012;8(3):131–139.

18. Koichiro O. Improving patient satisfaction in hospital care setting. *Health Serv Manage Res.* 2011;24:163–169.

19. Blanchard CG, Labrecque MS, Ruckdeschel JC, et al. Physician behaviors, patient perceptions, and patient characteristics as predictors of satisfaction of hospitalized adult cancer patients. *Cancer.* 1990;65:186–192.

20. Famiglietti RM, Neal EC, Edwards TJ, et al. Determinants of patient satisfaction during receipt of radiation therapy. *Int J Radiat Oncol Biol Phys.* 2013;87(1):148–152. doi:10.1016/j.ijrobp.2013.05.020.

21. Ubel PA, Silver-Isenstadt A. Are patients willing to participate in medical education? *J Clin Ethics.* 2000;11(3):230–235.

22. Porensky EK, Carpenter BD. Breaking bad news: effects of forecasting diagnosis and framing prognosis. *Patient Educ Couns.* 2015;99(1):68–76. doi:10.1016/j.pec.2015.07.022.

23. Morgans AK, Schapira L. Confronting therapeutic failure: a conversation guide. *Oncologist.* 2015;20(8):946–951. doi:10.1634/theoncologist.2015-0050.

24. Crookshank FG. The theory of diagnosis. *Lancet.* 1926;2:939.

25. Stewart M, Brown JB, Donner A, et al. The impact of patient-centered care on outcomes. *J Fam Pract.* 2000;49(9):796–804.

26. Divi C, Koss RG, Schmaltz SP, et al. Language proficiency and adverse events in U.S. hospitals: a pilot study. *Int J Qual Health Care.* 2007;19:60–67.

27. Lopez-Class M, Perret-Gentil M, Kreling B, et al. Quality of life among immigrant Latina breast cancer survivors: realities of culture and enhancing cancer care. *J Cancer Educ.* 2011;26(4):724–733. doi:10.1007/s13187-011-0249-4.

28. Taylor EJ. Spirituality, culture, and cancer care. *Semin Oncol Nurs.* 2001;17(3):197–205.

29. Weinberg AD, Jackson PM. *Cultural Competence in Cancer Care: A Health Care Professional's Passport.* Houston, TX: Intercultural Cancer Council of Baylor College; 2006.

30. Hicks D. *Dignity.* New Haven, CT: Yale University Press; 2011.

31. Chochinov HM, Hassard T, McClement S, et al. The patient dignity inventory: a novel way of measuring dignity-related distress in palliative care. *J Pain Symptom Manage.* 2008;36(6):559–571.

32. Gummadi S, Housri N, Zimmers TA, et al. Electronic medical record: a balancing act of patient safety, privacy and health care delivery. *Am J Med Sci.* 2014;348(3):238–243.

33. Shabason JE, Mao JJ, Frankel ES, et al. Shared decision-making and patient control in radiation

oncology: implications for patient satisfaction. *Cancer.* 2014;120(12):1863–1870. doi:10.1002/cncr.28665.

34. Eton DT, Fairclough DL, Cella D, et al. Early change inpatient-reported health during lung cancer chemotherapy predicts clinical outcomes beyond those predicted by baseline report: results from Eastern Cooperative Oncology Group Study 5592. *J Clin Oncol.* 2003;21:1536–1543.

35. Gotay CC, Kawamoto CT, Bottomley A, et al. The prognostic significance of patient-reported outcomes in cancer clinical trials. *J Clin Oncol.* 2008;26:1355–1363.

36. Maione P, Perrone F, Gallo C, et al. Pretreatment quality of life and functional status assessment significantly predict survival of elderly patients with advanced non–small-cell lung cancer receiving chemotherapy: a prognostic analysis of the multicenter Italian lung cancer in the elderly study. *J Clin Oncol.* 2005;23:6865–6872.

37. Montazeri A. Quality of life data as prognostic indicators of survival in cancer patients: an overview of the literature from 1982 to 2008. *Health Qual Life Outcomes.* 2009;7:102.

38. Sloan JA, Zhao X, Novotny PJ, et al. Relationship between deficits in overall quality of life and non–small-cell lung cancer survival. *J Clin Oncol.* 2012;30:1498–1504.

39. Kapur A, Potters L. Six sigma tools for a patient safety-oriented, quality-checklist driven radiation medicine department. *Pract Radiat Oncol.* 2012;2(2):86–96. doi:10.1016/j.prro.2011.06.010.

40. Kovalchuk N, Russo GA, Shin JY, et al. Optimizing efficiency and safety in a radiation oncology department through the use of ARIA 11 visual care path. *Pract Radiat Oncol.* 2015;5(5):295–303. doi:10.1016/j.prro.2015.05.001.

41. Kruskal JB, Reedy A, Pascal L, et al. Quality initiatives: lean approach to improving performance and efficiency in a radiology department. *Radiographics.* 2012;32(2):573–587. doi:10.1148/rg.322115128.

42. Strong K, Kunst AE. The complex interrelationship between ethnic and socio-economic inequalities in health. *J Public Health (Oxf).* 2009;31:324–325.

43. Goss E, Lopez AM, Brown CL, et al. American Society of Clinical Oncology policy statement: disparities in cancer care. *J Clin Oncol.* 2009;27:2881–2885.

44. Crawley L, Kagawa-Singer M. *Racial, Cultural, and Ethnic Factors Affecting the Quality of End-of-Life Care in California: Findings and Recommendations.* Oakland, CA: California Health Care Foundation; 2007. http://www.chcf.org/~/media/MEDIA%20LIBRARY%20Files/PDF/PDF%20C/PDF%20CulturalFactorsEOL.pdf.

45. Sabin J, Nosek BA, Greenwald A, et al. Physicians' implicit and explicit attitudes about race by MD race, ethnicity, and gender. *J Health Care Poor Underserved.* 2009;20:896–913.

46. Agénor M, Bailey Z, Krieger N, et al. Exploring the cervical cancer screening experiences of Black Lesbian, Bisexual, and Queer women: the role of patient-provider communication. *Women Health.* 2015;55(6):717–736. doi:10.1080/03630242.2015.1039182.

47. National Patient Safety Foundation. *Patient Safety: Your Role in Making Healthcare Safer.* North Adams, MA: National Patient Safety Foundation; 2002.

48. National Patient Safety Foundation. *National Patient Safety Foundation at the AMA: Public Opinion on Patient Safety Issues, Research Findings.* North Adams, MA: National Patient Safety Foundation; 1997.

49. Arora NK, McHorney CA. Patient preferences for medical decision making: who really wants to participate? *Med Care.* 2000;38:335–412.

50. Beaver K, Luker KA, Owens RG, et al. Treatment decision-making in women newly diagnosed with breast cancer. *Cancer Nurs.* 1996;19:8–19.

51. Degner LF, Kristjanson LJ, Bowman D, et al. Information needs and decisional preferences in women with breast cancer. *JAMA.* 1997;277:1485–1492.

52. Adams RJ, Smith BJ, Ruffin RE. Patient preferences for autonomy in decision making in asthma management. *Thorax.* 2001;56:126–132.

53. Catalan J, Brener N, Andrews H, et al. Whose health is it? Views about decision-making and information-seeking from people with HIV infections and their professional careers. *AIDS Care.* 1994;6:349–356.

54. Radiation Oncology UCLA. Medical physics: letter from the medical physics team. http://radonc.ucla.edu/body.cfm?id=301.

55. Davis RE, Jacklin R, Sevdalis N, et al. Patient involvement in patient safety: what factors influence patient participation and engagement? *Health Expect.* 2007;10(3):259–267.

23 The Impact of Incidents: Reporting, Investigating, and Improving

Jennifer L. Johnson and Suzanne B. Evans

INTRODUCTION

A medical physicist uses an inadequate chamber size to calibrate small field dosimetry for stereotactic radiation; 145 patients are treated using micro-multileaf collimators with a maximum overdose of approximately 200% (1). The radiation oncology team makes a small error in localizing the target of an early-stage inoperable lung cancer patient undergoing hypofractionated stereotactic body radiation therapy (SBRT), leading to potentially 20% underdosing of the tumor and unintended overdosing of adjacent organs at risk (2). In the Therac-25 incidents, two different computer software errors in a computerized linear accelerator resulted in massive radiation overdoses that injured six people and killed two more (3).

How can incidents like these happen? The impact of harmful incidents on patients is sometimes immediate and life changing. They may be so egregious that family members, the health care facility, or governments demand answers as to how such incidents could happen. When scenarios like these are made public, other practices not involved in the incidents look at their own processes and try to assess whether they could have the same incident, or cause the same patient harm.

These clinical examples are shocking and devastating, and, unfortunately, the occurrence rates nationally or internationally are not well known. They are estimated to be rare (4). The rare ones, however, are not the only ones that impact the patient. Other clinical scenarios may include localizing to the wrong vertebral body for a thoracic spine irradiation for one fraction; treating an electron field with the wrong electron cone insert; or inserting a physical wedge into the treatment machine with the wrong orientation. This chapter explores the impact of all manner of radiotherapy incidents, and comments on the role of reporting, methods of investigation, and the path to meaningful improvement.

THE IMPACT OF INCIDENTS ON THE RISK OF THERAPEUTIC FAILURE

"Minor" incidents, although potentially not devastating in dosimetric or medical severity, may still affect the patient's treatment outcome. They are much more common than the catastrophic errors previously described. As radiation biology teaches us, radiation works by logarithmic cell kill. If the prescribed dose is not delivered as intended, this may result in clonogens remaining at the conclusion of treatment, with an escalated chance of recurrence. While there has never been and never should be a randomized trial on the impact of error, the process of clinical trial quality assurance is quite informative. Protocol variations typically include incorrect segmentation, incorrect field design, and incorrect dose, meaning either geometric miss or improper dosing to cancer target structures. Likewise, errors in radiation therapy typically involve errors in dose or targeting. These sorts of protocol variations are actually quite common, even among common diseases very familiar to the radiation oncology team. The results of the European Organisation for Research and Treatment of Cancer (EORTC) dummy-runs quality assurance program demonstrated major deviation rates of 70% in the setting of salvage radiation for prostate cancer (5), 20% for EORTC 22042 for meningioma (6), and 50% in a breast cancer trial (7). Furthermore, major protocol deviations were statistically significant for an increase in the observed hazard ratios for death, including 1.336 for pancreas (8), 1.99 for head and neck (9), and 1.74 for a meta-analysis of 8 separate trials (10). This suggests that however the incorrect dose to the target structure occurs, it may have a very real impact on the chance of therapeutic success.

THE IMPACT OF INCIDENTS ON PATIENTS

The impact of process deviations and protocol deviations on patients may be difficult to ascertain. Although the physical impact of incidents on patients can be direct, immediate, and known for certain incidents, they are more commonly unknown. Underdosing all or part of the tumor does not cause normal tissue damage, and therapeutic failure can occur without radiotherapy error. This makes an underdosing incident difficult to detect. Likewise, there is often a range (albeit narrow) of acceptable doses for a given cancer, so an underdose according to the prescription may still result in a clinically acceptable delivered dose. Conversely, it may take years or decades to see radiation injuries related to an overdosing incident. They may be obscured by a variety of other potential contributing factors not related to an incident. These include the nonzero incidence of complications in correct delivery and fastidious adherence to normal tissue constraints; the ability of a cancer regression to result in deformity to the body (e.g., soft palate obliteration after successful treatment for oropharyngeal cancer); the ability of recurrent disease to cause profound morbidity, which can nonetheless coexist with radiation-induced injury; the ability of chemotherapeutics or biologic agents to enhance typically small incidences of radiotherapy toxicities; and the patient's comorbidities, health history, and general physical condition. This all makes a radiation overdose difficult to discern from any number of events/circumstances that can lead to a radiotherapy-associated toxicity. Thus, sometimes an error is undetected and does not have an attributable psychological impact on the patient due to its obscurity.

The psychological impact of known incidents on patients is typically profound. Patients may lose confidence in a provider or a treatment team that does not address an incident. For example, a patient experiences a close call in a linac gantry clearance. The radiation therapists try to reassure the patient. The patient is exasperated and tells the radiation oncologist during the weekly visit; there is little that can be done to reassure the patient about his or her safety after such a close call. Error disclosure to a patient is more accepted because it shows respect to the patient and the transparency in care. If the incident did not cause severe patient harm, patients at a minimum appreciate being told by the radiation oncologist what happened, why it happened, and what steps the practice is taking to prevent it from happening to another patient. The readers are directed to Chapter 24 on medical error disclosure and Chapter 22 on the patient perspective on quality and the role of the patient in safety for a more robust discussion of these issues.

THE IMPACT OF INCIDENTS ON THE CLINICAL TEAM

The impact of error on the clinical team is quite different with "insignificant errors" than with significant errors. Normalization of deviance (11) occurs when repeated deviation from a quality or safety process does not result in harm and becomes the new normal process. Because the original process was designed for quality and safety, it is likely that the deviated process may not sufficiently provide the same protections. Usually, signals and evidence of the deviation are available, and it is up to the organization to recognize and act upon them before the deviation leads to a significant error. However, process deviations in the absence of consequence are likely to be adopted and result in a drift of the behavior of the staff from the procedural ideal, lowering safe behavior and predisposing to incidence as the new "norm."

Similarly, individual responses to close calls can go two ways: an increase in risk awareness and becoming risk averse, or a loss of vulnerability and reinforcing the risk-taking behavior (12,13). Dillon et al describe human behavior toward risk in relation to threats of major weather incidents, and present scenarios as "vulnerable near misses" and "resilient near misses." A "vulnerable near miss" is one in which an undesirable outcome almost occurs, but, through some chance of fate, is narrowly avoided. This sort of perception decreases risk-taking behavior. A "resilient near miss" occurs when those involved in the incident perceive that the same narrowly avoided undesirable outcome was avoided owing to some skill, characteristic, or protection possessed by those involved. This resilient near miss increases risk-taking behavior. Being more risk averse fosters quality and safety initiatives in the organization, whereas more risk taking puts the organization and the patients at greater risk. Part of the role of organizations investigating incidents is to ensure that their staff view these sorts of events as vulnerable near misses! Too many incidents perceived as resilient near misses can lead the therapy team into actually increasing risk-taking behavior. This is a pattern seen in human behavior in other settings as well, even at great personal consequence—survivors of military combat exhibit postcombat invincibility (14), wherein they adopt risky behaviors from a false sense of invulnerability caused by many near misses. This is a human tendency that must be guarded against, and is part of the reason why open discussions of near misses are essential to a strong safety culture in a radiation department.

Without a doubt, serious incidents have a profound impact on the clinical team. The sense of failure to ensure the safety of a patient's care delivery can greatly affect any team member involved in the incident, either directly or indirectly. Some involvement in significant errors can lead to feelings of being a "second victim" (15) and experience of grief. They may also lead to worry about judgment and decreased trust, impacting the team dynamics and professional relationships, or lead to burnout (16). The mistakes that are made or the occurrence of severe near misses weighs heavily and has a long-lasting impact. Experienced individuals will remember them as though they had occurred just the previous day, even years after the event. Sometimes, the clinician involved may be so overwrought as to request time away from his or her duties, a practice that is routine in other industries (17). There is evidence, however, that involving clinicians in investigation of the error and allowing them to still be seen as valued members of the clinical team can be helpful in their recovery following an incident (18).

INVESTIGATING INCIDENTS: BEGINNING WITH THE FRAME

When embarking on an investigation of an incident, it is helpful to know how to frame the investigation. Is this the work of one "bad apple"? Or is the situation more complex? Consider the structure of the radiotherapy treatment team. The responsibility for radiation treatment is diffused throughout the roles of the team members, each with their specialty knowledge and understanding. The care is so complex that it would be impossible for one person to do it all, and for only one person to be responsible. The physician, in essence, delegates the technical understanding and safety to the medical physicist; he or she delegates the actual treatment plan details to the dosimetrist; and he or she delegates the actual patient set-up and beam delivery to the radiation therapists. Instead of focusing on the actions of a single individual at the sharp end of the error, a systems view of both treatment and incidents reflects the reality. The reader is directed to Chapter 5 for a deeper discussion on the nature of error.

USING INCIDENT LEARNING SYSTEMS TO INVESTIGATE INCIDENTS

The airline and the nuclear power industries (19,20) are now described as high-reliability organizations because of their low frequency of catastrophic events. They became highly reliable because they report any incident, near miss or close call, or unsafe condition that they encounter. They have a reporting culture and utilize incident learning systems, which are covered in detail in another chapter. Reporting incidents into an incident learning system is the first step in process and organizational improvement.

However, collecting the information is the beginning, and merely collecting the information is insufficient. If the organization does not take action on what is reported, then people stop reporting. In addition, the opposite is true: if people find that reporting improves their working conditions or processes, then people believe reporting is worth their time and effort and so will increase their reporting. It might seem counterintuitive that the number of reported incidents, near misses, and unsafe conditions actually increases with an improved safety culture; however, the severity of incidents goes down (21–23). Increased reporting reflects an interest in learning, the importance of transparency, and the value of active participation in making things better for oneself as well as others. It reveals that engagement outweighs the fear of retaliation for reporting, although fears of blame and litigation can persist (24,25).

Improvements can happen only if the organization looks at the incidents and near misses and tries to find ways to take positive actions to resolve them. Therefore, organizations that are highly reliable are so not just because they report these things, but also because they learn from them. They have a learning culture about their processes, which keeps the actual number of events as low as possible. Learning can come from examining both major and minor incidents. Organizations should examine high-frequency incidents or near misses. A large number of similar minor incidents or near misses highlights some problem in the process or the organization, creating a huge learning opportunity for the organization. The organization then has time to incorporate a safety barrier before something more severe happens, in addition to decreasing the occurrence rate. Organizations clearly should examine cases of high severity to find root causes contributing to the incident. Organizations with a strong safety culture understand that individuals do not work in a vacuum, but rather in a system that creates conditions for the incident to happen.

TENETS OF INCIDENT INVESTIGATION

The airline and nuclear power industries study their incidents using a root cause analysis (RCA) technique (26), developed for investigating industrial accidents. The goal of conducting an RCA is very simple: to determine what happened, why it happened, and what to do to prevent it from happening again. Clearly, these industries' tragedies are public events, and they use many resources to investigate. In an effort to become more highly reliable in their care, radiation oncology practices also have moved toward a more formal approach in incident learning and examination of actual incidents. Resource availability within a radiation oncology practice is local and limited, but investigating a single severe incident or a high-occurrence type of incident is doable and valuable even within those constraints.

There are basic tenets of incident investigation. The first involves a foundational understanding of why errors occur. There are underlying problems in the practice that increase the likelihood of errors. Errors can be of two types: active, where the individual interacts with the complex system; and latent, where problems are hidden until the conditions are right for them to occur (27). As such, an RCA is really a "systems analysis," where relationships between the different layers of the system are examined as well as other aspects of system design (26).

A second tenet is choosing the team to complete the investigation. First, none of the primary team members should have been directly involved in the incident. This is important in order to keep an impartial view of the events while collecting the data. However, this does not mean that once the investigation is complete and the causes are understood, one should not turn to those involved in the incident for potential solutions to future prevention. Doing so can actually help reinforce the personal and professional worth of team members involved in error, and is encouraged. It is preferred that none of the investigation team members have direct supervision over the involved team members, to avoid implications of blame or retribution. The team leader needs to have knowledge of how to conduct an RCA as well as of the subject area. If possible, the RCA team should include a facilitator who has RCA expertise. Lastly, the team should include content experts who have knowledge of the subject area. Individuals have different backgrounds, knowledge, experience, and understanding of processes based on their role in the practice, and so would look at the incident from their viewpoints. The radiation oncologist, medical physicist, dosimetrist, and radiation therapist are experts in their delivery roles and have specific knowledge of processes and responsibilities. The team in the practice may not always be the same for every incident, however. For example, if the incident involved prior records of previous radiation treatment, the team may include a representative from medical records, nursing, midlevel providers, and administration.

A third tenet is to form the language of the incident investigation. The language helps team members and the practice have a consistent understanding and meaning of words, as well as to help shape the tone of the investigation. For example, there are differences in a blame culture, a blame-free culture, and a just culture. A nonretaliation policy of reporting incidents is not the same as a blanket nonretaliation policy. Additionally, those conducting the investigation should be very careful about how questions are asked. Those involved in an incident are often very sensitive to any perception of wrongdoing or errors in judgment. Language should be chosen gingerly to avoid the perception of blame or consternation, and to reinforce the purpose of learning and prevention of reoccurrence.

DATA COLLECTION AND INCIDENT CHRONOLOGY

An investigation of an incident is a bit like detective work, where evidence is reviewed to piece together what happens. The RCA team looks at the case records to piece together what happened in the incident. This may include medical records and record-and-verify system data. However, this tells only part of the story in uncovering what happened. Therefore, the team needs to conduct interviews to understand the conditions or reasons why involved members of the incident acted in the manner that they did. The interview questions should be open-ended, to allow the individual to freely provide useful information. The purpose is to minimize the chances of a team member introducing any potential bias; likewise, the investigating team can ask questions to consider other, less explicit contributing factors owing to their worldview to help expand the range of possibilities. The entire purpose of gathering evidence is to find out what exactly happened, in what particular chronology.

Additionally, it is meant to find out how the incident happened. The Therac-25 incidents were infamous because the newly designed computer-controlled treatment machine could not handle the speed with which the therapists entered keystrokes (3). Similar issues occur with other hardware and software bugs that are inadvertently uncovered. Uncovering the order of specific actions is also important in human-to-human interactions. For example, it may help to understand when peer reviews of contours and treatment plans occur, either before or after the patient has begun treatment; or it may be useful to know when a prescription change was communicated, starting a chain of events.

Lastly, the investigation is meant to get at the root causes as to why an incident happened. One way to do this is to utilize the "five why's" (28) until you get to something fundamental that you can control or correct. The technique works well at getting at certain issues. Imagine a situation where an on-call calculation is for SSD when the set-up is SAD treatment. An example plays out like the following:

- *Why was the patient set up for an SAD treatment technique?*
  - ○ Because the physician changed his mind midstream.
- *Why did the physician change his mind midstream?*
  - ○ Because he was uncertain which treatment technique he wanted to use.
- *Why was he uncertain which treatment technique he wanted to use?*
  - ○ Because he doesn't do clinical set-ups very often.
- *Why doesn't he do clinical set-ups very often?*
  - ○ Because we usually get notified early enough to go ahead and CT our emergent patients and follow regular treatment planning processes.
- *Why didn't we get notified early enough?*
  - ○ Because no one picked up the referral order when it came in.

In an example like this, different useful information becomes available that is helpful in identifying a root cause that contributed to the incident. The process is repeated about other key actions in the incident, such as specific questions regarding the SSD calculation itself. The goal is to find upstream factors that triggered the events in order to then make improvements in the radiation oncology treatment processes and practice environment to have higher quality and safely delivered care. The final answer cannot be something that cannot be controlled, such as the weather.

There are many versions of conducting an RCA that can be intimidating when first implementing the process properly. Firstly, the process seems very formal, lengthy, and intimidating. Depending upon the severity of the incident, this need not be the case. Certainly, a misadministration or reportable event to the state should be more formal, involving risk management and other institutional members with experience in conducting RCAs. However, other incidents may benefit from conducting an RCA internally without such intimidation. A mini-RCA can be done in as little as five to ten minutes. RCAs can be a very successful technique if the process is consistently followed and approached in as unbiased a manner as possible.

INCIDENT INVESTIGATION APPROACHES

Two such methods that are useful in the clinical environment include approaches known as the London Protocol (29) (Figures 23.1 and 23.2) and the Vincent methodology (30). Charles Vincent et al (30) applied James Reason's organizational accident model (27) for the clinical setting. Conditions and health care organization factors are combined into "factors influencing clinical practice," which includes the following types with specific contributing factors in each: institutional context, organizational and management factors, work environment factors, team factors, individual (staff) factors, task/technology factors, and patient factors. It is worth exploring each of these terms for clarity. The *institutional context* refers to the nature of the institution in which the department lives; for example, the institution is subject to certain regulations, and perhaps is slow to adopt new technology. *Organizational and management factors* relate to the existing policies, safety culture, and constraints of a given department; for example, the department perhaps is a blame culture that has unrealistic expectations in a financially constrained environment. *Work environment factors* relate to staffing levels, skill levels of the team, equipment status, and physical environment; for example, Spanish-language translators are scarcely available and often late, and an overworked department running extended hours skips their time-out and site confirmation with a Spanish-language speaker. *Team factors* refer to the working dynamics of the group; for example, there is a long-standing feud between dosimetry and therapy, which results in poor communication and reluctance to call each other for assistance. *Individual (staff) factors* relate to the individual's own intrinsic situation and skill set; for example, the physician is going through a divorce and is preoccupied while doing her contouring, resulting in a geometric miss. *Task and technology factors* relate to the sort of "human factors" things that can affect the likelihood of error; for example, the therapists are asked to look at five different monitors simultaneously. *Patient factors* refer to the characteristics of the patient that can contribute to a given incident; for example, the patient is extremely impatient and demanding, so rather than wait for dosimetry to come to the unit to confirm a treatment parameter in question, the patient is treated, and the parameters in question are later discovered to be in error.

Reason's "unsafe acts" of human behavior become Vincent et al's "care delivery problems." The term *care delivery problem* refers to any number of "unsafe acts":

lapses in judgment, slips, or departures from safe operating procedures. *Care delivery problem* is a more appropriate term because it is neutral, and encompasses the reality that a care delivery problem cannot be defined as one singular, isolated act. For example, the scenario of an inpatient not being monitored appropriately while within the department encompasses something that is likely a chronic problem over many days, by many individuals. The care delivery problem of inadequate monitoring may include the lack of communication of transport to nursing upon arrival/departure, therapy to nursing and vice versa, physician to nursing about completion of the weekly visit, management to administration about what equipment is needed for proper monitoring, or even the physical layout of the department, which may make monitoring more difficult. For each incident, after completing the chronology, the care delivery problems are individually identified, and the related clinical context and other patient factors are identified. Additionally, for each care delivery problem, contributing factors are identified. In general, the method recognizes that unsafe acts will occur in an environment that contributed to the situation.

The London Protocol is the revised, broader version of the Vincent methodology, originally devised for incidents in acute medical care. Additionally, the London Protocol emphasizes the response to incidents, such as making recommendations for improvement and creating an action plan. The original version was intended for individual risk managers, which was common practice at that time.

MAKING IMPROVEMENTS BASED ON INCIDENT INVESTIGATION

After completing an incident investigation, the practice should consider implementing improvements. From a variety of options to correct a single incident, the practice should choose no more than three to correct the system at a time. How to decide which three? For each proposed corrective action, the following must be answered:

- Does it effectively address the problem?
- How soon can it be implemented?
- What resources does it require?
- How can its effectiveness be monitored?
- Are there any downsides or unintended consequences?

The decision depends upon the effectiveness, timeliness, resources, monitoring, and unintended consequences.

There is a hierarchy of action effectiveness (27) based on the science of human behavior. Strong actions are those that make it difficult to deviate from. An example may be to introduce an engineering control or interlock, such as requiring physician prescription approvals in the record-and-verify system before turning on the radiation beam;

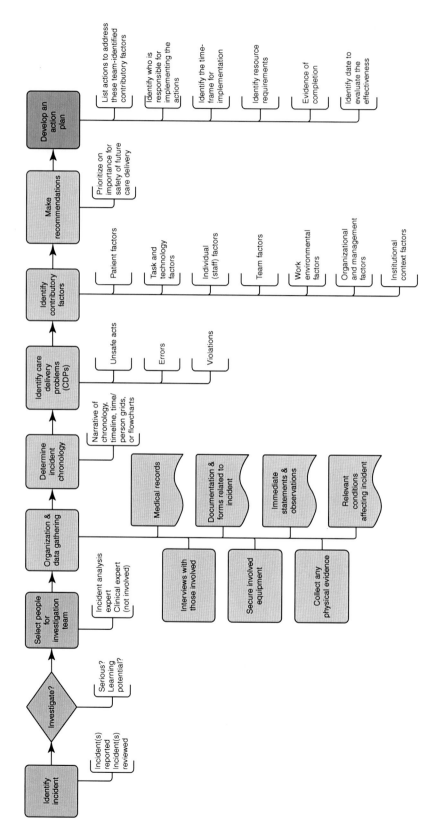

FIGURE 23.1 A schematic for incident investigation. (*Source*: Adapted from Ref. (29). Taylor-Adams S, Vincent C. Systems analysis of clinical incidents: the London protocol. *Clin Risk*. 2004;10(6):211–220.)

For each interviewee:

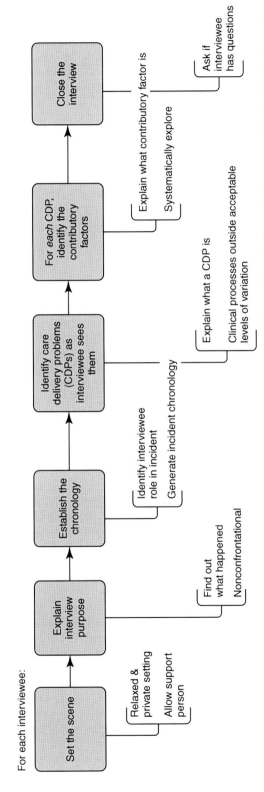

FIGURE 23.2 Key components of incident investigation interviews. (*Source*: Adapted from Ref. (29). Taylor-Adams S, Vincent C. Systems analysis of clinical incidents: the London protocol. *Clin Risk*. 2004;10(6):211–220.)

the information transfer to the delivery system becomes blocked. Other strong actions include simplifying the process wherever possible without affecting quality and safety, so that eliminating unnecessary steps minimizes normalization of deviance to the process. When strong actions cannot be identified, then the next lower effectiveness level should be considered. These are less effective because they are not as foolproof, as they rely on human behavior to follow; however, they have proven to be more effective than other remedial actions. Intermediate actions such as increasing staffing levels or decreasing the workload are useful and effective. Additional steps, such as implementing checklists, read-back procedures, and redundancy checks are also intermediate action examples. The weaker actions are usually the cheapest and quickest to implement, but are the least reliable in preventing errors. A weak action in response to an incident is to implement a new procedure or policy, without effectively addressing the causes of the incident. Training, although it has its value for new procedures, if completed the same way as it was initially may not resolve the issue, and it can be perceived as punishment.

When safety barriers are implemented into the process, they should be measured for effectiveness. The strategy should be tested to see if it works—that it actually prevents what it meant to. Then the practice should decide on timeliness to implement immediately or complete a pilot test for acceptability. Some solutions may be acted upon immediately but imperfectly, buying time until a more robust solution can be developed and rolled out. Some solutions should be tested in a pilot study, to see if a solution then should be adopted and transferable. Although not all solutions need to be pilot-tested, those that are intermediate and weaker actions could be, such as checklists that get refined over time. Error-preventative actions also should be monitored for effectiveness. This may be more easily done with high-frequency incidents or near-miss occurrences, where the number of related incidents reported is reduced. For less frequent, more serious incidents, proxies may have to be considered. Proxies can be electronic documentation where compliance can be pulled, such as an electronic time-out documentation completed daily. Electronically monitored options are preferred in terms of resources available for monitoring. Nonelectronic means may include using observation tracers on a routine basis to observe the adoption of better practices, such as for handwashing in and out of the treatment rooms or time-out procedures.

SUMMARY

Effective implementation of incident investigation, monitoring for effectiveness, and support for staff involved in error can result in the development of a true learning organization. When a practice becomes a learning organization, it adopts a continuous improvement approach to quality and safety. Leadership understands that its organization is a system to provide high-quality patient care, and that active and latent errors are always possible. The goal is to minimize the severity as much as possible, and to use both actual events and near misses to learn. Despite the need for leadership commitment and the dedication of resources, the end result will be higher quality care and a higher quality organization.

REFERENCES

1. Lopez PO, Cosset JM, Dunscombe P, et al. Preventing accidental exposures from new external beam radiation therapy technologies. *Ann ICRP.* 2009;39(4):1–86.

2. Solberg TD, Balter JM, Benedict SH, et al.. Quality and safety considerations in stereotactic radiosurgery and stereotactic body radiation therapy: executive summary. *Pract Radiat Oncol.* 2012;2(1):2–9.

3. Patton GA, Gaffney DK, Moeller JH. Facilitation of radiotherapeutic error by computerized record and verify systems. *Int J Radiat Oncol Biol Phys.* 2003;57(5):1509.

4. Macklis RM, Meier T, Weinhous MS. Error rates in clinical radiotherapy. *J Clin Oncol.* 1998;16(6):551–556.

5. Sassowsky M, Gut P, Hölscher T, et al. Use of EORTC target definition guidelines for dose-intensified salvage radiation therapy for recurrent prostate cancer: results of the quality assurance program of the randomized trial SAKK 09/10. *Int J Radiat Oncol Biol Phys.* 2013;87(3):534–541.

6. Weber DC, Poortmans PM, Hurkmans CW, et al. Quality assurance for prospective EORTC radiation oncology trials: the challenges of advanced technology in a multicenter international setting. *Radiother Oncol.* 2011;100(1):150–156.

7. Hurkmans CW, Borger JH, Rutgers EJ, et al. Quality assurance of axillary radiotherapy in the EORTC AMAROS trial 10981/22023: the dummy run. *Radiother Oncol.* 2003;68(3):233–240.

8. Abrams RA, Winter KA, Regine WF, et al. Failure to adhere to protocol specified radiation therapy guidelines was associated with decreased survival in RTOG 9704—a phase III trial of adjuvant chemotherapy and chemoradiotherapy for patients with resected adenocarcinoma

of the pancreas. *Int J Radiat Oncol Biol Phys.* 2012;82(2):809–816.

9. Peters LJ, O'Sullivan B, Giralt J, et al. Critical impact of radiotherapy protocol compliance and quality in the treatment of advanced head and neck cancer: results from TROG 02.02. *J Clin Oncol.* 2010;28(18):2996–3001.

10. Ohri N, Shen X, Dicker AP, et al. Radiotherapy protocol deviations and clinical outcomes: a meta-analysis of cooperative group clinical trials. *J Natl Cancer Inst.* 2013;105(6):387–393.

11. Banja J. The normalization of deviance in health-care delivery. *Bus Horiz.* 2010;53(2):139.

12. Dillon RL, Tinsley CH, Burns WJ. Near-misses and future disaster preparedness. *Risk Anal.* 2014;34(10):1907–1922. doi:10.1111/risa.12209.

13. Dillon RL, Tinsley CH, Cronin M. Why near-miss events can decrease an individual's protective response to hurricanes. *Risk Anal.* 2011;31(3):440–449.

14. Killgore WD, Cotting DI, Thomas JL, et al. Post-combat invincibility: violent combat experiences are associated with increased risk-taking propensity following deployment. *J Psychiatr Res.* 2008;42(13):1112–1121.

15. Wu AW. Medical error: the second victim: the doctor who makes the mistake needs help too. *Brit Med J.* 2000;320(7237):726.

16. Prins JT, van der Heijdenb FM, Hoekstra-Weeberscd JE, et al. Burnout, engagement and resident physicians' self-reported errors. *Psychol Health Med.* 2009;14(6):654–666.

17. Stiegler M. What I learned about adverse events from Captain Sully: it's not what you think. *JAMA.* 2015;313(4):361–362.

18. Plews-Ogan M, May N, Owens J, et al. Wisdom in medicine: what helps physicians after a medical error? *Acad Med.* 2016;91(2):233–241.

19. Fiorino F. CAST-ing a safety net. *Aviat Week Space Technol.* 2005;163:72–73.

20. Bernard-Bruls X. Nuclear power plant operating experience. IAEA/NEA International Reporting System for Operating Experience 2005–2008. 2010:1453. www-ns.iaea.org/downloads/ni/irs/npp-op-ex-05-08.pdf.

21. Arnold A, Delaney GP, Cassapi L, et al. The use of categorized time-trend reporting of radiation on-cology incidents: a proactive analytical approach to improving quality and safety over time. *Int J Radiat Oncol Biol Phys.* 2010;78:1548–1554.

22. Bissonnette JP, Medlam G. Trend analysis of radiation therapy incidents over seven years. *Radiother Oncol.* 2010;96:139–144.

23. Clark BG, Brown RJ, Ploquin J,et al. Patient safety improvements in radiation treatment through 5 years of incident learning. *Pract Radiat Oncol.* 2013;3:157–163.

24. Leape LL. Error in medicine. *JAMA.* 1994;272:1851–1857.

25. Wachter RM, Pronovost PJ. Balancing "no blame" with accountability in patient safety. *N Engl J Med.* 2009;361:1401–1406.

26. *RCA: Improving Root Cause Analyses and Actions to Prevent Harm.* Boston, MA: National Patient Safety Foundation; 2015.

27. Reason J. Understanding adverse events: human factors. *Qual Health Care.* 1995;4(2):80–89.

28. Serrat O. *The Five Whys Technique.* Washington, DC: Asian Development Bank.

29. Taylor-Adams S, Vincent C. Systems analysis of clinical incidents: the London protocol. *Clin Risk.* 2004;10(6):211–220.

30. Vincent C, Taylor-Adams S, Chapman EJ, et al. How to investigate and analyse clinical incidents: clinical risk unit and association of litigation and risk management protocol. *Brit Med J.* 2000;320(7237):777.

24 | Medical Error Disclosure

John Banja and Suzanne B. Evans

INTRODUCTION

Errors in providing radiation treatment usually incorporate some form of "wrongness"; for example, a patient's receiving the wrong dose of radiation, or the administration of treatment to a wrong anatomical site or to a wrong patient (1). Fortunately, such errors occur relatively infrequently (2,3), and even when they do, the majority tend not to cause serious harm. Nevertheless, catastrophic error is well documented in the annals of radiation oncology (4,5), and all treatment-related errors—whether they cause harm or not—deserve risk management attention as to their causal and systemic factors.

This chapter focuses on disclosing medical errors in radiation oncology and discusses current policies and practices on (a) characterizing the language of medical error; (b) the growing consensus favoring the disclosure of medical errors; (c) obstacles to disclosing errors in a patient-centered way; (d) organizational policies bearing on safety practices, error reporting, and error disclosure; and (e) communication strategies and recommendations in disclosing errors to patients or their family members. Our goal is to provide readers with ethical considerations and practical strategies that figure prominently in error disclosure so that when the need for these usually unpleasant conversations arises, the expectations of patient-centered care will be realized and respected.

THE LANGUAGE OF ERROR

Defining error

An obvious place to begin a discussion of error disclosure is to define *error*. A familiar and still current definition, offered by Lucian Leape more than 20 years ago, is "an unintended act, either of omission or commission, or an act that does not achieve its intended outcome" (6). The Institute of Medicine's definition is virtually identical: "[T]he failure of a planned action to be completed as intended (i.e., error of execution) or the use of a wrong plan to achieve an aim (i.e., error of planning)" (7, p. 28). Despite the popularity of this definition, some authors have pointed out that a health professional might not intend for X to happen, but because of certain unpredictable or unusual

factors, X may occur but still not have been associated with or caused by error. Consider patients who receive health care that leaves them worse off in ways that none of their providers "intend." As long as the treating professional exercises clinical judgment and skill that accords with the professional standard, however, it seems incorrect as well as unfair to say he or she "erred" in instances of suboptimal or "unintended" outcomes. For example, an instance of radiation myelopathy or radiation necrosis is always unintended; however, these complications can occur even when normal tissue dose constraints have been strictly adhered to.

Consequently, we urge a definition of error that uses the language of the standard of care and propose that "When a mistake in reasoning, judgment, or action does involve erring from standards of due care . . . it is a genuine error" (8). Obviously, health professionals should only be held to performance standards that are "reasonable," that is, standards according with what a professional's decisional and practice obligations are in a given clinical context. As long as the health professional's actions accommodate those expectations or obligations—that is, as long as they comply with the practice standards that the professional's relevant clinical community adopts in the given situation—health professionals should refer to any untoward or unintended sequelae of treatment not caused by error as "complications" or "unpreventable adverse events."

These grammatical considerations are important insofar as a professional's admitting "error" to a patient or family member implies fault, meaning that the errant behavior should not have occurred or would not have occurred had the agent been practicing "reasonably" (9). Also, because every patient has the right to expect that his or her treating professional will act reasonably, once the health professional admits fault, he or she assumes legal liability for any "damages" that the faulty behavior has caused. This is why informed consent conversations, at least from a risk management perspective, serve as a "risk transfer" mechanism from professional to patient. By communicating the risks and the possibility of adversities that can happen before an intervention and securing the patient's consent, the health professional is not only educating the patient as to the potential for harm, but also securing the patient's agreement that he or she will shoulder the discomforts or burdens of any adverse events that occur, *assuming that the professional renders care reasonably or in an ordinary and prudent fashion* (10). Harm that is caused by error, in contrast, is something that patients do not "consent" to because they have the right to care that accords with professional standards rather than care that unreasonably deviates from them. A key recommendation in disclosing error, then, is that reasonable clinical certainty should be present indicating that error has indeed occurred. If that certainty does not exist, the professional might tell the patient or family that "we don't know why X happened, but we're investigating it and will certainly reveal to you what we learn." More will be said about this in the following section on conducting an error disclosure discussion.

Intentional versus unintentional error

Root cause analyses often reveal the degree to which health professionals intentionally and knowingly commit "technical" errors by virtue of their failure to follow their own or established policies, procedures, and standards (11). Within radiation oncology, failure to comply with pretreatment time-out procedures, failure to utilize pre-scribed beam modifiers, patient misalignment, or errors in planning can occur. Additionally, the high-tech field of radiation oncology is also subject to many insidious errors, for example, planning on the incorrect CT dataset, errors in machine calibration, or failure of multileaf collimator (MLC) transfers in a given radiotherapy plan. In many instances, the primary "error" in patient safety is simply the failure to exercise vigilance, especially by way of professionals checking on one another or correcting one another's rule or care standards deviations (12). In the tragic case of Scott Jerome Parks (4), a transfer error occurred, resulting in the absence of MLCs in his treatment plan and his eventual death from radiation-induced toxicity. Additionally, in the case of Alexandra Jn-Charles (4), a radiation therapist programmed a computer for "wedge out" rather than "wedge in," which the plan required. Over the patient's next 27 treatments, staff repeatedly failed to catch the error, as well as failing to notice that during treatment, the wedge was missing. The overdose caused a wound in the patient's chest that would not heal despite several surgeries. By the time the wound finally healed, Jn-Charles's cancer had returned and eventually took her life.

A challenge that these system failures present for error disclosure conversations lies in adequately explaining to patients and families what happened when multifactorial, complex, and elaborate causational factors enabled the harm occurrence to happen. Table 24.1 offers a list of common system failures that enable disasters and catastrophes in health care to occur. These factors are especially relevant to the delivery of radiation therapy where radiation oncologists, medical physicists, dosimetrists, radiation therapists, and nurses regularly work in tandem to deliver the intended treatment. Interprofessional communications and handoffs, however, are known to be among the most worrisome moments in maintaining patient safety, as the clinician who receives the patient will sometimes not receive important information that keeps the patient's treatment plan on course, or may be too busy to check the safety profile or parameters of the care the patient has been receiving—that is, to ensure that it does not reflect error such as what occurred in the Parks or Jn-Charles cases (13).

When patients request an explanation of what happened in a complex instance of harm-causing error, we suggest that the discloser be psychologically and informationally prepared to answer all the questions and not rationalize by omitting certain facts because they are thought to make the conversation too complex, vague, or embarrassing. This is a particular challenge in the instance of radiation oncology, where the truth is that many of the details of the error are indeed technologically complex, and verbiage must be carefully chosen to be "patient level." Hence, the practice of using a disclosure coach can be particularly helpful. The clinician should not try to form the words for the disclosure spontaneously, in front of the patient, but rather form them to a colleague or coach, who can give feedback as to the technical nature of the terms and the clarity of the message (14). Many patients or families will want a seeming overabundance of information while they are trying to make sense out of what happened, and may often harbor suspicions that the health professionals are leaving something out. Health professionals should also consider that when serious harm-causing error occurs that may prompt a patient or family to resort to litigation, their lawyer will probably acquire all the relevant medical records and study them intensely. Professionals should therefore consider that any attempt on their part to obfuscate or hide relevant information on harm-causing error may ultimately fail, given an aggressive legal effort to accommodate the patient's right to learn about what happened and seek compensation (15). Consequently, we believe that health professionals should be prepared to respond to patients' inquiries truthfully and comprehensively as they are asked and regardless of the discomfort they cause. Resisting such requests might very well result in an expensive and time-consuming retrieval and study of the medical records, a needlessly prolonged and expensive period of legal machinations and actions, the never-pleasant process of deposing individuals who figured in the event, and the possibility of trial.

DISCLOSING ERROR: REASONS AND BENEFITS

It seems fair to say that the overwhelming response of 20th-century medicine to the commission of medical

Table 24.1 Familiar Practice Failures in Health Care That Increase the Chance of Disaster

Failure to:		
Wash hands	Secure required consents	Perform handoff/shift change communications
Use infection control measures	Store or disperse medications appropriately	Notice or question incomplete information
Change instruments appropriately	Assess patient fall risk	Learn new procedures or technology
Resist temptation to take shortcuts	Implement fall procedures	Investigate errors
Perform equipment safety checks	Monitor patient condition in timely fashion	Clarify orders
Gather sufficient data	Deliver care on time	Secure a second opinion
Work Environment Factors Encouraging Error:		
Long patient waits	Unfamiliar technology	Multitasking
Many sick patients to be seen	Unworkable policies	Violence
Phone-call interruptions	Poor work area design (cramped, dim lighting)	Goal ambiguity
Uncertain expectations	Unavailable expertise/consult services	Technology failures
Stress	Absent supervision	Haste
Noise	Fatigue	Constant interruptions
Hunger	Trainees (especially new)	Conflicting priorities
Inadequate staff	Inadequate reminder systems	Inaccessible medical records

Source: From Ref. (36). Banja J. Alcohol and drug testing of health professionals following preventable adverse events: a bad idea. *Am J Bioeth.* 2014;14(12):25–36.

error was to conceal it from patients and families (16). The reasons consist of a mix of factors, such as an unjustified lack of moral sensitivity to the right of persons who have been wronged by medical error to receive an explanation of what happened; a morally problematic but largely unquestioned acceptance of the defense bar's position that the burden of proof in a medical error case is on the plaintiff—meaning that the defendant professionals are not legally required to incriminate themselves or make "admissions against interest"; and the power of rationalization among health professionals that persuades them they can be excused from disclosing errors. Given that error disclosure conversations are often extremely unpleasant and that most professionals would prefer to avoid them, rationalizing concealment can be very tempting, as professionals might want to convince themselves that disclosure will unduly upset patients and families and thus harm them further; the error might not have changed the eventual outcome of care; the error was due to many factors, with its harm sometimes exacerbated by the patient's own actions; the error was God's will, and so on (16). This can be particularly problematic within cancer care, as local radiation does not always have a bearing on eventual distant metastasis, can sometimes result in complications or morbidity despite excellent care, and is often given in palliative situations where the outcome is a foregone conclusion.

While it seems morally obvious that disclosing a serious error to the harmed party is the ethically right thing to do, that belief exists alongside the entrenched right of U.S. citizens not to incriminate themselves and is buttressed by tort law's position that the burden of proof in medical error cases is on the plaintiff. While professionals may feel guilty over concealing errors, their ethical obligation to reveal error might rest on little more than a society's moral intuitions about what virtuous professionals should do.

There are, however, at least three very practical reasons that urge disclosure. One looks to the possibility that the patient's learning about an error to which he was subjected might cause him to seek care from another provider. Such a decision would be perfectly reasonable, especially in a culture that extols a marketplace economy and a consumer's right of choice, and especially in instances where a consumer must shoulder burdens or unpleasantries caused by incorrectly delivered services. Disclosure respects the patient's autonomy to choose care providers, and, additionally, respects the patient's inarguable right not to be harmed by lapses in the delivery of care, while the professional who discloses exhibits moral character in being honest and truthful (17).

A second reason looks to the experience of many patients and family members who suspect that something has gone wrong but are not receiving a satisfying explanation of what happened. The patient safety literature capaciously attests to how "stonewalling" on the part of professionals can cause immense suspicion and anguish among patients and families (18). Concealing error sometimes imposes an additional layer of suffering onto health consumers who, without an explanation or information as to what caused the harm, are unable to effect a psychological closure of the adversity and so remain bewildered, depressed, and frustrated.

Those disrupted feelings invite a third reason for disclosure, which is now familiar to many health professionals: Research on medical malpractice claim frequency and severity has consistently shown that organizational policies insisting on disclosure of harm-causing error invariably result in fewer claims and lower expenditures associated with malpractice-related costs (19). These findings are buttressed by others indicating that patients and families often sue health professionals and hospitals simply to find out what happened. One does not have to read deeply into that literature to come upon patients and families asserting that "all we wanted was an explanation and an apology for what happened." Anger is known to be a powerful stimulus for initiating litigation, while communications that are apologetic, empathetic, and respectful of a patient's right to know the circumstances of any unjustifiable harms that occurred to her will often contain or soothe ruptured feelings as well as heighten the patient's respect and goodwill (20). Consequently, even if a health professional feels no particularly compelling moral reason to disclose error, certain very pragmatic considerations bearing on the financial and emotional costs of adverse litigation resulting from error concealment strongly argue for consideration.

Finally, health care members involved in error have reported a benefit to error disclosure as well. Individuals involved in error may have tremendous guilt about the error, which can be compounded by concealing it from the patient (21). The ability to disclose this error to the patient and to be true to one's moral self may reduce stress and burnout related to medical error (22).

COMMUNICATION STRATEGIES FOR DISCLOSING ERROR

The literature on conducting "bad news" conversations is voluminous, and disclosing a medical error is an iconic example of a bad news communication. We cite some of that literature in what follows, in addition to suggesting

that the following considerations figure prominently in the preparation and delivery of an error disclosure.

Learn what happened in as detailed a way as possible

Harm-causing error trajectories can be so enormously complex that it is often tempting to speculate on certain facets of what happened. See the following Case Study for an example of this complexity. In disclosure conversations, however, the conveyor of information must stick to the facts and resist guessing (23). It is extremely easy for a layperson listener to interpret a professional's surmising as fact—so much so that if that surmising later turns out to be wrong, it might be very difficult to take certain statements back, as doing so might provoke the listener's suspicions or distrust. Professionals should not dismiss any of the listener's questions, however, but confess that as yet, the investigation has not produced answers but when it does, the listener will be informed. Obviously, much of this preparation and study should be done with risk management, who can often coach the disclosers in numerous, helpful ways.

Ensure that all professionals are in agreement as to what occurred

A devastating moment in error disclosure (or subsequent litigation) occurs when professionals disagree among themselves on what happened. In preparing for error disclosure, then, the disclosers must meet beforehand and ensure that they have very similar, if not identical, versions of the events that transpired (24). This will also point out which portions of the story are unknown or uncertain. Again, support from risk management is crucial.

Resist blaming

While the identities of the error perpetrators might seem obvious (for example, the therapist who treated patient A with patient B's treatment plan), explaining why an error occurred can be sheer guesswork, as multiple factors can be at work that caused its happening. For instance, imagine a scenario where the therapist aide brought the improper patient to the treatment unit because the patient was hard of hearing and responded to the incorrect name, where an identifying photograph was

A Case Study: The Multifaceted Nature of Error

A 68-year-old man is diagnosed with a left upper lobe T1 N0 lung cancer. He has two separate nodules—one biopsy-proven cancer measuring 2.2 cm in the right upper lobe, and one granuloma measuring 1.5 cm in the left upper lobe (stable since 2006). The patient is medically inoperable and has transportation difficulties. Because of these factors, a course of stereotactic body radiation therapy (SBRT) is chosen with a dose of 10 Gy × 5. During simulation, the therapists are interrupted, and they fail to follow protocol and verify the site and side through their established time-out procedure. Contours are done by the physician, and the left upper lobe nodule, which abuts the esophagus, is contoured as the target area. The right-sided cancer is not contoured.

Although departmental procedure calls for the treatment planner and physicist to review site and side with a review of the pathology report, the dosimetrist who performs treatment planning only reads the history and physical report, which inconsistently mentions both the right- and left-sided lesions.

Martha, the dosimetrist, wants to ask the treating physician, Dr. Evans, about this, but as Dr. Evans has a volatile personality and hates being questioned, Martha refrains and trusts in the physician's contours without mentioning her concerns to the team.

The plan is approved. No esophageal contour is performed, and Dr. Evans does not notice this omission. The second-check physicist does not check laterality despite independent verification of laterality being required per institutional protocol; and the lack of an esophagus contour is unnoticed. At the treatment machine, the therapist check fails to validate laterality by reviewing the path report.

On treatment day, the therapists perform a time-out. The patient responds, "Right lung." The therapists question, "You mean left lung?" and the patient replies, "You would know better than me; I thought it was the right side." The therapists proceed to treatment without verification. Cone beam computed tomography (CBCT) used for localization also images the right-sided lesion, and Dr. Blind, who is covering, notices the opposite lesion but does not question the treatment site. The patient tolerates treatment well, but 3 months later, he presents with chest pain and is found to have an esophageal perforation. A diagnostic CT scan at the time of admission reveals fibrotic RT-related changes around the granuloma, with no fibrotic changes around the right upper lobe lesion, which has now increased in size to 2.8 cm. Additionally, there are now innumerable liver and bony metastases, consistent with explosive, widespread metastatic disease. The patient is admitted to the ICU with mediastinitis, and dies within 48 hours from the mediastinitis.

The Disclosure: Radiation Oncology is called at the time of admission to alert them of suspected esophageal perforation. Dr. Evans is in clinic that day, and responds to the consult. In reviewing the case, she understands that the wrong lung nodule was treated, and that this has led to esophageal perforation. She immediately contacts risk management and her chairperson.

Risk management and Dr. Evans review the case. From here, several things happen simultaneously. With the help of the radiation team members, an incident learning system report is filed, and in accordance with her state's rules, a report is made to the department of public health. A root cause analysis is begun by the incident learning system team, and interviews are conducted using the London Protocol.

Meanwhile, Risk Management gives Dr. Evans "just-in-time" disclosure coaching. Dr. Evans speaks with the family within 4 hours of confirmation of esophageal perforation and explains that the esophageal perforation resulted from medical error. She also explains that there is not a full investigation at this time, but she will follow up the next day with further details. She explains that this mediastinitis is a result of the radiation. She also explains that it is unclear whether properly treating the lung cancer 3 months earlier would have prevented metastasis, although, clearly, that would have been ideal treatment. Dr. Evans specifically apologizes that this happened to this man. Medical Oncology is also following the patient, and considers the lung cancer highly aggressive, with a high risk of metastasis from diagnosis, which does give the family a small amount of peace.

After the disclosure, Dr. Evans seeks help from her hospital peer support ("second victim") organization. She has a colleague cover the rest of her clinic day, and she spends 2 hours with a close colleague, discussing the event and her feelings. That evening, she goes home and seeks support from her spouse. After careful consideration, she speaks to her chair and asks to be removed from clinical duties for 3 days so that she might deal with this properly and attend to the needs of this family, as well as her own. Likewise, the therapists and physicists involved seek second victim support through the hospital.

The next day, Dr. Evans meets with the family (as the patient is intubated and sedated), who reacts angrily now that this news has had time to sink in. Dr. Evans does not get defensive, but slowly explains to the family the steps that were missed in this case, leading to error. Dr. Evans explains that as a result of this error, her department is immediately instituting segmentation rounds, where contours are reviewed for accuracy and consensus before treatment planning takes place. She explains that the multiple individuals who failed to follow site and side procedure receive verbal warnings for failure to follow policy. She also explains that the hospital will be speaking with them shortly about a compensation offer. She asks social work to meet with the family and direct them to support organizations like Medically Induced Trauma Support Services (MITSS).

The next day, the patient dies. One week later, the hospital meets with the family and offers them a generous compensation package, accompanied by a letter of apology. The family signs documentation preventing future legal action surrounding this incident.

The family does engage with MITSS, and finds it a great comfort. With time, the family releases their anger and appreciates the honesty and integrity with which this event was handled.

missing from the chart, and the physician was unable to come to the treatment unit to verify a large shift at filming. Health professionals should remind themselves that error-caused harms are rarely the work of one person doing something inexplicably unwise (25). They generally reflect the intersection of all-too-human imperfections in environments that never run perfectly and thus often fail to intercept the error and contain its harm potential. Ideally, disclosure should admit collective blame for harm-causing error, because multiple people are virtually always involved in enabling harm-causing error to occur. Nevertheless, if the patient or family demand to know who was involved in the error trajectory, it is virtually certain that they will find out, especially if they secure an attorney and file suit. Although health professionals might feel a moral obligation to protect their peers, it is unlikely that the anonymity of persons involved in error will be maintained once the legal process of discovery begins.

Rehearse what you are going to say

It is amazing what human beings will say when they are nervous or upset. Especially in instances of serious, harm-causing error, the professional should meet with risk managers and agree on what the content of the disclosure will be. Facts should be distinguished from conjecture; knowns and unknowns should be identified and elaborated; and the likelihood of patients or families raising uncomfortable questions should be anticipated. If the patient or family asks what has been done to ensure that the error they experienced does not reoccur, professionals should be prepared with a thoughtful response rather than "We just told everyone to be more careful" (26). As already mentioned, does the organization's error disclosure policy allow revealing the names of the professionals involved in the error if the listeners ask? Very importantly, professionals should anticipate that listeners will likely think of more questions to ask after the initial meeting—such that the index conversation may be the first of many—and so should supply the patient or family with contact information of professionals who will respond to any further questions they have. Additionally, the proper corrective actions to policy, procedure, or additional safeguards cannot possibly be known at the time of the initial incident, and this is often what patients are most interested in: making sure this never happens to anyone else again. A follow-up meeting will be needed to share what changes were made as a result of this incident (23).

Prepare to feel uncomfortable if not wretched

The professional who waltzes into an error disclosure feeling extremely confident that he or she will be able to control the conversation may be headed for disaster. As soon as the conversation takes an anxious turn, this person may be tempted to regain control by steering the conversation to something different, by dominating the conversation, by minimizing the error, or by arguing with listeners. Probably the best attitude or conversational tone to assume is one of pronounced humility and regret for what has happened (27). The professional who is acting defensively and is blaming others, who is dismissing or ignoring pointed questions, and who seems intent on ending the conversation as quickly as possible will likely not impress the listeners with his or her compassion or regret over what happened. Although the primary error discloser should be someone in authority with pronounced familiarity with what happened—an individual who is usually the attending physician—persons with good empathetic skills are ideal disclosers of error, as some professionals may be poor communicators, or too upset or fearful over what has happened to speak coherently, let alone empathetically. In instances of serious error, it is probably wise to have a second professional accompany the primary communicator, not only for moral support but also in case the conversation gets sidetracked and the primary communicator is at a loss to handle it artfully (26). All individuals should be introduced to the patient and/or family, with their role clearly stated. For example, "This is Dr. Doe, and she is here today to help me give you a clear description of what happened."

Handling emotional outbursts

Emotional outbursts, especially involving angry, threatening patients or family members, can be very challenging even among highly skilled and empathetic communicators. In fact, the best response from the professional should simply be an accepting, humble, nondefensive one, assuming that the listener is not becoming violent. This includes being mindful of body language and avoiding hostile postures. The professional should appear contrite and match his or her feeling behaviors to the gravity of the situation, bearing in mind that it is very difficult for an individual to remain angry at someone who takes responsibility for wrongdoing and expresses genuine sorrow over it (27). Professionals should remind themselves that they will likely feel tempted to diminish or minimize the gravity of what happened (because they are unconsciously seeking to soothe their anxious feelings of incompetence or failure). Short of a physical attack, however, virtually any and all of the listeners' reactions are appropriate. The professional who tells the listener that his emoting is somehow "inappropriate" or who demands that the listener "get control of herself" invites enormous trouble, since it may cause the listener to feel dismissed or put down by someone who thinks himself or herself superior (but who is very paradoxically admitting that a serious error occurred in the course of a patient's care) (28,29). Regardless of how uncomfortable it is for the professional, whenever listeners emote in an unsettling way, the best strategy is

Table 24.2 Helpful Things to Say in Bad News Conversations

* "This must be . . . [dreadful, awful, depressing, frightening] . . . for you to hear."

* "This is obviously making you feel very . . ."

* "I hear you."

* "Tell me how you'd like me to proceed."

* "I wonder what you're feeling right now."

* "What is it about that . . . that [worries, upsets] . . . you?"

* "What is it about talking about that . . . [you don't like? Makes you anxious? Makes you want to talk about something else?"]

* "What would you like to have happen from this?"

* "Anything else?"

* "We need to decide together where we go from here."

* "Now let me make sure I'm understanding you. You're asking me . . . [whether or not, how it is that]. . . . Is that correct?"

* "So, what you're saying is that . . ."

* Repeat the other's last three or four words.

* "Is this making sense? Do you see what I mean?"

* Validate questions: "That's an excellent question." "You raise a very important point."

to just sit there and "take it"—perhaps offer tissues to a weeping listener or murmur variations of "I'm sorry," but surrender the urge to take over the conversation (which can nevertheless be very difficult to do).

What to say

Table 24.2 lists some useful communication techniques and responses to use in any bad news conversation. The point of these responses is to discern what the listener is feeling, respond appropriately, and maintain an emotional atmosphere where listeners feel respected, heard, safe, and supported. Health professionals who have an anxious need to always make things better may find the error disclosure conversation extremely challenging, because there may be no way to accomplish these objectives. The best one can do is admit and describe the error, answer questions truthfully and honestly, and support listeners as they grapple with their feelings and try to make sense out of what has happened. As already noted, judgmental responses such as "You shouldn't feel that way" or "Try to control yourself" or "That's a very inappropriate thing to say" have no place in such conversations, even if they may be objectively true (27). Communicators must remember that the point of the error disclosure conversation is to serve the listener's needs according to the listener's understanding of them, while the success of the disclosure will be measured by how much the listener feels respected and supported (3). Admittedly, however, mastering what to say in the midst of emotionally charged scenarios and

navigating a listener's feeling world in an artful, respectful way can take a lifetime of study and practice.

Body language, touching, and talking

One should always sit rather than stand when delivering bad news, and deliver the news in a private rather than public setting. Do not speak medicalese, and try hard not to dominate the conversation. Instead, be guided largely by the patient's or family's questions and responses. Empathetic body language recommends sitting forward and "leaning" into the conversational zone with shoulders slumped and elbows resting in one's lap. Some experts advise that the speaker try to get his or her eye level lower than the listener's, which feels to listeners as though the speaker is "looking up" to them (increasing the chances that they will feel respected). Good eye contact is essential except among cultures that are affronted by it. If the speaker has great difficulty looking at listeners, he or she might stare at a spot on the listener's nose or forehead (27,30).

The vocal tone should be gentle but firm. Most difficult for many health professionals, however, is to regulate and control their urge to explain and describe. This is not to say that the health professional should omit important details of what happened; it is to say that it is better to answer the listener's questions with a minimum of gloss and to let listeners guide the conversation. Periods of silence may feel excruciating to some health professionals, but they should understand them as part of emotionally difficult conversations where listeners may be stunned or deeply saddened at what they are hearing. Another important consideration is to speak slowly, which may be very challenging in instances when the speaker feels agitated or vulnerable. Nevertheless, the best conversational posture is a humble one, where the professional readies himself or herself to absorb very painful projections of psychical material from listeners and respectfully tolerates and sympathizes and empathizes with their distress (23).

Beginning and navigating the conversation

If at the end of an error disclosure conversation, listeners are befuddled at what they heard—for example, they are not sure whether the speakers did or did not commit error or how, exactly, their loved one wound up requiring additional care that was thoroughly unanticipated—then the "disclosure" of "error" was ethically unsuccessful. Still, many health professionals will be loath to use the word "error" and want to say instead "incident," "problem," "unfortunate event," or some more benign, less incriminating term or label (31). If the professional, however, is intent on an ethically ideal disclosure of medical error, he or she might begin with something like, "Ms. Smith, the reason we asked you to meet with us today is to tell you that we've learned that an error occurred in the course of your father's care while he was here at our hospital. I'm prepared to tell you what happened and I'm wondering how you'd like me to proceed." Most likely, the listener will want to learn the details, but some may request a postponement until they can call additional persons to hear the disclosure, or they might want to record the conversation with their smartphones. Health professionals often wonder about whether or not listeners should be allowed to record such conversations. We suggest that a sincere patient-centered conversation would not balk at such a request, unless the institution prohibits it. Resisting a family's wish to record a conversation might give them the impression that the professional is planning to be dishonest. After all, why would the request be denied? Is the professional intending to dissemble or hedge on embarrassing questions that he or she does not want recorded? Nevertheless, it would also be wise for the professional to record the conversation as well, in order to ensure the accuracy and reliability of the recording should it be entered into evidence at some future malpractice action.

There is no secret or magical way to deliver bad news (27). The speaker might fire a warning shot like "This is difficult for me to tell you, Mrs. Jones," but should proceed to tell the truth directly and briefly: "We discovered that your father received a significant overdose of radiation at his last treatment session. That was our mistake and it has doubtlessly caused the problems we're now seeing. We're indescribably sorry this happened." At that point, the professional should stop talking and wait for a response. Indeed, most of the conversation should be guided by response cues from the listener to which the empathetic

communicator will be keenly and artfully attentive. If the patient registers sadness or anguish, the speaker might empathetically acknowledge it with "This must be awful for you to hear." Do not say things like "Please know that we feel much worse about this than you do" or "You say you can't imagine how this happened? How do you think we feel?" The point is that the conversation must maintain the empathetic and supportive spotlight on the listeners' feelings—perhaps with a response like "Of course, we're very upset over what happened, Mrs. Smith, but this must be utterly horrible for you to hear and absorb" (24). If the listener makes a threatening response, for example, by screaming, "Let me tell you something, by the time this is over I'm going to own this clinic!" the listener should accept the outburst and humbly respond: "I cannot express my regret over what happened enough. And I can understand your refusal to forgive us." Speakers should remember that listeners will likely review the index conversation many times. If the speaker remained empathetic, contrite, respectful, and truthful throughout, listeners may find themselves impressed by exactly that and moderate their feelings of anger and, often, desire for revenge (23).

Follow-up

Frequently, and especially in instances of serious, harm-causing error, the index disclosure of error will not be the last conversation to occur. There are at least two points to take from this. One is that the speaker who remains empathetic throughout the disclosure conversation, regardless of the listeners' responses, may improve the chances of forging a positive relationship with the listeners, who may be impressed with the speaker's contriteness, truthfulness, and so on (27). The second is to anticipate the likelihood of listeners' requesting multiple meetings and to therefore supply them with names and contact information of health professionals who can discuss their issues anytime. Indeed, when confronted by patients or family members who seem to want an endless quantity of information and sympathizing, professionals should appreciate the human tendency to fixate on and even maximize feelings of being wronged (because it is hard to ignore deep violations of the self) along with the tendency of the wrongdoer to minimize the deed (so as to relieve oneself of guilt feelings) (18). Some health care organizations have adopted early settlement strategies when they are certain that error occurred. The idea is to head off an expensive and prolonged litigation process and allow everyone involved to move on with their lives as best as they can.

PATIENT RESOURCES

Being a victim of a serious medical error is extremely stressful. Families and patients who exhibit considerable need should be directed to appropriate resources (18). Support groups exist within hospitals, but also within external organizations, such as the MITSS group (32). Patients and families can find great comfort in such organizations, and they should be directed to seek them out to help with the healing process. It is part of the institution's care for these individuals to help them move beyond this event to find peace.

RESOURCES FOR CLINICIANS INVOLVED IN ERROR

A full discussion of the second-victim phenomenon is beyond the scope of this chapter. However, clinicians involved in serious medical error may require significant emotional or psychological support (33,34). Where possible, the institution should seek their help in obtaining solutions to prevent reoccurrence of the problem. Additionally, after a serious medical error, the clinician may request time away from the clinic (35) to process the error and recover from it.

CONCLUSION

While the most familiar response to medical error during the 20th century was concealment, it is impossible to ethically condone that practice today. The old saw of "not upsetting patients" with disclosure information is abandoned in favor of the honest disclosure of error, which leads to reduced malpractice costs, promotes healing of the relationship between patients and caregivers, and respects ethical practice.

Nevertheless, disclosing serious harm-causing error can be very difficult, and may stand as the most challenging "bad news" conversation a physician can conduct. Perhaps one cannot know too much about it; indeed, the more one learns about the empathetic stance, the wiser and more tolerant he or she becomes. Acquiring performative excellence in these practice domains may well require a lifetime. But it is very likely to be work well worth doing.

REFERENCES

1. World Health Organization (WHO). *Radiotherapy Risk Profile: Technical Manual.* Geneva, Switzerland: World Health Organization; 2008. http://www.who.int/patientsafety/activities/technical/radiotherapy_risk_profile.pdf.

2. Ford EC, Terezakis S. How safe is safe? Risk in radiotherapy. *Int J Radiat Oncol Biol Phys.* 2010;78(2):321–322. doi:10.1016/j.ijrobp.2010.04.047.

3. Macklis RM, Meier T, Weinhous MS. Error rates in clinical radiotherapy. *J Clin Oncol.* 1998;16(2):551–556.

4. Bogdanich W. Radiation offers new cures, and ways to do harm. *New York Times.* Jan 23, 2010. www.nytimes.com/2010/01/24/health/24radiation.html.

5. Bogdanich W, Rebelo K. A pinpoint beam strays invisibly, harming instead of healing. *New York Times.* Dec 28, 2010. www.nytimes.com/2010/12/29/health/29radiation.html.

6. Leape L. Error in medicine. *JAMA.* 1994;272:1851–1857.

7. Institute of Medicine, Committee on Quality of Health Care in America. *To Err Is Human: Building a Safer Health System.* Washington, DC: National Academy Press; 2000.

8. Sharpe VA, Faden AI. *Medical Harm: Historical, Conceptual, and Ethical Dimensions of Iatrogenic Illness.* Cambridge, UK: Cambridge University Press; 1998: 137.

9. King JH. *The Law of Medical Malpractice in a Nutshell.* St. Paul, MN: West; 1986.

10. Lo B. *Resolving Ethical Dilemmas: A Guide for Clinicians.* 3rd ed. Philadelphia, PA: Lippincott Williams & Wilkins; 2005.

11. Vaughn D. The dark side of organizations: mistakes, misconduct, and disaster. *Ann Rev Soc.* 1999;25:271–305.

12. Reason J. *Human Error.* Cambridge, UK: Cambridge University Press; 1990.

13. Reason J. *The Human Contribution.* Washington, DC: Arena Press; 2008.

14. Gallagher TH, Denham C, Leape L, et al. Disclosing unanticipated outcomes to patients: the art and the practice. *J Patient Saf.* 2007;3(32):158–165.

15. Robbennolt JK. Apologies and legal settlement: an empirical examination. *Mich Law Rev.* 2003; 102:460–516.

16. Banja J. *Medical Errors and Medical Narcissism.* Sudbury, MA: Jones and Bartlett; 2005.

17. Smith ML, Forster HP. Morally managing medical mistakes. *Camb Q Healthc are Ethics.* 2000;9:38–53.

18. Woodward HI, Mytton OT, Lemer C, et al. What have we learned about interventions to reduce medical errors? *Ann Rev Public Health.* 2010;31:479–497.

19. Boothman RC, Blackwell A, Campbell D Jr, et al. A better approach to medical malpractice claims? The University of Michigan experience. *J Health Life Sci Law.* 2009;2(2):125–159.

20. Mazor KM, Simon SR, Yood RA, et al. Health plan members attitudes regarding the disclosure of medical errors. *JAMA.* 2003;289(8):1001–1007.

21. Christensen JF, Levinson W, Dunn PM. The heart of darkness: the impact of perceived mistakes on physicians. *J Gen Intern Med.* 1992;7:424–431.

22. Wu AW, Cavanaugh TA, McPhee SJ, et al. To tell the truth—ethical and practical issues in disclosing medical mistakes to patients. *J Gen Intern Med.* 1997;12:770–775.

23. Truog RD, Browning DM, Johnson JA, et al. *Talking With Patients and Families About Medical Error.* Baltimore, MD: The Johns Hopkins University Press; 2011.

24. Banja J. Why, what and how ought harmed parties be told? The art, mechanics, and ambiguities of error disclosure. In: Hatlie M, Youngberg B, eds. *The Patient Safety Handbook.* Sudbury, MA: Jones and Bartlett; 2003: 531–548.

25. Chassin MR, Becher EC. The wrong patient. *Ann Int Med.* 2002;136(11):826–833.

26. Gallagher, TH. A 62-year-old woman with skin cancer who experienced wrong-site surgery. *JAMA.* 2009;302(6):669–677.

27. Buckman R, Kason Y. *How to Break Bad News.* Baltimore, MD: Johns Hopkins University Press; 1992.

28. Chan DK, Gallagher TH, Reznick R, et al. How surgeons disclosure medical errors to patients: a study using standardized patients. *Surgery.* 2005;138(5):851–858.

29. Gallagher TH, Waterman AD, Ebers AG, et al. Patients' and physicians' attitudes regarding the disclosure of medical errors. *JAMA.* 2003;289(8):1001–1007.

30. Stone D, Patton B, Heen S. *Difficult Conversations.* New York, NY: Penguin Books; 1999.

31. Gallagher TH, Garbutt JM, Waterman, et al. Choosing your words carefully: how physicians would disclosure harmful medical errors to patients. *Arch Intern Med.* 2006;166(15): 1585–1593.

32. Medically Induced Trauma Support. www.mitss .org.

33. Waterman AD, Garbutt J, Hazel E, et al. The emotional impact of medical errors on practicing physicians in the United States and Canada. *Jt Comm J Qual Patient Saf.* 2007;33(8):467–476.

34. Berlinger N. *After Harm: Medical Error and the Ethics of Forgiveness.* Baltimore, MD: Johns Hopkins University Press; 2005.

35. Stiegler MP. A piece of my mind. What I learned about adverse events from Captain Sully: it's not what you think. *JAMA.* 2015;313(4):361–362. doi:10.1001/jama.2014.16025.

36. Banja J. Alcohol and drug testing of health professionals following preventable adverse events: a bad idea. *Am J Bioeth.* 2014;14(12):25–36.

25 | Error Identification and Analysis

Yan Yu, Laura A. Doyle, and Amy S. Harrison

ACCIDENT, ERROR, EVENT: NOMENCLATURE FOR DEVIATIONS FROM INTENDED TREATMENTS

"Accidents happen" is a simple statement of truths. Regrettably, in health care, "accidents or errors" affect the health care provided to patients, and sometimes health care harms the patients it was intended to help. What is an accident? According to the Merriam-Webster online dictionary, an *accident* is "an unforeseen and unplanned event or circumstance or an unfortunate event resulting especially from carelessness or ignorance" (1). Alternate terminology for medical accident includes *error*, which is defined as "an act or condition of ignorant or imprudent deviation from a code of behavior or the quality or state of erring or something produced by mistake or a variation in measures" (2). Thus, to discuss "errors or accidents," there has to be a common nomenclature.

Both accident and error imply some level of individual fault, and in a culture of safety, fault and blame should be cast aside for a more productive review of how a deviation from the intended plan of care occurred. To encourage this philosophical shift from blame to prevention and remedy, many institutions as well as accrediting bodies have switched the negative labels of "error" or "deviation" reporting to phrases such as "medical events" or "treatment incidents," so that discussing these events can be perceived in a nonnegative light and staff can start the process of discussing events and improving care within a culture-of-safety mindset. The Nuclear Regulatory Commission changed its nomenclature from "misadministration" to "medical event" in 1998 (3). Having a less intimidating nomenclature also encourages open reporting, as the submission now looks at the entire process or event as opposed to just the end point. *Event reporting* is the nomenclature used for this chapter to discuss any deviation from intended treatments.

International standards for nomenclature have been defined by the World Health Organization (WHO), the European Society for Radiotherapy and Oncology (ESTRO), Radiation Oncology Safety Information System (ROSIS), and the International Atomic Energy Agency (IAEA). All agencies use independent classifications for patient safety reporting (4). All groups use either "incident" or "event" as their reporting nomenclature and only use negative-connotation words, such as *incorrect, error,* and *failure,* in the description of the events (Figure 25.1). Much of this terminology has been incorporated by the American Association of Physicists in Medicine (AAPM), and subsequently, the AAPM–ASTRO supported radiation oncology incident learning system (RO-ILS) as a common taxonomy for event reporting (4).

Medical events, as with all accidents, have varying severity levels and reporting infrastructures. In general, in the United States, there are three levels of treatment events that have different names and categories according to the defined oversight and reporting structure provided: Sentinel Events (SEs) or Medical Reportable Events (MREs), Patient Safety Events (PSEs), and Near Miss Events (NMEs). Similar to motor vehicle accidents, radiation event classification can be determined by both severity of injury and the mandatory documentation of the event with respect to who is notified, timing of notification, and the actions that follow the event. In a multivehicle car accident, the police and, possibly, the fire department would be notified; a medical team would be called if injuries occurred, families would be notified, and traffic patterns might be adjusted in the short term and possibly in the long term after the accident was reviewed. In the case of hitting a tree at a slow speed on a quiet country road, the occurrence might cause a small injury, the police may be notified, the car owner would be informed as well as the tree owner, repairs might be made to the car, and, possibly,

ESTRO-ROSIS	WHO	IAEA
• Incident = the incorrect delivery of radiation	• Patient Safety Event = event or circumstance that could have resulted or did result in harm to a patient • Adverse Event = incident that results in harm to a patient • Error = failure to carry out planned action as intended; may be an error or failure	• Incident = any unintended event, including operator errors, equipment failures, accidents, near misses, unauthorized acts that are not negligible from the point of view of safety

FIGURE 25.1 International nomenclature.

to the driver's driving habits in that area. If you took your car to the shop and the mechanic found that your brakes were bad, he would report it to you, and together you would decide how much it would cost to fix, how to repair it, and whether you needed to fix the vehicle. These three examples are similar to the levels in radiation oncology.

MREs (Figure 25.2) were defined by the Nuclear Regulatory Commission (NRC) to clearly define radiation events that must be reported to the NRC and the patient, how they must be reported, the time frame for reporting, and what the event report must include for descriptive

purposes (5). Most agreement states have copied the NRC requirements and terminology verbatim for MREs, as it is a requirement to have this reporting process in place. Similarly, The Joint Commission (TJC), an accreditation body for health care–related organizations and hospitals, has requirements for reportable medical events. For institutions to receive TJC accreditation, they must comply with tracking and reporting SEs (6,7). Although it is not mandatory to report to TJC, it is necessary to internally document and address these events according to TJC policy. Both MREs and SEs tend to carry more severity or potential to cause harm,

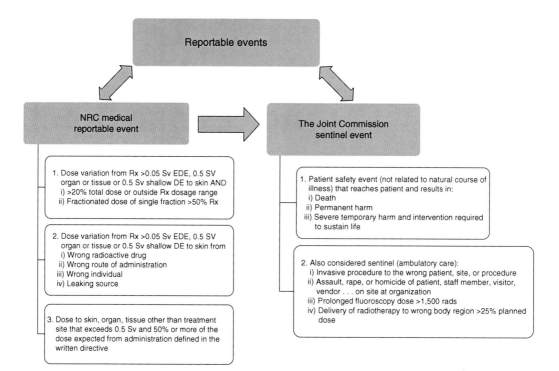

FIGURE 25.2 Reportable events in the United States.

as compared with the type of events discussed in the next section.

PSEs are events that could have caused or did cause harm to a patient. PSEs encompass NMEs as well as unsafe conditions. NMEs are frequently segregated from PSEs so that proactive corrections can be made to processes or systems to prevent future events. NMEs are often called "good catches," "close calls," or "near collisions" (8). *Unsafe conditions* are defined by the Agency for Healthcare Research and Quality as "a hazardous physical condition, circumstance or work environment that has the potential to directly lead to an incident" (8). In view of the number of organizations that classify any type of medical event, a PSE may have crossover to the level of an SE or MRE.

Although regulating bodies such as the NRC, TJC, and others may make recommendations on what types of errors must be reported, each institution is faced with generating the common taxonomy a department needs to establish an internal reporting structure. Some institutions may have existing programs or procedures for reporting, collecting, and tracking events of any level; however, radiation oncology departments must have special reporting procedures for dealing with MREs that must be reported to the state or NRC based on defining criteria. Almost all event reporting is voluntary, which is why a culture of safety and trust must be established between the frontline staff, managers, and administration. This culture of safety must ensure a blame-free and nonpunitive structure for event reporting. What departments must strive to create is an environment in which treatment events are utilized to improve quality of care and limit errors while maintaining individual and institutional accountability. One technique to help create this environment is to recognize staff members when they submit a near-miss event and acknowledge their efforts in improving patient care when they submit a treatment event.

In 2008, Farley et al (9) sought to review existing event reporting systems. Their criteria for assessment were four previously published features of effective reporting systems (Figure 25.3). Their survey reported an 81% response rate from 2,050 hospitals, with results indicating that broad staff involvement in reporting was limited, and that only 32% of institutions had environments supporting event reporting.

Traditionally, in radiation oncology, an adverse treatment event would trigger event documentation through verbal communication to a manager or physicist, who would then complete written event or incident forms. Preferably, these forms would document the details of the event, include a review of any dose or technical analysis, and engage all members of the care team by requiring signatures as formal acknowledgment. This paper trail allowed each clinician (physician, therapist, dosimetrist, and physicist) to narrate their portion of the event and describe factors that might have influenced workflow and patient care, creating the environment in which the treatment event occurred. This process allowed the completion of a formal root cause analysis (RCA) when necessary.

Since the Institute of Medicine's report, *To Err Is Human*, many institutions have focused on quality initiatives to improve patient care and learn from treatment events (10); hospitals have created in-house, electronic incident learning systems to improve the process of event reporting, and devised more accessible incident learning systems. These institution-wide computerized systems are designed to provide anonymous submissions, facilitate managerial interdepartmental reviews, and generate aggregate data analysis for the institution. Through this overview, the institution can see trends in infrastructure, processes, and care delivery that can be addressed at the highest level. Aggregate analysis and reporting through incident learning systems can promote safety by notifying the field about new hazards, innovative solutions for the prevention of errors, and giving early notification of error trends in the field or specific new hazards, as well as shared best practices based on the analysis of events (11).

The Patient Safety and Quality Improvement Act of 2005 authorized the creation of Patient Safety Organizations (PSOs) to improve the quality and safety of U.S. health care delivery (12). The Patient Safety Act encourages clinicians and health care organizations to voluntarily report and share quality and patient safety information at a national level without fear of legal discovery. There are currently two radiation oncology–specific incident learning systems in the United States and several internationally. The Radiation Oncology Incident Learning System (RO-ILS) is supported by ASTRO and AAPM and uses Clarity to

---

1. Protective of privacy of staff reporting events

2. Broad reporting by a range of staff (physicians, nurses, staff, others)

3. Timely distribution of report summaries and follow-up actions for prevention of future adverse events

4. Senior-level review and discussion with key departments and committees for policy decisions and development of follow-up actions or prevention strategies

FIGURE 25.3 Features of effective reporting systems. (*Source*: Adapted from Ref. (9). Farley DO, Haviland A, Champagne S, et al. Adverse-event-reporting practices by U.S. hospitals: results of a national survey. *Qual Saf Health Care.* 2008;17:416–423.)

facilitate its PSO. The Radiation Incident Reporting and Learning (RIRL) system is supported by the Agency for Healthcare Research and Quality (AHRQ) and utilizes AHRQ as the PSO for the system. Internationally, incident learning systems include ROSIS, which was established in 2001, IAEA, and WHO; at the national level, systems such as the Australian state-based Department of Radiation Oncology annually collect incident reports for review (13). Results from ROSIS analysis since 2001 showed an over-view of the 150-department equipment, quality assurance practices, and a summary of 1,074 events. The majority of events were minor in scope, but the process of reporting created an overview of international treatment event reporting with respect to detection of events, magnitude or severity of events, percentage of fractions delivered incorrectly, and the quality assurance tool that detected the event (14). National incident learning systems, RO-ILS and RIRL, provide reports back to the departments with aggregate and local data tabulated, as well as a review of anonymized reported events to use as a teaching tool for all departments. A review of 43 published studies on ILS summarized that ILS showed evidence of changes in clinical process or settings, but that there was limited evidence in publication of cultural change generated from ILS (15). Additionally, the study concluded that more explicit event criteria and department-level ownership of the ILS participation could have a greater impact on wider safety programs.

Part of this ownership includes review and analysis of event reports to look for patterns in care that could be improved to eliminate the probability of the same event occurring in the future. Sometimes, this review requires a quick analysis by an individual (physician, physicist, quality team member, chief therapist) to gauge severity and make immediate corrective actions. This quick review may be sufficient for minor events until the event is reviewed in the departmental quality forum/committee format, where representatives from the entire care team discuss and review severity and solutions of all treatment events. In the case of significant treatment events (reportable or high-risk near-miss cases), a lengthy review to establish all details, timelines, roles, and par-ticipant feedback is necessary; in general, this is done through an RCA (4). An RCA is a problem-solving tool that helps find the primary causes of faults or problems; it has its basis in engineering and is discussed in full in subsequent chapters.

Ultimately, creating a culture of safety where em-ployees feel safe in reporting events allows departments to analyze all events and near-miss events, in order to learn from the past to improve future care. The ability to review and reflect on historical events creates both a proactive and a reactive environment that can both nimbly recover from treatment events as a team, and approach new clinical situations from the foundations of learning from past mistakes.

REFERENCES

1. Accident. 2015. www.merriam-webster.com/dictionary/accident.

2. Error. (n.d.). www.merriam-webster.com/dictionary/error.

3. NRC SECY-98-054. http://pbadupws.nrc.gov/docs/ML9929/ML992910060.pdf.

4. Thomadsen BR, Dunscombe P, Ford E, et al, eds. *Quality and Safety in Radiotherapy: Learning the New Approaches in Task Group 100 and Beyond.* Madison, WI: Medical Physics; 2013.

5. U.S. NRC. 2014. Subpart M—reports. www.nrc.gov/reading-rm/doc-collections/cfr/part035/part035-3045.html.

6. The Joint Commission. Sentinel event policy and procedure. 2014. www.jointcommission.org/Sentinel_Event_Policy_and_Procedures/.

7. Comprehensive Accreditation Manual for Ambulatory Care Update 2, January 2015. www.jointcommission.org/assets/1/6/CAMAC_22_SE_all_CURRENT.pdf.

8. DHHS, AHRQ. Common formats for patient safety data collection and event reporting. *Federal Register.* 2009;74(169):45457–45458.

9. Farley DO, Haviland A, Champagne S, et al. Adverse-event-reporting practices by US hospitals: results of a national survey. *Qual Saf Health Care.* 2008;17:416–423.

10. Kohn LT, Corrigan JM, Donaldson MS, eds. *To Err Is Human: Building a Safer Health System.* Washington, DC: National Academy Press; 1999.

11. Leape LL. Reporting of adverse events. *N Engl J Med.* 2002;347(20):1633–1638.

12. Patient Safety and Quality Improvement Act of 2005. Pub. L. No. 109-41, 119 Stat. 424 (2005).

13. Shafiq J, Barton M, Noble D, et al. An international review of patient safety measures in radiotherapy practice. *Radiother Oncol.* 2009;92(1):15–21.

14. Cunningham J, Coffey M, Knoos T, et al. Ra-diation Oncology Safety Information System (ROSIS)—Profiles of participants and the first 1074 incident reports. *Radiother Oncol.* 2010;93(3):601–607.

15. Stavropoulou C, Doherty C, Tosey P. How effec-tive are incident-reporting systems for improving patient safety? A systematic literature review. *Milbank Q.* 2015;93(4):826–866.

26 Introduction and History of Patient Safety Organizations: The Formation of a National Safety Program

Tom Piotrowski

Patient safety organizations (PSOs) were created under the Patient Safety and Quality Improvement Act of 2005 (PSQIA) (1). The PSQIA statute was passed in order to advance national learning about errors in health care delivery, and to do this learning in an environment that is free from the customary punitive measures that occur in liability and/or adverse employee actions. The question, then, is how to create this in a national program and apply it to essentially every type of health care provider?

To understand the structure of PSOs and how they operate, we need to consider why such a program was initiated in the first place. Most notably, this was a response to the release of the Institute of Medicine (IOM) report published in 1999 (2). This publication gathered statistics on the number of deaths that occur as a result of medical errors and the number of dollars spent on medical errors each year in the United States. The report sparked a call to action that led Congress and other stakeholders to implement a program(s) that addresses medical errors and how to reduce that impact on care delivery. One answer was the passage of the PSQIA, which mandated the creation of PSOs.

THE UNDERLYING PRINCIPLES OF THE PATIENT SAFETY ORGANIZATION PROGRAM

After the release of the IOM report in 1999, many folks began identifying possible reasons for such a gap in the self-regulation of medical errors—meaning the reporting of those errors, analyzing their pathways, and fixing the problem. It did not take long to understand that we live in a litigious society that often punishes us for making mistakes, particularly in health care delivery. Additionally, the response by health care institutions has often been that the mistake must have been due to the person or health care provider who was involved in the patient's care. So again, the thinking is that there must be punishment for mistakes, as if, somehow, health care providers are meant to be perfect and there is no room for mistakes. The result of this punitive environment has been an unwillingness and a fear to be more proactive in identifying error publicly, because of the negative backlash that was certain to occur. There is no incentive to learn from or fix the problem—only to viscerally or emotionally respond to the mistake, partly because perhaps we do not know what else to do, and yet there are pressures to find and fix whatever is broken.

Another principle that underscores the PSO program and is related to the historical punitive/negative culture is the lack of information or data about errors in care delivery. As noted previously, there is no incentive to publicly report medical errors. So then, how do we learn? There has to be an environment, with guidance, that supports reporting of this sort of safety information. Traditionally, health care providers look at safety information in silos, so the learning that may prevent a similar situation in another facility is stifled—again, because of the fears and likelihood that there will be a negative or legal backlash. Now, we do recognize that there are state statutes allowing specific quality data to be subject to privilege and/or confidentiality protections, so as to support this kind of work. We also recognize that there are other voluntary means to report information, such as registries or other databases whose primary focus is to analyze and learn from opportunities to optimize the best patient outcomes. However, it is arguable that a national program focused on safety and error prevention does not exist—or at least did not exist before the passage of the PSQIA. This is clear when we consider that the PSQIA offers a federal protection that is intended to lay the groundwork for providers to be willing to report information in a secure and safe manner, with the primary aim of improving quality and safety of care delivery. Hence, the true aim of the PSQIA is to foster a culture of safety. That is, we remove the fear of litigation and punitive measures and focus on how to make the system of care better and safer.

WHAT IS A PATIENT SAFETY ORGANIZATION?

PSOs are entities that work with health care providers to receive and share sensitive information about the quality and safety of care delivery. PSOs and health care providers work together to analyze and then implement changes to care delivery, which will provide for safer care. In turn, the information reported to a PSO is subject to strong federal protections. Here is where we start to see the research and thought that went into the Final Rule regulations for participating in the PSO program (3). In other words, the PSQIA statute and, subsequently, the PSO program were ultimately designed to support the absolute need for a safety culture.

The Final Rule regulations point out that the information reported to a PSO is protected information, called patient safety work product (PSWP). PSWP offers dual protection. On the one hand, and taken directly from the Final Rule regulations, PSWP is privileged information and shall not be subject to (a) federal, state, local, or tribal civil, criminal, or administrative subpoena or order, including in a disciplinary proceeding against a provider; (b) discovery in connection with a federal, state, local, or tribal civil, criminal, or administrative proceeding, including a disciplinary proceeding against a provider; (c) disclosure under the Freedom of Information Act (Section 552 of Title 5, United States Code) or similar federal, state, local, or tribal law; (d) admitted as evidence in any federal, state, local, or tribal governmental civil proceeding, criminal proceeding, administrative rulemaking proceeding, or administrative adjudicatory proceeding, including any such proceeding against a provider; or (e) admitted in a professional disciplinary proceeding of a professional disciplinary body established or specifically authorized under state law. As can be seen, the privilege protections of PSWP are what is adjudicated in the courts. To date, there are not very many court cases where the challenges have

been asserted. However, there are a growing number of them, and they will create the interpretation of the details of the privilege protections. As will be seen in a later section, protecting your protections is largely, but not entirely, dependent on how you work with and engage the PSO in the first place. The PSO should assist you in structuring your participation so that you may leverage the strengths and benefits of the protections.

The second part of the protections of PSWP holds that it is confidential and shall not be disclosed by anyone holding the PSWP, except as permitted or required to under the rule. There are 10 permissible disclosures to the confidentiality provisions under the Final Rule. The permissible disclosures are intended to provide some flexibility to health care providers so that they can manage PSWP information and still carry out other business operations if needed, should there be a crossover or other need to share the PSWP.

HOW PROVIDERS WORK WITH A PATIENT SAFETY ORGANIZATION TO GAIN PROTECTIONS AND IMPROVE SAFETY: THE PATIENT SAFETY EVALUATION SYSTEM

Up to this point, we have noted some of the definitions and principles of the PSO program, and the depth of the protections that health care providers have available to them through this program. With respect to operationalizing the PSO program, there is one key principle to be addressed at length here. This refers to the development of a patient safety evaluation system (PSES). The PSES is the vehicle by which information becomes protected, because it is the reserved mechanism by which PSWP (the protected information) is transferred to and from provider and PSO. It is a requirement for both the health care provider and the PSO because without it there can be no PSWP. Think of the PSES as a box containing whatever you have identified as protected information for reporting to the PSO. From the regulatory perspective, there really is no specific guidance on how a PSES is structured. The thought here is that if it were too stringent, providers would not participate. Additionally, the PSO program allows essentially any type of health care provider to participate. A *health care provider* is defined as anyone or any entity licensed or otherwise authorized to delivery health care services. So, to encourage participation from all types of providers, there has to be variety with respect to PSES construction. Factors to consider when structuring your PSES include:

1. What type of organizational structure do you have?

2. In what type of health care setting do you practice?

3. What sort of data do you wish to have protected and reported to the PSO?

4. What activities do you want the PSO to do with you?

5. Do you have other reporting obligations, such as to the state or other agencies?

Generally, there is a small group or committee that determines the appropriate fit for your organization and that will serve as the "gatekeeper" of the PSES as well as the liaison to the PSO. See Figure 26.1 for a generic PSES structure.

In both the provider's PSES and the PSO's PSES, there are activities relating to information identification, usually in the form of a safety event or an incident. Once this event is identified, the provider will go through its process of investigation and analysis. Then the information is reported to the PSO. The ultimate goal of both the provider and the PSO is to create solutions that will help to prevent or at least reduce future errors. See Figure 26.2.

The PSES structure and function are critical to success in the PSO program, and your PSO is required to help

you. Beyond the requirements, it should be leveraged to be your "learning laboratory." The learning laboratory is essentially the place (your PSES) where providers can freely explore, analyze, and test various data sources and methods that help improve the quality and safety of care delivery.

BUILDING A SAFETY PROGRAM: WHAT IS REQUIRED FOR SUCCESS

Understand your environment

Radiation oncology is a very complex field that entails a higher degree of coordination than is normally required, particularly in relation to technology and equipment. If you think about and map out all the different steps in the radiation therapy treatment process, it quickly becomes clear that there are many modes of possible failure and many opportunities to identify and develop

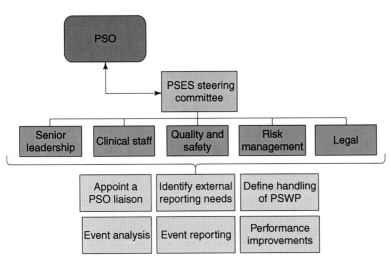

FIGURE 26.1 Generic PSES structure.

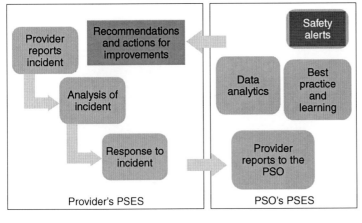

FIGURE 26.2 PSES Workflow Process.

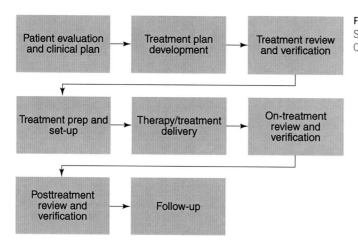

FIGURE 26.3 Model for Typical/Standard Radiation Care Pathway as Created by ASTRO.

fail-safe processes so that patients are not harmed. See Figure 26.3, which is a simplified derivative of the radiation treatment process through the safety work from American Society for the Radiation Oncology (ASTRO) (4).

Recognize the need for a safety culture

Understanding the framework within which care is delivered is the first step to building a strong safety program. You will see that the levels of care complexity become irrelevant to some degree—meaning that we all face the same underlying issues and challenges with error detection and prevention. It is seldom the person that is the true causative factor in a failed process. Rather, it is most often the process itself that is broken and has to be fixed. Further, the better we recognize how we need to layer our defenses, the better we will be able to mitigate errors that find their way through the breakdowns or "swiss cheese" holes in our systems (5).

The practice of focusing on process fixes versus fixing or changing the person is inherently a great deal of work done under the banner of a safety culture. In creating a safety culture, we are not only finding our way to the true intent of the PSO program and its statutory regulations, but are also aligning ourselves to expect that we can eliminate all preventable errors and harm. Although we have a fair amount of work to do in health care to achieve a true national safety culture, we do have the conceptual frame for how to accomplish this work. Many thought leaders, such as Sidney Dekker (6,7), point to the key elements in this cultural transformation. In part of his work, Dekker essentially points out that it takes an entire organization to move the culture and that it must be grounded in three things: (a) culture of safety; (b) culture of learning; and (c) culture of justice (see Figure 26.4).

First, a culture of safety. This is simply defined as the willingness to talk about and discuss bad things that happen. We need to be able to allow our frontline providers to step forward and tell us when things go wrong. That empowerment is the basis for replacing a culture of fear with a health culture of safety. Second is a culture of learning. This is defined as the elimination of finger-pointing. When an error or mistake occurs, there are two questions that are historically asked: the first is what happened, and the second often is who did it? In a learning culture, the two questions asked are what happened, and how do we prevent this from happening again? The focus is shifted to the process rather than the person. Third is a culture of justice. Once you have created an environment in which you can talk about and analyze mistakes, the energy and efforts of the organization should be aimed at mobilizing the resources and hold ourselves accountable to build the fail-safe process so that we may protect our patients as well as our providers.

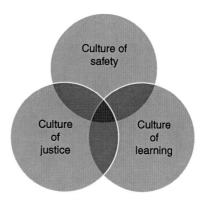

FIGURE 26.4 Elements of Creating a Safety Culture.

Engage your staff

As mentioned, building a safe culture is absolutely fundamental to a successful safety program, for without it you cannot adequately engage your staff openly and honestly. Provider engagement becomes the means by which you operationalize your safety program. Your frontline providers then become your true owners of safety; in the ideal world, this is a shared responsibility and is *everyone's* role in health care delivery. One of the most productive ways to engage staff is rooted in the safe culture philosophy described earlier. That is, when mistakes are found and reported, it is far more important to ask how we can prevent them or similar mistakes rather than to point a finger at and punish providers. So, if you transform the question(s) a bit, you can give direction to the providers involved in the mistake to become part of your solution; instead of punishing them, you treat them as experts or champions.

Identify common elements that you may benchmark and learn from

Providers who review and analyze data often fall into the data silo trap. For example, you may trend a particular safety element over time, and in its isolation, you may notice a downward trend in prevalence, meaning that it appears that you have improved an aspect of your practice. However, what does it look like if you compare yourself with other, similar providers? There really is no way to gauge what the standard of care is unless you expand your comparison to providers beyond your immediate environment of care. To accomplish this, you need to identify standard or common data elements by which you will be compared. There are established standards and templates. For the PSO program, in particular, the Agency for Healthcare Research and Quality (AHRQ) has created a set of Common Formats. Although largely applied in the overall hospital setting, there are elements that can be utilized in any practice environment, such as severity/level of harm, contributing factors, and types of events (patient event vs. near miss). In fact, today there are PSOs that have a radiation oncology focus (namely, ASTRO-Clarity PSO RO-ILS: Radiation Oncology Incident Learning System®, and Center for Assessment of Radiological Sciences [CARS] PSO) and that have created derivatives of the AHRQ Common Format—in essence, a "Common Format" for radiation oncology. In this way, those PSO programs work with radiation oncology providers to set up safety event collection systems, analysis, safety alerts, and benchmarking on common matters.

Create learning

Once you have established some of the foundational principles (such as the ones already described), the ongoing activities are really the heart of the work to implement safety improvements. The findings and recommendations for improvement derived from PSO analysis can vary greatly. These can range from trend reports to statistical significance testing to rate comparison and case study review. As can be seen, this is not unlike safety work that has existed for many years. Remember, the difference here is that we can break down silos and encourage more robust reporting because we have focused our beginnings on the safety culture, including the protections of the PSQIA.

PSO reports specific to radiation oncology are in fact being produced and can be found in deidentified form; see ASTRO's website for an example of a Radiation Oncology Incident Learning System (RO-ILS) report. These types of reports become the basis and catapult for specific and focused analysis that are both general in scope as well as provider specific, which support the ability to avoid the data silo trap.

PSO safety activities can also range in terms of the span of process analysis. As highlighted in Atul Gawande's work (8) as well as Donald Berwick's philosophy, there is a need for safety activities that allow providers to examine and test how all the parts of a complex system can work together better. This true systems approach is seen in PSO project work that focuses on tools such as simulation and systematic checklists. The great work of these thought leaders and the application of their principles is relevant to every health care setting, including the field of radiation oncology.

THE HISTORY OF PATIENT SAFETY ORGANIZATIONS IN SPECIALTIES

Since their inception in 2008, PSOs have had various focuses in terms of safety activities. Some PSOs have taken a global safety approach, whereas others have taken a specialty approach. Notable successes have included safety work in the fields of anesthesia, renal care/dialysis, vascular surgery, and, of course, radiation oncology. There is a wide range and scope of what these PSOs have been able to do with regard to advancing care. Some have included registry data whose main data source is patient outcomes; others have included anonymous free-text reporting of safety events. Still others have included a more structured reporting system that narrows and focuses on error reporting. Certainly, all of these examples fall within the purview of the PSO program. It is critical to stress that in the PSO program, the fundamental premise is that we need to focus on ultimately creating a national error reporting system. Today, this is in the form of a database called the Network of Patient Safety Databases (NPSD), which is now beginning to be developed by AHRQ and a few of the innovative and early-adopter PSOs.

The history of PSOs specific to radiation oncology is a relatively short story. As mentioned earlier, to date there are two PSOs that have specialized programs designed for the field of radiation oncology. Although both have the common goal of making radiation oncology care safer, their structure and genesis are somewhat different. A fair amount of flexibility is given to both PSOs and providers participating in the program, which is seen in the creation of PSESs as well as in how patient safety activities are carried out. These programs allow for anonymous event reporting as well as specific and detailed provider reporting.

REDEFINING OUR CULTURE

As described earlier, the culture of health care delivery is in desperate need of significant attention. If you were to approach your organizational leaders and ask them, "Do you think we have a safe culture here?" the chances are they would say yes. Then ask them to describe it to you and then show it to you. The chances here are that you would get a "deer in the headlights" look and type of response. That is not to say that there are no leaders in the radiation oncology community (or in any health care setting) who have formally adopted a safety culture ; it is merely to point out that the majority of providers cannot clearly articulate this effort because it is incomplete. The culture exists in pockets at both the organizational and national levels, and until we leverage the strengths of programs such as the PSO, we will fall short of creating that learning laboratory and, most importantly, in reducing preventable harm to our patients. The work of James Reason, Sidney Dekker, Marcus Buckingham (9), and many others lay the groundwork for us, from describing systems approaches to understanding the difference between great leadership and management. After all, a healthy safety culture is a complete circle that operates an equally distributed top-down as well as a bottom-up approach.

Safety is translational. Whether you are in radiation oncology or neuroendovascular surgery, human factors that affect safety and create errors/mistakes are manifested in the same way. In one sense, this makes a specialty not so special, because we are not immune to any of the failures in a care delivery system. For example, consider the following case study:

Safety event summary
The patient came into the facility for a scheduled treatment. Upon treatment follow-up, one of the health care providers realized that there was an error that resulted in an overdose of the prescribed treatment.
Investigation of the event:
How many times has this happened?
Do you believe the event is reproducible?

Are you aware of this happening at another institution?
Was equipment related? If so, what follow-up have you received from the vendor?
What do you believe were the contributing factors to the event?
Was the patient harmed?
Findings:
There was a misuse of the technology involved, that is, there was a preset default on the treatment device that went undetected until after the treatment was completed.

Now, in this event, a radiation oncology provider would probably race through all the different checkpoints related to treatment planning review, on-treatment review, and so on. That would be very logical given the information provided. However, the event just described was a medication event of a home infusion therapy not involving radiation delivery. It also happened to be the basic premise of an error that occurred and was reported to a PSO in a radiation therapy treatment. Interestingly, a radiation oncology subject matter expert provider who was provided the information on the radiation oncology treatment safety event derived almost the same investigatory process, as well as the general findings and underlying root causation, as the medication therapy event that was analyzed by a pharmacy subject matter expert. The underlying assumptions and overall findings were nearly identical, meaning that safety is translational: the types of fail-safes, as well as the practice of a safety culture, generally apply to every aspect of care delivery and in every type of health care setting. Focusing on the process and fundamental pathways of error production is the key to finding and applying necessary changes in an error-prone system.

CONCLUSION

The amount of change that has occurred in health care over the past few decades has been unprecedented. Technology and the speed with which health care advances often create unsafe situations. Health care is one of the few professions where we will implement a completely new process with zero testing (for example, electronic medical records). Additionally, regulators and stake-holders continue to place pressure on the health system to improve, produce more data, and meet additional standards of care. Although these are all noble aims and are necessary in advancing the possibilities, and certainly what we all want to do, it begs the question: as health care providers, have we self-regulated our profession enough and in the right ways? One need only look at the immediate work required to transform our current safety culture in the U.S. health care delivery system to know that more remains to be done.

REFERENCES

1. Patient Safety and Quality Improvement Act of 2005. Pub. L. No. 109-41, 42 U.S.C. 299 et seq (July 29, 2005).

2. Institute of Medicine. *To Err Is Human: Building a Safer Health System.* Washington, DC: National Academy Press; 1999.

3. Federal Register. Patient Safety and Quality Improvement Final Rule: 42 CFR Pt 3. Washington, DC: Department of Health and Human Services; 2008.

4. American Society for Radiation Oncology. *Safety Is No Accident.* Reston, VA: ASTRO; 2012.

5. Reason J. *Managing the Risks of Organizational Accidents.* Burlington, VT: Ashgate; 1997.

6. Dekker S. *Just Culture: Balancing Safety and Accountability.* Burlington, VT: Ashgate; 2012.

7. Dekker S. *The Field Guide to Understanding Human Error.* Burlington, VT: Ashgate; 2014.

8. Gawande A. *The Checklist Manifesto: How to Get Things Right.* New York, NY: Picador; 2009.

9. Buckingham M, Coffman C. *First, Break All the Rules: What the World's Greatest Managers Do Differently.* New York, NY: Simon & Schuster; 2009.

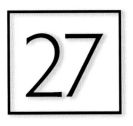

27 Quality Assurance and Safety Requirements for Clinical Trials

Ying Xiao, Stephen F. Kry, and David S. Followill

THE NCI NATIONAL CLINICAL TRIAL NETWORK (NCTN)

For more than four decades, the National Cancer Institute (NCI) has provided a critical infrastructure through the Clinical Trials Cooperative Group Program to promote large-scale cancer clinical trials, many of which have resulted in the standard of care offered today and life-prolonging treatments for patients. Facing rapid scientific advances in medicine and the need to ensure that the cooperative groups live up to their potential to carry out timely, large-scale, innovative clinical trials that result in improved patient care, the NCI invited the Institute of Medicine (IOM) (1) to assess the state of NCI-funded cancer clinical trials. The IOM provided recommendations to the NCI leadership on how to modify and improve the national clinical trials system.

As a result of the IOM's recommendations, the NCI created and funded the National Clinical Trials Network (NCTN) on March 1, 2014 (2). The NCTN represents the NCI's reformulated research network that aims to more efficiently conduct cancer clinical trials focused on state-of-the-art research questions. The new streamlined network features five clinical trial groups, down from 10, plus a Canadian network group, each with its own operations and statistical center (Figure 27.1). In addition to the trial groups, other core support groups were established to serve the entire NCTN network (2).

Imaging and Radiation Oncology Core (IROC)

One of the core service groups established was the Imaging and Radiation Oncology Core (IROC) cooperative. This group's mission is to provide integrated radiation oncology and diagnostic imaging quality control as well as clinical, scientific, and technical expertise in support of the NCTN. Through these activities, they ensure high-quality data for NCTN trials (3).

QUALITY ASSURANCE FOR NCTN CLINICAL TRIALS

The five core service operations offered by the radiation therapy and imaging quality assurance (QA) centers are shown in Figure 27.2. This unification of the five key core services between the imaging and radiation therapy (RT) QA centers is a major achievement of IROC. One of the key services, data management, is shown twice because it happens before and after the patient case reviews.

Site qualification

The site qualification service will verify and qualify NCTN participating sites' site imaging and radiotherapy capabilities.

Trial design support

The trial design support service ensures the review of new protocol concepts and development of protocols to provide feedback to the NCTN group. During a concept review, the IROC group will assess the needed QA requirements and resources needed to accomplish the QA activities based on protocol specifications listed in an IROC concept questionnaire. The IROC protocol review will be communicated back to the NCTN groups in a timely manner by the key contact QA center so as not to hinder the efforts of the Operational Efficiency Working Group (OEWG). Protocol assistance and education activities to participating institutions will be coordinated by this service.

Credentialing

The credentialing service will develop and implement appropriate tiered credentialing processes and analysis

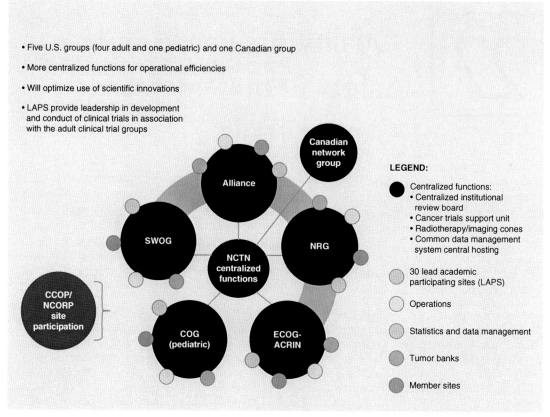

- Five U.S. groups (four adult and one pediatric) and one Canadian group

- More centralized functions for operational efficiencies

- Will optimize use of scientific innovations

- LAPS provide leadership in development and conduct of clinical trials in association with the adult clinical trial groups

LEGEND:

Centralized functions:
  • Centralized institutional review board
  • Cancer trials support unit
  • Radiotherapy/imaging cones
  • Common data management system central hosting

30 lead academic participating sites (LAPS)

Operations

Statistics and data management

Tumor banks

Member sites

FIGURE 27.1 NCTN structure.

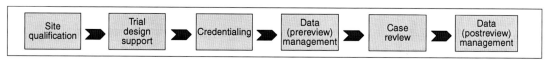

| Site qualification | Trial design support | Credentialing | Data (prereview) management | Case review | Data (postreview) management |

FIGURE 27.2 IROC's five general NCTN program QA approaches.

tools to ensure that before a patient is entered on a specific protocol, a site can implement a new imaging or therapy technology and/or technique. Credentialing will further ensure that a qualified site clinician and/ or physicist has the knowledge and ability to ensure protocol compliance.

Data (pre- and postcase review) management

The data management service will review and validate data acquisition methods, provide for facile data archiving/ retrieval, and serve as a platform for post hoc data analysis. In collaboration with the information technology (IT) subcommittee, robust and efficient imaging and RT data transfer methods will be developed according to recognized data transfer standards.

Case review

The case review service will interact with the NCTN groups and protocol Principal Investigators (PIs) to conduct patient case reviews. Timing of reviews will vary according to trial needs, and may include eligibility/staging confirmation, posttherapy imaging assessments, and pre-, on-, or post-RT treatment/imaging patient case reviews. This IROC service will facilitate the reviews in a timely and efficient manner and may assist NCTN group personnel who are responsible for conducting the clinical reviews.

REQUIREMENTS FOR ADVANCED RADIATION ONCOLOGY TECHNOLOGY

One of the goals of clinical trial quality assurance in radiation oncology is to reduce the variability and uncertainties related to treatment planning and beam delivery. A well-established and comprehensive QA effort is essential for the successful conduct of multicenter clinical trials so the trials are not compromised by poor quality, such as undesired variability in delivered doses (4–7). Minimizing trial uncertainty translates directly into fewer patients needed to reach statistical significance for a certain endpoint, reducing the cost of the trial and bringing optimal results to light more quickly (8,9).

Advances in radiotherapy technologies make it essential to develop appropriate QA tools in sync. Robust and efficient QA methodologies have to be optimized for implementation into a multicenter clinical trial setting for maximum benefit. The efficacy of novel QA must be demonstrated in terms of both trial outcome and resources needed to conduct trials. The research and development of clinical trial QA should answer the following questions: (a) Are our QA processes of the highest standard, and how can we best manage rapidly changing radiotherapy technologies? (b) How can we best focus our QA efforts to have the largest impact, via evidence-based practice, both on the QA processes themselves and on the radiation therapy community in general? (c) Can we perform our QA functions more efficiently (for example, which of our QA processes can we automate)? (d) By how much can we reduce the overall clinical trial cost by reducing uncertainties and thereby reduce the number of patients required? How does QA affect the health economics of cancer patient treatments?

To answer these extremely important questions, we will need to engage expertise and knowledge from different scientific areas. Collaboration across and beyond the entire NCTN network will be an essential component of QA research and development.

For example, as new radiotherapy technologies are being introduced, QA tools that can be used to accommodate the new features must be developed and evaluated for their efficacy and cost-effectiveness (10,11). For example, 2D/3D registrations are introduced in proton centers for the IGRT process. We need to develop processes and tools to address the QA of these new technologies. Image-guided radiotherapy (IGRT) is being implemented widely in clinical practices to detect, evaluate, and reduce interfraction set-up errors and monitor the intrafraction target motion for various disease sites. IGRT credentialing is a crucial component of clinical trial QA to improve treatment consistency and data quality, and covers many aspects such as immobilization, in-room image acquisition, and registration. The outcome may vary, largely depending on the implementation, as there are accumulated uncertainties that occur at various steps in the process. Image registration is mostly carried out automatically by the treatment software system, which is a major source of uncertainty. Because of the limitation of rigid registration for deformable objects and the variation in implementation of registration techniques, uncertainty exists during the procedure of image registration between planning and daily online IGRT data sets. Quantitative information on the differences between image registration results from multiple systems is needed as guidance for establishing an IGRT credentialing procedure. Because there is no absolute ground truth in the evaluation of registration accuracy, the deviation of registration results between different IGRT systems and software systems may provide a useful estimate of that uncertainty. This may be particularly useful to the radiation therapy community in the studies that allow margin reduction based on IGRT proton radiation, which is an emerging therapy that is being sought with increasing frequency by patients. Compared with photon therapy, proton therapy spares more critical structures because of its unique physics. However, the novelty and unique characteristics of proton beams also introduce a host of novel challenges regarding QA for such treatments. New tests of institutional competency are required, complete with hurdles such as new plastics being identified to serve as tissue surrogates (12). Additionally, protons are more sensitive to organ motion and anatomy changes compared with photons. Image guidance with greater accuracy is needed in proton treatment delivery. However, different image sets are often used in proton therapy, requiring different IGRT processes that must be verified (13). As with all new tools, it is mandatory that a detailed and standardized validation process be carried out to study the overall accuracy of the process. Such a validation test would necessarily include design of validation data sets, the definition of corresponding ground truth and its accuracy, the validation protocol, and the design of a validation metric.

EVIDENCE-BASED QUALITY ASSURANCE

To answer the question as to how best to focus our QA efforts so as to have the largest impact, via evidence-based practice, both on the QA processes themselves and on the radiation therapy community in general, we can perform studies that retrospectively correlate QA score with outcome, or prospectively include these aspects in the trial design stage (14). One such retrospective study investigated unacceptable deviations in radiotherapy data from RTOG 0933 (15). RTOG 0933 was a phase II trial of hippocampal avoidance during whole brain radiation therapy for patients with brain metastases. The results demonstrated improvement in short-term memory decline, as compared with historical control individuals, and preservation of quality of life. The QA processes include pre-enrollment credentialing and pretreatment centralized review of enrolled patients. Although more than 95% of the cases passed the pre-enrollment credentialing, the pretreatment centralized review disqualified 5.7% of reviewed cases, prevented unacceptable deviations in 24% of reviewed cases, and limited the final unacceptable deviation rate to 5%. Pretreatment review is found to be necessary in this hippocampal avoidance trial.

Similar studies should be conducted for more trials with varieties of radiotherapy technologies, and the value of these results should be tied to study outcomes.

Because of the multi-institutional and independent nature of the IROC review processes, IROC has unique knowledge and a unique perspective on radiation oncology practice. This unique knowledge is key to performing optimal, meaningful, and efficient reviews of clinical trial patient cases. However, this knowledge and the QA process have the potential to be relevant well beyond the clinical trial, improving the quality of radiotherapy for all patients. Although the scope of IROC is clearly clinical trial support (16), strategic design of the QA process could provide the maximum benefit to the radiation oncology community at no extra cost. This information could include feedback on target delineation during a pretreatment review, feedback on a linear accelerator calibration issue identified on an output check, or a CT calibration error identified with a credentialing phantom. All of these issues have the potential to change practice and thereby improve radiotherapy quality for other patients as well. Although these examples are institution-specific, there is also the potential for systematic radiotherapy issues to be identified and improved upon. Pencil beam algorithms have been identified as calculating substantially inaccurate and inconsistent dose estimates for lung tumors (17–19). Different combinations of treatment-planning systems (TPS) and linac have been shown to produce better or worse agreement in the setting of intensity-modulated radiation therapy (IMRT) credentialing phantoms (20,21). Even more generally, there are indications that the number of linacs in a hospital, and potentially the number of physicists per machine, can affect the quality of IMRT delivery based on credentialing phantoms (21). These sorts of findings have the potential to programmatically steer the practice of radiation oncology. Although the mission of IROC is, first and foremost, support of clinical trials, there is clear opportunity to have this benefit a broader patient base at no extra cost. This context should be used to help IROC develop and optimize QA procedures and information dissemination.

QUALITY ASSURANCE EFFICIENCY

To increase QA efficiency, we are constantly evaluating our QA processes to identify where we can automate.

One example is the introduction of automated structure verification during the data submission process. An integral component of IROC data management is the Transfer of Images and Data (TRIAD) system designed for imaging and radiation therapy digital data transmission. The TRIAD system is now being used for digital radiation therapy and imaging data transmission for NCTN (and other) clinical trials. The TRIAD system includes built-in functions that can be used to automate digital data QA during the transmission process. In particular, it includes an automated evaluation of the consistency between the submitted structure names and protocol requirements. To use a single set of consistent structure names, we develop and maintain a uniform radiation therapy structure name library. This library is based on common clinical radiation oncology practice, guidelines from prior publications and other material on this topic (22). Validation profiles are implemented from this structure name library. The added benefit from implementation of a uniform structure naming convention for radiotherapy practice is the capability of safety enhancement in the workflow of patient treatment planning and delivery, adding to the impact from our QA processes on the general radiotherapy community practice as a collateral benefit, as illustrated in the previous section. MiMsoftware, a component of the IROC data management system, is used for performing case review. We have built scripts and extensions in MiMsoftware to automate the dose volume histogram (DVH) analysis process.

REDUCTION OF UNCERTAINTY AND QUALITY ASSURANCE COST-EFFECTIVENESS

How much can we reduce the overall clinical trial cost by reducing uncertainties and thereby reducing the number of patients required? How does QA affect the health economics of cancer patient treatments?

Answering these questions directly demonstrates the value of the activities performed by the IROC QA core group. Indications have highlighted that such QA procedures actually reduce the cost of conducting clinical trials by requiring fewer patients enrolled in a given study, offsetting the resources needed for maintaining these QA functions (8,9). Moreover, even though trial QA has a cost (both clinical trials and RT delivery become more complicated because of the human and financial resources involved in the verification of the planned RT), by reducing the risk of tumor recurrence or treatment-induced toxicity, QA procedures may also decrease the overall health care costs (7,23). Health economics evaluations are helpful by assessing cost-effectiveness of the overall process. Decision analytic models can be used for these cost-effectiveness studies. QA reviews may be cost-effective in the long run because they will result in a greater cure rate with improved quality of life. Although QA of clinical trials is continually shown to be a financially worthwhile investment, this question requires continuous evaluation, particularly as radiotherapy and the corresponding QA processes evolve.

SUMMARY

Radiation oncology is a rapidly changing field with important and nontrivial requirements for the QA of clinical trials. It is important that the QA processes provide the highest impact while being cost-effective. Ensuring this optimal QA is a challenging question, particularly as radiotherapy advances, but it is one that must be addressed. Proper consideration of the issues discussed in this chapter will yield QA programs that streamline the clinical trial process, maximize outcomes, save money, and, both in the short term and in the long term, help cancer patients

ACKNOWLEDGMENT

This project was supported by NCI grants U24CA180803, U10CA180868, and PA CURE grant.

REFERENCES

1. Institute of Medicine. *A National Cancer Clinical Trials System for the 21st Century: Reinvigorating the NCI Cooperative Group Program.* Washington, DC: National Academies Press; 2010.

2. http://read.uberflip.com/i/321978-am-2014-daily-news-sunday-a.

3. Fitzgerald TJ. A new model for imaging and radiation therapy quality assurance in the National Clinical Trials Network of the National Cancer Institute. *Int J Radiat Oncol Biol Phys.* 2014;88(2):272–273. www.ncbi.nlm.nih.gov/pubmed/24411600.

4. Fairchild A, Straube W, Laurie F, et al. 2013. Does quality of radiation therapy predict outcomes of multicenter cooperative group trials? A literature review. *Int J Radiat Oncol Biol Phys.* 2013;87(2):246–260. www.ncbi.nlm.nih.gov/pubmed/23683829.

5. Ohri N, Shen X, Dicker AP, et al. Radiotherapy protocol deviations and clinical outcomes: a meta-analysis of cooperative group clinical trials. *J Natl Cancer Inst.* 2013;105(6):387–393.

6. Peters LJ, O'Sullivan B, Giralt J, et al. Critical impact of radiotherapy protocol compliance and quality in the treatment of advanced head and neck cancer: results from TROG 02.02. *J Clin Oncol.* 2010;28(18):2996–3001.

7. Weber DC, Hurkmans CW, Melidis C, et al. Outcome impact and cost-effectiveness of quality assurance for radiotherapy planned for the EORTC 22071–24071 prospective study for head and neck cancer. *Radiother Oncol.* 2014;111:393–399. www.ncbi.nlm.nih.gov/pubmed/24861631.

8. Doot RK, Kurland BF, Kinahan PE, et al. Design considerations for using PET as a response measure in single site and multicenter clinical trials. *Acad Radiol*. 2012;19(2):184–190. doi:10.1016/j.acra.2011.10.008

9. Pettersen MN, Aird E, Olsen DR. Quality assurance of dosimetry and the impact on sample size in randomized clinical trials. *Radiother Oncol.* 2008;86(2):195–199. www.ncbi.nlm.nih.gov/pubmed/17727987.

10. Cui Y, Galvin JM, Straube WL, et al. Multisystem verification of registrations for image-guided radiotherapy in clinical trials. *Int J Radiat Oncol Biol Phys.* 2011;81(1):305–312. www.pubmedcentral.nih.gov/articlerender.fcgi?artid=3129475&tool=pmcentrez&rendertype=abstract.

11. Cui Y, Galvin JM, Parker W, et al. Implementation of remote 3-dimensional image guided radiation therapy quality assurance for radiation therapy oncology group clinical trials. *Int J Radiat Oncol Biol Phys.* 2013;85(1):271–277. www.ncbi.nlm.nih.gov/pubmed/22541964.

12. Grant RL, Summers PA, Neihart JL, et al. Relative stopping power measurements to aid in the design of anthropomorphic phantoms for proton radiotherapy. *J Appl Clin Med Phys.* 2014;15(2):121–126.

13. Pawiro SA, Markelj P, Pernus F, et al. Europe PMC Funders Group Validation for 2D/3D Registration I: a new gold standard data set. *Med Phys.* 2011;38(3):1481–1490.

14. Bekelman JE, Deye JA, Vikram B, et al. Redesigning radiotherapy quality assurance: opportunities to develop an efficient, evidence-based system to support clinical trials: report of the National Cancer Institute Work Group on Radiotherapy Quality Assurance. *Int J Radiat Oncol Biol Phys.* 2012;83(3):782–790. www.pubmedcentral.nih.gov/articlerender.fcgi?artid=3361528&tool=pmcentrez&rendertype=abstract.

15. Gondi V, Cui Y, Mehta MP, et al. Real-time pretreatment review limits unacceptable deviations on a cooperative group radiation therapy technique trial: quality assurance results of RTOG 0933. *Int J Radiat Oncol Biol Phys.* 2015;91(3):564–570. http://linkinghub.elsevier.com/retrieve/pii/S0360301614043600.

16. Deye JA. Evidence based quality assurance for radiation therapy clinical trials. *Int J Radiat Oncol Biol Phys.* doi:10.1016/j.ijrobp.2015.02.033.

17. Aarup LR, Nahum AE, Zacharatou C, et al. The effect of different lung densities on the accuracy of various radiotherapy dose calculation methods: implications for tumor coverage. *Radiother Oncol.* 2009;91(3):405–414. doi:10.1016/j.radonc.2009.01.008.

18. Davidson SE, Popple RA, Ibbott GS, et al. Technical note: heterogeneity dose calculation accuracy in IMRT: study of five commercial treatment planning systems using an anthropomorphic thorax phantom. *Med Phys.* 2008;35:5434–5439.

19. Knoos TE, Wieslander E, Cozzi L, et al. Comparison of dose calculation algorithms for treatment planning in external photon beam therapy for clinical situations. *Phys Med Biol.* 2006;51(22):5785–5807.

20. Kry SF, Alvarez P, Molineu A, et al. Algorithms used in heterogeneous dose calculations show systematic differences as measured with the Radiological Physics Center's anthropomorphic thorax phantom used for RTOG credentialing. *Int J Radiat Oncol Biol Phys.* 2013;85(1):e95–e100. doi:10.1016/j.ijrobp.2012.08.039.

21. Molineu A, Hernandez N, Nguyen T, et al. Credentialing results from IMRT irradiations of an anthropomorphic head and neck phantom. *Med Phys.* 2013;40(2):022101. http://scitation.aip.org/content/aapm/journal/medphys/40/2/10.1118/1.4773309.

22. Yu J, Straube W, Mayo C, et al. Radiation therapy digital data submission process for national clinical trials network. *Int J Radiat Oncol Biol Phys.* 2014;90(2):466–467. http://linkinghub.elsevier.com/retrieve/pii/S0360301614033252.

23. Retèl VP, van der Molen L, Hilgers FJ, et al. A cost-effectiveness analysis of a preventive exercise program for patients with advanced head and neck cancer treated with concomitant chemo-radiotherapy. *BMC Cancer.* 2011;11(1):475. www.biomedcentral.com/1471-2407/11/475.

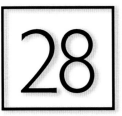

28 Incident Learning Systems

Gary Ezzell, Stephanie Terezakis, and Courtney Buckey

INTRODUCTION

Incidents in radiation therapy can have dramatic consequences. Fortunately, most incidents are minor and the majority are preventable. Mitigation strategies can be developed after understanding the nature, frequency, and potential severity of such events through the process of incident learning (1). Prospective utilization of methods such as failure modes and effects analysis (FMEA) and analysis of event root causes can identify areas for systematic improvement that can lead to enhanced patient safety (2). The incorporation of advanced technologies such as intensity-modulated radiation therapy (IMRT) and stereotactic radiation hold the promise of therapeutic ratio improvement. However, it is known that the implementation of such technologies can be associated with an increased risk for error, particularly if not properly evaluated and quality assured (3).

As our field advances, it becomes increasingly important that appropriate systems to report and learn from incidents and errors be implemented both intradepartmentally and intrainstitutionally, as well as nationally. Intradepartmental and hospital-wide reporting systems can aid in uncovering specific process errors that may be unique to a departmental culture or workflow. Incident learning systems are in place in many institutions throughout the country (4–6). It is feasible to use a hospital patient safety reporting system for reporting, but the complexity of the radiation oncology process often cannot be captured in a generic hospital system. A radiation oncology–specific system has the advantage of capturing relevant field-specific information that can be used for unique quality improvement (7).

Patients are at risk for events regardless of the type of center in which they are being treated. National and international reporting systems facilitate the collection of data across a range of sites, including both community and academic settings, to determine the common elements that may put patients in harm's way. The Radiation Oncology Incident Learning System (RO-ILS), a centralized national reporting system in the United States, allows input of data from radiation treatment centers across the United States and was established to facilitate the reporting of events nationally (8). In this way, safety standards can be derived on the basis of those incidents occurring on the ground.

An international reporting system (Radiation Oncology Safety Information System [ROSIS]) has been online for years, collecting information through a voluntary reporting structure (9). The International Atomic Energy Agency (IAEA) is also spearheading the development of an incident learning system named SAFRON (Safety in Radiation Oncology). Consensus recommendations for incident learning database structures in radiation oncology have been published by the American Association of Physicists in Medicine (AAPM) Work Group on the Prevention of Errors (WGPE) (10). Incident learning has the potential to improve patient safety and quality by facilitating knowledge sharing that can lead to incorporation and prioritization of process improvement initiatives and quality assurance program evaluation.

Incident reporting systems can also potentially be used to identify treatment-related factors that may increase the risk of radiation safety events. Patient- and disease-specific risk factors could be identified and used for error prevention prospectively at the time of treatment plan review and during the course of treatment delivery. The treatment process may then be modified for those patients thought to be at higher risk for errors. However, voluntary incident reporting systems are not without their pitfalls. The potential for large variability in the nature and frequency of reports received when incident reporting is voluntary is well described. Ultimately, reports that are submitted are subject to the biases of the observers reporting; thus, reports could represent a limited sample of the events actually occurring in the care setting (11). Therefore, incident reports may not include all areas that pose risk for patients. Despite this issue, incident reporting systems still provide an objective means for evaluation of actual events occurring during the workflow or to patients themselves. Ultimately, these incidents provide us with a way in which we can prioritize and develop mitigation strategies to reduce the incidence of events.

INCIDENT LEARNING SYSTEMS

Incident learning systems have been used in individual radiation oncology departments for many years. Here we distinguish between *incident learning systems* and *event reporting systems,* which have been part of radiation oncology practice for decades. Every department reacts, formally or informally, when it is recognized that a patient has been treated contrary to plan. The staff deals with the issues associated with that particular patient, which may involve making adjustments to the patient's subsequent treatments (or not), reporting to risk managers or regulators (or not), and making changes to processes (or not). A true incident learning system (ILS) formalizes the process by which the organization recognizes and responds to events in order to make treatments safer. Several steps characterize that process:

1. Identifying that something has happened that should be addressed

2. Reporting the issue

3. Investigating the circumstances

4. Analyzing the issue for proximate and underlying causes

5. Designing corrective actions

6. Implementing corrective actions

7. Evaluating the effectiveness of the corrective actions

An effective ILS must accomplish each of these steps. A number of authors have published their experience in designing, implementing, learning from, and evaluating the effectiveness of an institutional ILS, and we will refer to those as we consider each of these steps in turn.

Identifying that something has happened

What should be reported to the ILS? It is generally understood that any delivery of a therapeutic radiation dose contrary to the intended plan constitutes an event that should be reported. Similarly, an intervention that discovered and prevented a misapplied dose, that is, a "near miss," should be reported. Several authors comment that it is also important to recognize and respond to the "various hassles that practitioners experience in their everyday clinical work" (12). Ford et al (7), chose to use the term *incident*

> mainly to highlight the fact that all deviations are potentially of interest even those that do not necessarily impact the patient. Other terms could be used equally well such as "variance," "event," or "condition." Incidents also include deviations or variations to expected workflow, conditions that would impede the smooth completion of a task without a workaround of the standard process.

Reporting and responding to all such process variances, not just those clearly related to safety, has a number of benefits. One is that it promotes a culture of reporting and expecting that things can be made better, so that

staff are more likely to report issues that are clearly related to safety. Another is that eliminating hassles and workarounds and improving efficiency also improves safety. This is Reason's well-known Swiss cheese model of how errors come about (13). "In this way, information is gathered from frontline staff about contributory factors that might at some point lead to patient harm if left unaddressed" (12).

Authors have published the frequency of incidents reported in their ILS, and the numbers have varied widely. Those that encourage staff to report all process variances have seen 1 (14) to 0.6 (4) to 0.14 (15) events per patient, whereas lower numbers are more common, e.g., 0.1 to 4.7 per 100 patients treated (5,16–22). Mutic et al (4), who reported 0.6 events per patient, classified 7.8% of them as of high or critical importance (see following text), corresponding to 4.7 per 100 patients treated. Others have seen ratios on the order of 1:10:30:600 for critical:major:serious:minor categories of incident (23). These data support an expectation that a robust ILS could see on the order of 0.1 to 1 report per patient, some 60% to 90% of which will be of low or minor immediate significance. This has ramifications for the system required to analyze and respond to the reports.

Reporting the issue

The reporting mechanism should be readily accessible and easy to navigate. Several authors have reported significant increases in the number of reports submitted after shifting from a paper-based system to an electronic system, ranging from factors of 1.8 (20) to 4 (4) to 9 (14), although that effect has not been universally seen (17). In fact, introduction of an unwieldy electronic system was found to decrease reporting (24).

If the desire is to have frontline staff members routinely report all manner of incidents, then it is important that the link to the reporting tool be ubiquitous within the department and that the initial report require a minimal amount of information. The frontline reporter must feel few barriers to reporting. Submitting that initial report should then flag others who have the responsibility to dig into the details and contributing causes, flesh out the narrative description, and classify the incident according to the chosen taxonomy. That two-step workflow has been used by institutionally designed systems (4,25,26), recommended by an AAPM Working Group (7), and used by the national ILS for Radiation Oncology (RO-ILS) sponsored by the American Society for Radiation Oncology (ASTRO) and AAPM (8).

In order to promote reporting, making the system easy to use is necessary but not sufficient. Other key strategies include ensuring that the response to reports is supportive and nonpunitive (27); rewarding reporters, as with a "Good Catch" award (28, 24); and providing reliable feedback to the individual reporters and to all the staff about the changes made in response to the reports (27–29). In addition, it is necessary to provide training to staff on when and how to use the system. Using standardized, hypothetical events in the training can promote consistent and effective use (10). Even institutions with sophisticated internal reporting systems can experience reluctance to report, especially among physicians, who have expressed more concerns than other staff about getting colleagues in trouble, liability, effect on departmental reputation, and embarrassment (30). In the long term, it will be helpful to incorporate into medical residency training the expectation to report concerns in the ILS.

Investigating the circumstances; analyzing the issue for proximate and underlying causes

The initial report will rarely provide sufficient information to permit a useful response to be determined. Those charged with reviewing the report will need to augment the initial narrative with a fuller description of the incident and surrounding circumstances. The narrative is key; effective corrective action can be designed only after a deep understanding of the incident, relevant circumstances, and contributing causal factors has been achieved. It can be a challenge to condense that description into a succinct narrative, but necessary if the report is to be the basis for later review. Furthermore, if the report is intended to be useful and comprehensible to people outside the department (e.g., if it will be reported to a national system), then the authors of the narrative need to keep that target audience in mind and avoid department-specific jargon.

The reviewers will also need to classify aspects of the incident in order to enable statistical analysis of the population of reports. Such analysis is useful in at least two ways. One is to help identify patterns of failure so that attention can be effectively focused, and the other is to help measure the effectiveness of the ILS. As an example of the former, it can be useful to see what types of errors in treatment planning are caught by the physics plan check (often the first available safety barrier) and what types are not caught until the first treatment (after having gotten through some checks). Having data elements that keep track of where the error occurred and where it was found can help sort that out. As an example of the latter, authors have reported a decrease in the average severity of reported incidents over time, even as the number of reports has increased (29) or in the frequency of actual treatment deviations as compared with near misses (23). Designing a classification scheme that is comprehensive, robust, and manageable is a difficult task. The consensus document published by the AAPM Working Group (7) offers one approach.

A particularly tricky issue is estimating the severity of the incident. Because of the latency of radiation effects, both beneficial and detrimental, assigning severity nearly always entails a degree of speculation and subjectivity. There is no standard accepted scale. Most systems use a 4 or 5 scale; as an example, that proposed by Mutic et al (4) is summarized here:

1. Low: Not a dose delivery–related event but an inconvenience to the department or patient. These are events that result in inefficiencies and repeat or unnecessary work.

2. Medium: Limited toxicity (may not require medical attention) or minor underdose to the planning target volume. These are events that have the potential to result in minor deviations of delivered doses. Minor deviations are considered to be less than 10% or 10 mm in magnitude.

3. High: Potentially serious toxicity or injury (may require medical attention) or major underdose to the target. These events have the potential for significant deviations from the intended treatment and are all greater than 10% or 10 mm in magnitude.

4. Critical: Selecting this option causes the software to immediately send alpha pages to the involved area supervisors; it is intended for use only in urgent situations.

The AAPM working group consensus document (10) uses a 10-point scale for dosimetric severity and medical severity. Carefully designing the severity scale, educating the staff who do the scoring as to its use, and testing the consistency of its application are very important, especially when the number of reports requires some prioritization as to which receive the most attention, such as a root cause analysis.

Further complicating the issue of severity is the problem of near misses. If the error was avoided, or was caught very early in the treatment, then does one score what happened or what might have happened? The proper answer may be to score both (15). Only scoring what actually happened would discount a potentially catastrophic near miss, but imagining the worst possible scenario for every potential error can dilute the focus on the most concerning incidents.

There is value in having an intradepartmental team review the reports to look for underlying causes and to design corrective action (25). Very often, the underlying issues will involve workflows and communication channels affecting multiple sections of the department, and insights will come from multiple areas. The relevant supervisor should do an initial investigation to ascertain the details of the event so that the committee will have good information to work with. This implies a multiple-step workflow: the frontline person puts in a report, the supervisor looks into the situation, and then the intradepartmental committee discusses those reports requiring broader review.

NATIONAL AND INTERNATIONAL REPORTING SYSTEMS

Expanding from using a local incident learning or practice improvement system to a national or international one makes intuitive sense. Learning about incidents, near misses, and unsafe conditions from other institutions offers substantially greater opportunities than a single internal system can provide. One caveat, however, is that the heterogeneous nature of the training, technology, resources, infrastructure, staffing, and workflows at other facilities, and in other countries, can make applying the lessons learned to your own department more challenging. Another issue to confront is the potential lack of uniformity, or interreviewer reliability, of reports from different organizations within the same reporting system. Analyses of this variability have been done, and multiple groups have shown that results from reviews are divergent—with suggestions that longer narratives and improved taxonomies will lead to more consistent scoring results (31–33).

Many national and international groups have waded into this arena, and in this section, we report on some of the more well-known efforts—some which have been in existence for years and others that are in the more nascent stages of development. Unfortunately, at the time of this writing, although the need for national and international systems has been well recognized, experiences with the systems have not yet been well published.

Radiation Oncology Safety Information System

The ROSIS was established in 2001 by the European Society of Therapeutic Radiology and Oncology (ESTRO) as a patient safety tool with exclusive emphasis on radiation oncology. It is a voluntary reporting system for both incidents and near misses, with an international focus. Reports related to linear accelerators, cobalt-60 units, and brachytherapy devices are accepted. As of early 2014, more than 150 departments had registered with ROSIS; initially registered departments were located within Europe, but there is now a more diverse global distribution of departments in ROSIS (34).

ROSIS classifies incidents into two broad areas: process-related (where the occurrence is related to a failure in the process), and non–process-related (including hardware and software failures, falls, etc.). The process-related activities are further divided into subgroups related to the point at which they occurred.

At the time of initial registration, a departmental profile is established related to equipment, staff, and environment. However, clinic details are confidential, are stored separately from the incident information, and are not searchable. Incident reports can be made through a variety of methods: transfer via local ROSIS patient safety module, direct input via the website, transfer and translocation via web service (cross-organizational system), and transfer and translocation via web service (local system) (34).

The incident reports are anonymized and stored in a searchable database, and made available to participants on the ROSIS website in their original text. As a further means of communication and engagement, ROSIS has published six themed newsletters to date, some with spotlight reports. Annual workshops are also held, which focus on generalized quality and safety topics, as well as ROSIS updates. The most up-to-date information about ROSIS can be found at http://rosis.info.

Safety in Radiation Oncology

The SAFRON system was developed by the Radiation Protection of Patients (RPOP) unit at the IAEA and piloted in 2012 by an international group of health care professionals from Argentina, Australia, Canada, Ireland, Malaysia, Nigeria, Sweden, United Kingdom, and the United States. It was designed to be both a facility-specific system and a support for an international error reporting system. As of June 2013, there were more than 1,100 reports, including both incidents and near misses—although not all of those were entered prospectively; some were from past reports to the IAEA and to ROSIS (35). The integration of prospective risk analysis together with retrospective reporting enables the system to be proactive, which is of value when considering the rapid development of new medical technology (36).

Facilities wishing to participate in SAFRON must first register with NUCLEUS, the agency's information resource catalog, and then separately register with SAFRON through a web portal. Currently, only external beam reports are accepted. SAFRON is searchable, and sorts incidents by such details as where in the process the incident was discovered, who discovered the incident, how it was discovered, and any word in the free-text fields (e.g., summary and description of incidents). It is possible to use these criteria in any combination as search filters. Another search feature permits searching on the basis of incidents from the home institution, or the database at large. The identifying information for facilities that are not your own remains anonymous. Participants can review causality information and what corrective actions have been taken by the reporting institution in order to build a resilient system and reduce the likelihood of having a similar incident at their institution. SAFRON publishes themed newsletters that share tips for using SAFRON, and spotlight cases. Aggregate data about types of reports are also offered. The newsletters are e-mailed, but only the most recent edition is currently available. The most up-to-date information about SAFRON can be found at https://rpop.iaea.org/SAFRON.

National System for Incident Reporting in Radiation Treatment

The Canadian Partnership for Quality in Radiotherapy (CPQR) has partnered with the Canadian Institute of Health Information (CIHI) on the National System for Incident Reporting in Radiation Treatment (NSIR-RT) project. The NSIR-RT is still under development, but it aims to be a dynamic tool that will include a searchable database. Events are expected to relate to "learning about, and reporting events arising along the RT delivery continuum, from the decision to treat to treatment completion" (37). The system looks at data for events within Canada, in three areas: actual incidents that reach the patient, near misses, and reportable circumstances (hazards not involving a patient). It is designed for use as a national event reporting system in conjunction with a local system, or to serve as the local system in facilities that do not have one of their own.

During the development of the system, existing incident reporting systems, including WHO, ASTRO, AAPM, and SAFRON, were reviewed to identify relevant elements and highlight their similarities, differences, and existing gaps in order to elaborate the key elements for the NSIR-RT. Efforts were made to maintain compatibility with those systems for future international collaboration. The taxonomy was launched in 2015, and a consensus process is under way. A published report about this consensus process indicated that 13 data elements were thought to warrant inclusion, and that near misses would be included in the implicit definition of an "incident" and not listed separately (38). The most up-to-date information about CPQR can be found at www.cpqr.ca/.

Radiation Oncology Incident Learning System

In June 2011, ASTRO approved a proposal to create a RO-ILS, and was later joined in the endeavor by AAPM. In 2013, a contract was signed with Clarity PSO, a patient safety organization, to afford special legal protections to participants. The patient safety work product (PSWP) entered into the system is privileged and confidential, allowing for analysis in a safe and protected environment. A beta test was executed between September 2013 and November 2014 among 14 sites from a variety of practice types.

As of February 24, 2015, 46 institutions had signed contracts with Clarity PSO; of these, 27 sites had entered 739 patient safety events into local database space, with 358 (48%) events pushed to the national database (39). The database accepts input related to both events and near misses, and functions as both a local reporting system (if desired) and a national database. Currently, the database is searchable only for reports from your own institution; because reports are not anonymized, they cannot be shared with all participants. The main method for dissemination of information is through quarterly newsletters. The most up-to-date information about RO-ILS can be found at www.astro.org/Clinical-Practice/Patient-Safety/ROILS/Index.aspx.

Other systems of note

Other systems do exist, and the motivated reader can find more information about them. These include, but are not limited to, STARSweb interface from the Health Service Executive (HSE) in Ireland (www.hse.ie); the National Health Service system in England and Wales, which is a collaboration between the National Patient Safety Agency, the Royal College of Radiologists, the Health Protection Agency, the Society and College of Radiographers, and other stakeholders, and based on *Toward Safer Radiotherapy* (40); RIRAS (Radiotherapy Incident Reporting and Analysis System) from the Center for Assessment of Radiological Sciences (CARS) with certification from the Agency for Healthcare Research and Quality (AHRQ) in the United States (www.cars-pso.org/); ROIRLS (Radiation Oncology Incident Reporting and Learning System) in the United States for Veterans Administration patients; two systems sponsored by the Conference of Radiation Control Program Directors (CRCPD) in the United States (www.crcpd.org/): a pilot tracking system for machine-based radiation medical events, and the Committee on Radiation Medical Events (H38) system to collect events reported to state agencies.

METHODS FOR CREATING AN EFFECTIVE FEEDBACK/LEARNING SYSTEM; MEASURES OF EFFECTIVENESS

Consensus recommendations on the development of incident reporting systems were recently published by the AAPM. This report includes process maps that list the key processes in the radiation oncology workflow to aid in the codification of incidents for both external beam therapy and brachytherapy (10). Severity scales are also discussed and categorized into a clinical/medical severity scale, as well as a dose deviations scale for dosimetric consequences that may have ultimately small or virtually no clinical impact. It is recommended that incidents be coded with both scales in the reporting system. The guidelines also include a taxonomy list of root causes and contributing factors to classify incidents, with the goal of identifying possible areas for improvement.

Additional factors must be considered in developing and maintaining an incident reporting system. The system itself may be relatively straightforward to develop from an information technology (IT) perspective, particularly as there are several models to use (4,6,23). However, the time, training, and resources required to evaluate the incidents submitted must be considered, particularly if the system is to be used for process improvement intradepartmentally.

Additionally, it is critical to provide feedback to the staff to incentivize departmental members to spend the time using the system, particularly if the system is voluntary (30). Thus, it is not enough to simply have an incident reporting system. To have a positive impact in the clinic, considerable resources must be directed toward maintaining the system, and conducting the analyses necessary to develop the corrective actions that will ultimately make patients safer.

In order for incident reporting systems to flourish, a safety culture must be encouraged. In a multi-institutional survey conducted to assess barriers to safety reporting, physicians and other staff felt it was their responsibility to report near misses and incidents (97% overall). Physicians were significantly less likely than other groups to report minor near misses ($P = .001$) and minor errors ($P = .024$). Physicians were significantly more concerned about getting colleagues in trouble ($P = .015$), liability ($P = .009$), effect on departmental reputation ($P = .006$), and embarrassment ($P < .001$) than their colleagues. Thus, even though all members of the radiation oncology team observe errors and near misses, physicians are significantly less likely to report events than other colleagues. Therefore, specific barriers to physician reporting should be investigated and analyzed to improve the systems in place today (30).

Ultimately, an effective incident reporting system should lead to mitigation strategies to prevent the same or a similar event from occurring, and thereby enhance patient safety. Several case examples have been previously published that describe effective changes that have led to improvement in processes (26). Although a mitigation strategy may be implemented, it is not always clear that the approach actually had its intended effect on improving safety or quality. The Plan–Do–Study–Act (PDSA) approach is one such method to qualitatively, and perhaps quantitatively, evaluate a new process to determine whether it succeeded in its intent. Although the PDSA approach has not been explicitly studied in radiation oncology, it is commonly used in health care for quality improvement. The PDSA cycle begins with the "plan," which involves the identification of the issue to be addressed. After the goal is set, the "do" step involves the actual implementation of the new process. Subsequently, the "study" step involves monitoring and collecting data on the outcomes after the new process has been implemented. New areas for improvement may be identified during the "study" step. Lastly, the "act" step completes the cycle and integrates the information learned from studying the outcomes to inform the next steps in meeting the goal of quality improvement. This may result in a change in the goal or methods that may be minor or major. The PDSA cycle is repeated with each of the four steps, in an iterative fashion, in order to provide effective feedback and continual improvement (41).

Ultimately, the value of an incident learning system depends on how effectively it contributes to making positive change happen. The staff must feel that the effort they put into reporting makes a difference in their lives and in the lives of patients; otherwise, that effort will not be sustained.

REFERENCES

1. Williams MV. Improving patient safety in radiotherapy by learning from near misses, incidents and errors. *Br J Radiol*. 2007;80(953):297–301.

2. Ford EC, Gaudette R, Myers L, et al. Evaluation of safety in a radiation oncology setting using failure mode and effects analysis. *Int J Radiat Oncol Biol Phys*. 2009;74(3):852–858.

3. Marks LB, Light KL, Hubbs JL, et al. The impact of advanced technologies on treatment deviations in radiation treatment delivery. *Int J Radiat Oncol Biol Phys*. 2007;69(5):1579–1586.

4. Mutic S, Brame RS, Oddiraju S, et al. Event (error and near-miss) reporting and learning system for process improvement in radiation oncology. *Med Phys*. 2010;37(9):5027–5036.

5. Bissonnette JP, Medlam G. Trend analysis of radiation therapy incidents over seven years. *Radiother Oncol*. 2010;96(1):139–144.

6. Cooke DL, Dunscombe PB, Lee RC. Using a survey of incident reporting and learning practices to improve organisational learning at a cancer care center. *Qual Saf Health Care*. 2007;16(5):342–348.

7. Ford EC, Fong de los Santos L, Pawlicki T, et al. The structure of incident learning systems for radiation oncology. *Int J Radiat Oncol Biol Phys*. 2013;86(1):11–12.

8. Evans SB, Ford EC. Radiation Oncology Incident Learning System: a call to participation. *Int J Radiat Oncol Biol Phys*. 2014;90(2):249–250.

9. Cunningham J, Coffey M, Knöös T, et al. Radiation Oncology Safety Information System (ROSIS): profiles of participants and the first 1,074 incident reports. *Radiother Oncol*. 2010;97(3):601–607.

10. Ford EC, Fong de los Santos L, Pawlicki T, et al. Consensus recommendations for incident learning database structures in radiation oncology. *Med Phys*. 2012;39(12):7272–7290.

11. Pham J, Girard T, Pronovost P. What to do with healthcare incident reporting systems. *J Public Health Res*. 2013;2(3):154–159.

12. Sujan M, Furniss D. Organisational reporting and learning systems: innovating inside and outside of the box. *Clin Risk*. 2015;21(1):7–12.

13. Reason J. Human error: models and management. *Brit Med J*. 2000;320:768–770.

14. Hasson B, Workie D, Geraghty C. WE-G-BRA-03: developing a culture of patient safety utilizing the national Radiation Oncology Incident Learning System (ROILS). *Med Phys*. 2015;42(6):3691.

15. Arnold A, Delaney GP, Cassapi L, et al. The use of categorized time-trend reporting of radiation oncology incidents: a proactive analytical approach to improving quality and safety over time. *Int J Radiat Oncol Biol Phys*. 2010;78(5):1548–1554.

16. Walker G, Johnson J, Edwards T, et al. Factors associated with radiation therapy incidents in a large academic institution. *Pract Radiat Oncol*. 2015;5(1):21–27.

17. Das P, Johnson J, Hayden SE, et al. Rate of radiation therapy events in a large academic institution. *J Am Coll Radiol*. 2013;10(6):452–455.

18. Yang R, Wang J, Zhang X, et al. Implementation of incident learning in the safety and quality management of radiotherapy: the primary experience in a new established program with advanced technology. *Biomed Res Int*. 2014;2014:392596.

19. Rahn DA III, Kim GY, Mundt AJ, et al. A real-time safety and quality reporting system: assessment of clinical data and staff participation. *Int J Radiat Oncol Biol Phys*. 2014;90(5):1202–1207.

20. Chang DW, Cheetham L, te Marvelde L, et al. Risk factors for radiotherapy incidents and impact of an online electronic reporting system. *Radiother Oncol*. 2014;112(2):199–204.

21. Macklis RM, Meier T, Weinhous MS. Error rates in clinical radiotherapy. *J Clin Oncol*. 1998;16:551–556.

22. Huang G, Medlam G, Lee J, et al. Error in the delivery of radiation therapy: results of a quality assurance review. *Int J Radiat Oncol Biol Phys*. 2005;61:1590–1595.

23. Clark BG, Brown RJ, Ploquin JL, et al. The management of radiation treatment error through incident learning. *Radiother Oncol*. 2010;95(3):344–349.

24. Clark BG, Brown RJ, Ploquin J, et al. Patient safety improvements in radiation treatment through 5 years of incident learning. *Pract Radiat Oncol*. 2013;3(3):157–163.

25. Gabriel PE, Volz E, Bergendahl HW, et al. Incident learning in pursuit of high reliability: implementing a comprehensive, low-threshold reporting program in a large, multisite radiation oncology department. *Jt Comm J Qual Patient Saf*. 2015;41(4):160–168.

26. Ford EC, Smith K, Harris K, et al. Prevention of a wrong-location misadministration through the use of an intradepartmental incident learning system. *Med Phys*. 2012;39(11):6968–6971.

27. Rashed A, Hamdan M. Physicians' and nurses' perceptions of and attitudes toward incident reporting in Palestinian hospitals. *J Patient Saf*. In press.

28. Mansfield JG, Caplan RA, Campos JS, et al. Using a quantitative risk register to promote learning from a patient safety reporting system. *Jt Comm J Qual Patient Saf*. 2015;41(2):76–81.

29. Nyflot MJ, Zeng J, Kusano AS, et al. Metrics of success: measuring impact of a departmental near-miss incident learning system. *Pract Radiat Oncol*. 2015;5(5):e409–e416.

30. Smith KS, Harris KM, Potters L, et al. Physician attitudes and practices related to voluntary error and near-miss reporting. *J Oncol Pract*. 2014;10(5):e350–e357.

31. Pappas D, Reis S, Ali A, et al. SU-E-T-511: interrater variability in classification of incidents in a new incident reporting system. *Med Phys*. 2015;42(6):3452.

32. Kapur A, Evans S, Ezzell G, et al. Data veracity in radiation medicine incident learning systems. In: *American Society for Therapeutic Radiology and Oncology (ASTRO) Big Data Workshop*. Bethesda, MD: NIH Campus; 2015.

33. Ekaette EU, Lee RC, Cooke DL, et al. Risk analysis in radiation treatment: application of a new taxonomic structure. *Radiother Oncol*. 2006;80(3):282–287.

34. Cunningham J, Holmberg O, Knöös T. *Reporting and Learning: ROSIS*. In *Introduction to Patient Safety in Radiation Oncology and Radiology: ROSIS Workshop*. Melbourne, Australia: Melbourne Convention Center; 2014.

35. Gilley D. Improving patient safety in radiotherapy: SAFRON. In: *ACCIRAD Workshop*. Poznań, Poland: International Atomic Energy Agency; 2013.

36. Holmberg O, Malone J, Rehani M, et al. Current issues and actions in radiation protection of patients. *Eur J Radiol*. 2010;76(1):15–19.

37. Marchand E, Drodge S, Liszewski B, et al. The national system for incident reporting in radiation therapy: a central repository for radiation therapy incidents in Canada. *J Med Imaging Radiat Sci*. 2014;45(2):172–173.

38. Liszewski B, Drodge CS, Marchand E, et al. A national system for incident reporting in radiation therapy: development of a taxonomy and severity

classification. *Int J Radiat Oncol Biol Phys.* 2014;90(1, suppl 1):S741.

39. Hoopes DJ, Dicker AP, Eads NL, et al. RO-ILS: Radiation Oncology Incident Learning System: a report from the first year of experience. *Pract Radiat Oncol.* 2015;5(5):312–318.

40. The Royal College of Radiologists, Society and College of Readiographers, Institute of Physics and Engineering in Medicine, National Patient Safety Agency, British Institute of Radiology. *Toward Safer Radiotherapy.* London, UK: The Royal College of Radiologists; 2008.

41. Donnelly P, Kirk P. Use the PDSA model for effective change management. *Educ Prim Care.* 2015;26(4):279–281.

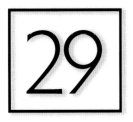

29 Quality and the Role of the Dosimetrist and Therapist in Radiation Oncology

Joumana Dekmak and Kathy Lash

When patients come to a heath care institution and are treated, they expect to leave in an improved condition. Although the science of teamwork has been around for more than 30 years, only in the last 10 years has it started to take hold as part of the health care organization. We continue to hear of the high percentage of errors that both result from and contribute to communication breakdowns and lack of effective teamwork (1). Communication failures have been identified by the Joint Commission as the primary root cause in more than 70% of sentinel events from 1995 to 2003. These failures continue as key factors in the occurrence of patient safety incidents (2). In health care, knowledge and skills are not enough for achieving excellent patient care; it is the combined efforts by all members of the team that make a difference. In order for teams to work effectively, team members need to have specific knowledge, attitude, and skill sets. Teamwork is critical for the delivery of health care, allowing health care professionals to work together to deliver safe and efficient patient care (23).

A *team* is defined as two or more individuals with complementary skills, who are committed and hold themselves accountable to a common purpose, set of performance goals, and approach (3). Teamwork is an essential component to achieve a high-performance team in any type of organization (19). The teamwork concept has been implemented in industries and management practices since the 1990s (4). Teamwork is most powerful when commitment and vision are shared between team members. Today, leaders are challenged to establish organizational cultures that foster a collaborative capacity. Team members of any organization should have the freedom to communicate with everyone, and work environments must be safe for everyone to offer ideas (5).

According to famous English poet John Donne, no man is an island. Each member brings a special gift or talent to strengthen a team (4). Donne's poem supports the fact that each member can have individual value, but when members come together, the overall quality and efficiency can be improved. Building a team could take months or even years. Letting a given team make high-level decisions can be of benefit to any given organization. Silo thinking is not team thinking. If people treat their internal identity as more important than their shared membership, they will always be protecting their turf, and large initiatives will be impossible (6).

Teamwork promotes success in any type of organization (20). If carried out correctly and shared effectively between team members, all can benefit with excellent outcomes (21). Research also indicates that team development has a lot to do with team management and leadership practices (7). Leaders play a significant role in empowering the team to work together. Leadership and teamwork are the glue that holds together and supports an excellent organization. Both components are achieved by skills that need to be practiced regularly. There should be a balance between leadership and teamwork to achieve a successful organization. Poor leadership cannot support a collaborative team. Similarly, strong leadership cannot achieve excellence with an incompetent, unmotivated team (8). Strong leaders build strong teams. They are known to actively listen, coach and mentor staff, support career development, and show interest in staff well-being (9). Excellent leaders not only influence and motivate teams, but also empower and delegate tasks as needed. To achieve teamwork, collaborative efforts from both the leader and team are needed to meet objectives (8). Leaders should not be decision makers, but decision facilitators. The best leaders usually motivate their followers to accomplish tasks and goals beyond their own expectations (6). Teams require continuous interaction to maintain high performance. By mentoring, motivating, and supporting a given team, excellent outcomes can be achieved. Shared leadership between team members and the leader can also aid in building a creative team. Senior team leaders assign leadership tasks to team members, and leadership roles change as new team members join the team. These results suggest that adaptive leadership enhances teams' ability to perform reliably in the face of dynamically changing task requirements (8).

Workload, time pressure, and job control were found to be associated with team member outcomes such as burnout, job satisfaction, and organizational commitment (22). For example, surveys of intensive care unit nurses showed that leadership styles that seek and value contributions from staff promote a climate in which information is shared effectively, and influence coordination of work to provide excellent care and in return increase nurses' intent to stay (10). Burnout symptoms such as emotional exhaustion, fatigue, and the inability to concentrate decreased clinicians' ability to ensure patient safety. Leadership and good team behaviors can help in creating an atmosphere where employees feel they can communicate and participate in decision making (11), which decreases the likelihood of negative team outcomes. For many years, three important leadership facts were shared when working with teams: work through others, recognize that you need subordinates more than they need you, and you get paid for what your subordinates do (12).

Indeed, leadership is important in achieving teamwork, but building and promoting peer-to-peer relationships is just as important. Team members are dependent on each other for success. Building a culture of respect, trust, and friendly behaviors between members is required. Forging solid relationships is the key for successful workplace collaboration (9). Attitude and behaviors of individual team members on any given team can enhance team performance. Whether peer to peer or supervisor to peer, we can improve teamwork by supportive communication, helping others, and acknowledging contributions from all members of the team (13).

In radiation oncology departments, there are many team members. The key players in the delivery and planning of accurate treatments are the radiation therapist and dosimetrist. They work best in a team work setting. The quality and efficiency are better developed in any field when a high-performance team is involved. Radiation therapist and dosimetrist work together with the proper physician's intent to ensure that patients receive safe and accurate radiation therapy treatments. For many years now, much effort has gone into exploring ways to compose high-performance teams in the radiation oncology setting. This is because poor coordination among providers at various levels of the organization appears to affect the quality and safety of patient care (e.g., delays in testing or treatment, conflicting information). Therefore, teamwork has become a focus of system-based interventions to improve patient safety and of medical education standards (2).

Even though teamwork increases patient safety and quality of care, this does not mean that variances from the direct physician's intent do not happen. In radiation oncology, institutional, departmental, and national variance reporting systems have been developed and implemented. These variance systems exist to track the types of variances that are identified by different members of the team. Aside from tracking variances, the system is also available to track near misses or "good catches." The team can learn from these types of variances. It is important that regular meetings be held with a representative from each team of the radiation oncology department to review the variances and write and implement policies and procedural changes as needed. These variances should also be shared in monthly meetings with clinical physicians, dosimetrist, physicist, clinical staff, and radiation therapists, to encourage feedback and look for root causes to make process improvements. This is an educational opportunity to help others perform more effectively and efficiently in order to deliver the best quality care to patients.

SIMULATION

Simulation is the first critical step in the planning process. At the University of Michigan, a team of therapists developed a safe and efficient simulation workflow using skills learned during Lean training and mentoring. Lean thinking is a process that maximizes customer value and minimizes waste. Lean means creating more value for customers with fewer resources but not necessarily less staff. A Lean organization understands customer value and focuses its key processes to continuously increase improvements. The ultimate goal is to provide perfect value to the customer through a perfect value creation process that has zero waste. Checklists and tasks were defined and implemented by a team of radiation therapist and dosimetrist.

Before checklists tasks were defined, driver (the person who is running the simulator) and nondriver (person who is working along with the person running the simulator) duties were shared without defining the responsibilities of each task. This created confusion and chaos for the team. For example, if the driver goes into the simulator between scans to make a mask and the nondriver does not complete other tasks, the workload might be repetitive or can increase for the driver. As we became paperless, electronic clinic flow generated more electronic documents that require immediate attention.

The following electronic flow was derived to create a more successful flow in the simulator. Before taking any patient to the simulator, the radiation therapy technologists (RTTs) should ensure that the following tasks are completed:

- Simulation directive (simulation directions) must be signed off by the physician

- Patient consent must be completed and signed

- IV contrast form must be completed

- Face photo was taken and downloaded by clinical staff

- Simulator room must be set up for the patient

- Nursing education has been completed before proceeding with patient to the simulator

Presimulation huddle is an important step in the process of patient safety. All simulation staff should be involved in the presimulation process of reviewing patient information, the simulation site, and treatment modality. Then one RTT (or two if possible) completes the time-out by greeting the patient, verifying his or her name and date of birth (DOB), and notifying the clinic that the exam room will be available for the next simulation patient.

It was suggested and proven that two therapists are essential to complete the required simulation duties. RTT, driver, and nondriver duties were written and displayed in the simulator room. Competencies were built for different radiation modalities and equipment.

In the simulator, for example, the driver and nondriver tasks can be split into two groupings:

Driver:

- Input or verify the patient information

- Straighten/realign patient if needed

- Before scanning, verify that the chain utilized for safety between the control room and the simulator is up and the simulator room is clear

- Scan patient

- Make sure physician approves the simulation directive

- Push the scan to treatment planning system

Nondriver:

- Electronic paperwork (set-up sheet, photo/dosimetry page, scheduling form)

- Page attending/resident when needed

- Billing

- Provide breathing instructions to patient if needed for scan

- Take photos of CT reference marks and final simulation position

- Straighten/realign patient if needed

- Postsimulation, take patient on tour of department

In the simulator, the RTTs:

- Communicate with patients and explain what they can expect to happen (Team)

- Position patient and set equipment as referenced in simulation directive (Team)

- Page physician (Nondriver)

- Start paperwork (set-up page, scheduling form, simulation photo/dosimetry move sheet, care path) (Nondriver)

- Input patient data into scanner or verify (Driver)

- Take the scout, realign if necessary (Driver)

- Page physician and resident (Nondriver)

- Update patient on procedure progress (Driver)

- After physician reviews and approves scan, have him or her sign off on simulation documents, and provide scheduling information (chemo/protocol, IMRT, volumes date) (Nondriver)

- Take photos of CT reference marks (Driver)

- Upload photos to simulation photo/dosimetry move sheet (Nondriver)

- Push the scan to treatment planning system (Driver)

- Pull the scan into treatment planning system (Driver)

- Tour patient through the department, and provide map of the department (Team)

- Patient or family member tour: Review a safety/x-ray brochure that they can read over before they start their treatments so they can better understand why imaging is required for treatment

An example of an imaging brochure is provided in Figure 29.1.

Dosimetry

The next step in the patient planning journey involves the dosimetrist review and planning process. Depending on the instructions from the physician, a dosimetrist might be requested to be on set for the simulation planning. When the simulation scan is transferred to dosimetry, the dosimetrist–physician communication begins. To continue implementing the Lean process, it is suggested that the dosimetrist also develop checklists and procedures to ensure safe patient treatment delivery. Each dosimetrist is responsible for a body site and works primarily with specific physicians. After receiving the physician-defined planning goals on the planning directive, the dosimetrist proceeds with planning. He or she will also discuss the directive with the physician's resident in order to give the latter an opportunity to learn. The residents have designated computer stations where they can draw contours around target and organ-at-risk volumes and send them back to the dosimetrist for review. During the dosimetrist planning process, it is important to "huddle" or discuss plan initiatives with medical physics and the prescribing physician. After the plan is completed, the review stage begins. To make sure the plan meets all goals and that any deviations from the planning directive are documented, a second dosimetrist performs a peer review. When a fellow dosimetrist reviews the plan, a scheduling task is dropped for the clinical staff

ABOUT X-RAY IMAGING

◊ **The type and frequency of imaging depends on the unique characteristics of your treatment plan.**

◊ **Imaging is used to analyze and confirm your position before we start your treatment.**

◊ **The imaging dose is 0.1 – 1% of your treatment dose.**

◊ **There may be a delay between when you are imaged and when your treatment begins while your treatment team reviews your imaging.**

DEFINITIONS

Imaging: A generic term for any type of x-ray imaging, may also be called *picture, film* or *x-ray.*

CBCT: An acronym for cone beam computed tomography. This is a type of imaging that is similar to the CT scan that you received before the start of your treatment. The imager travels all the way around you to make this image, but doesn't touch you.

kV image: An image made with low energy x-rays designed to highlight certain anatomy.

MV image: An image made with high energy x-rays designed to highlight certain anatomy.

FAQs ABOUT RADIOTHERAPY IMAGING

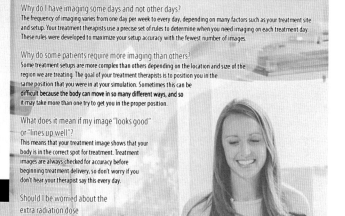

Why do I have imaging some days and not other days?
The frequency of imaging varies from one day per week to every day, depending on many factors such as your treatment site and setup. Your treatment therapists use a precise set of rules to determine when you need imaging on each treatment day. These rules were developed to maximize your setup accuracy with the fewest number of images.

Why do some patients require more imaging than others?
Some treatment setups are more complex than others depending on the location and size of the region we are treating. The goal of your treatment therapists is to position you in the same position that you were in at your simulation. Sometimes this can be difficult because the body can move in so many different ways, and so it may take more than one try to get you in the proper position.

What does it mean if my image "looks good" or "lines up well"?
This means that your treatment image shows that your body is in the correct spot for treatment. Treatment images are always checked for accuracy before beginning treatment delivery, so don't worry if you don't hear your therapist say this every day.

Should I be worried about the extra radiation dose from images?
The radiation dose that you receive from imaging is very small compared to the dose from your treatment. While we strive to limit the extra dose from imaging, our first goal is always to make sure you are positioned correctly.

FAQs (CONT.)

What can I do to help make the setup more accurate?
Your most important job during your radiation treatment is to try to stay as still as possible. Please let us know if at any time you are uncomfortable or you feel like you cannot stay still. Your treatment therapists can see and hear you at all times during your treatment and will watch for any signs of discomfort or motion.

At the dentist they use lead shielding for imaging, why don't you use any shielding?
Because of what we need to see in our images, we use stronger (higher energy) x-rays for imaging compared to your dentist. This means that a lead apron wouldn't be an effective shield.

Can you tell if my tumor is changing from imaging?
The images are not diagnostic quality, so rarely can your tumor be visualized on the image. The purpose of the images is to make sure you are in the correct position for treatment. A multidisciplinary team is evaluating your images throughout your treatment. You can talk with your doctor about their interpretation.

What if I have more questions about my treatment imaging?
Please let your treatment therapists know and they can help, or they can refer you to an additional member of your treat- ment team to give you more information. We always welcome your feedback.

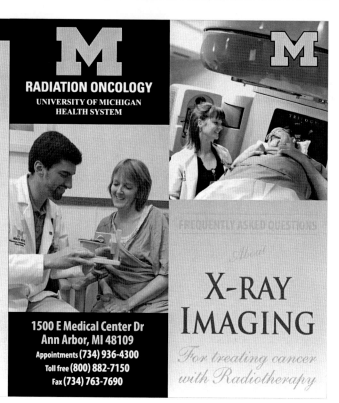

RADIATION ONCOLOGY
UNIVERSITY OF MICHIGAN
HEALTH SYSTEM

1500 E Medical Center Dr
Ann Arbor, MI 48109
Appointments **(734) 936-4300**
Toll free **(800) 882-7150**
Fax **(734) 763-7690**

FREQUENTLY ASKED QUESTIONS
About

X-RAY IMAGING
For treating cancer with Radiotherapy

FIGURE 29.1
X-ray Imaging brochure. Source: Reprinted with permission from the Radiation Oncology University of Michigan Health System

to call the patient and schedule the desired patient. As a second check, a software program can be created to catch some common errors, such as scheduling a treatment on a machine for which the patient is ineligible, or incorrect treatment field labels. When the dosimetrist peer review is complete, medical physics receives a notification to start the review process. At this point, the plan checker software is run again to catch common variances, and a manual check is also performed to ensure safe delivery.

Dosimetrists are required to work one on one with the physician to come up with the final plan for the patient. Sometimes, the dosimetrist needs to perform a plan revision, or might be working on a very complicated case requiring more attention and discussion. During this time, it is best to complete all the necessary planning steps before even scheduling the patient for treatment.

Radiation Therapy

Just as we created safety measures in the simulation and planning sessions, radiation therapists on the treatment units also have safety measures to check for variances from the physician's desired intent. Every day, the chief therapist looks ahead to ensure that new patient plans are ready for the following day. This will decrease the wait time for patients and ensure that all plans have been completed. If there are plans to be reviewed, dosimetrist and physicist are informed so the plan can be ready for the patient. From the safety team discussions, a new prestart quality assurance process has been implemented. The therapists are to do prestart quality assurance checks for those patients whose plans are ready (Figure 29.2). This is done to ensure safe delivery and to decrease delays or complications before the patient gets on the treatment table.

Once the quality assurance prestart check is completed, any variances from the physician's original intent that have been caught are logged in the department variance system as near misses. This allows the team to review the members' near misses so that they can be reduced in the future. The prestart check is a great tool that serves not only as a safety measure, but also as a continued educational measure for the radiation therapist. It allows the therapist to look beyond treating, and at the pretreatment phase of patient care. All the team members in radiation oncology share prequality check work to provide the patient the best quality care experience. It is critical to have standardization for the therapist and all staff members; an example of this is implementing tasks at different times throughout the treatment process.

For these reasons, checklists and detailed procedures are developed that assist the treatment team in performing their duties at all points along the patient care path. To perform excellent patient care and complete the process, driver and nondriver duties have also been written for the treatment unit team. All therapists are trained and competencies are built for safety reasons. From feedback and the variance reporting system, the University of Michigan Radiation

Oncology Department has decided to have a minimum of two to a maximum of three therapists involved with each patient's treatment. The checklist team works best at driving what is needed for the patient and what "huddles" and "discussions" should be done before and after treating the patient. Examples of information in these discussions are listed here and are located in each treatment area (Figure 29.3).

When the workload and checklist procedures are not followed, one will notice:

- Lack of communication
- Nonadherence to policies
- Rushing through treatment
- Near misses
- Incidents reaching the patient (treatment variances)

The following flowcharts (Figures 29.4 and 29.5) can be used to better help with the steps necessary for the radiation therapists to complete their tasks in simulation and on the treatment unit.

Organizations around the world have adopted programs to enhance quality and safety. Every organization should strive to create teams and build teamwork relationships. At the University of Michigan Radiation Oncology Department, the unit works toward building a safety culture. Employee competencies and daily huddles take place to promote safety. Competencies are built to make sure therapists are keeping up with radiation therapy policy and equipment changes; this also ensures standardization in processes and procedures. Huddles are time-outs that we take during the day to come up with ideas and problem-solve. In a health care organization, this has to start with hiring people who are naturally cooperative. A screening process that includes a short survey by the individual to evaluate behavior and team characteristics should be considered. The organization should create a 6-week workshop for new hires to help build strong relationships between team members. In this workshop, team members will share the vision, goals, and rewards that will be promoted by managers. After the 6-week program is completed, mentoring and helping team members grow with having a cooperative mindset can be done. Holding one-on-one meetings with subordinates can help build trust, respect, and unity. Peer-to-peer working relationships should be evaluated weekly to help people flourish and build trust, safety, and efficiency. In the world of radiation oncology, it is suggested to train the dosimetrists and therapists to be excellent patient caregivers. In addition, competencies and procedures are required in each group to ensure safe delivery. This should be done annually and as people are hired. Unless a safe culture is built, quality care cannot be achieved.

Methods used to ensure that the right staff are hired should include interviews, focus groups, and safety surveys. The latter can provide useful diagnostic information relating to the perception of teamwork and safety behavior.

Plan #'s checked	▦	▦	▦	▦
Script linked to and matches plan	▦	▦	▦	▦
Clear set-up instructions (photo, bolus, cutout, consent)	▦	▦	▦	▦
Present and clear IGRT document	▦Yes ▦N/A	▦Yes ▦N/A	▦Yes ▦N/A	▦Yes ▦N/A
Clear plan revision instructions	▦Yes ▦N/A	▦Yes ▦N/A	▦Yes ▦N/A	▦Yes ▦N/A
Treatment-related patient alerts and journal notes clear	▦Yes ▦N/A	▦Yes ▦N/A	▦Yes ▦N/A	▦ Yes ▦N/A
Laterality consistent on all documentation	▦	▦	▦	▦
Set-up fields appropriate and labeled correctly	▦	▦	▦	▦
Correct match anatomy	▦	▦	▦	▦
Correct treatment field labeling and order				
No clearance issues, or noted if clearance is a concern	▦	▦	▦	▦
Correct imaging templates attached	▦	▦	▦	▦
Correct machine scheduling	▦	▦	▦	▦
Correct appointment type and length	▦	▦	▦	▦
Initials Date				
Notes:				

IGRT, image-guided radiation therapy

FIGURE 29.2 Pre-start quality assurance checklist.

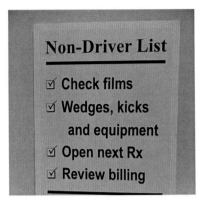

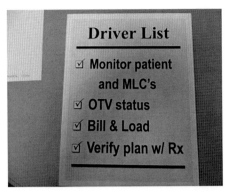

FIGURE 29.3 Therapists treatment checklists.

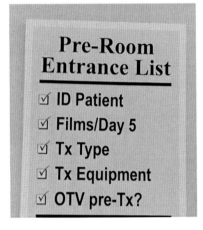

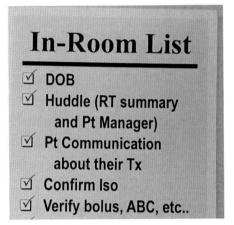

A number of health care surveys that evaluate what safety means to the individual should be considered. Methods used to describe and assess team relationships should include observation studies of patient care teams. This can provide information on effective team behaviors such as coordination and leadership. Team performance can be improved through teamwork and collaboration. For example, doctors, nurses, and allied health workers should come together to work on issues or problems that are raised in a heath care setting. In these meetings, it is important for each member to be held accountable to gather data, help analyze the data, plan actions, and implement and evaluate outcomes. The more the teams become involved, the better the outcome will be. If conflicts are recognized early by leaders, more efforts can be put in to help the overall success of the team.

Dosimetry and radiation therapy teams should work together to accomplish results. Regardless of whether it is a production unit, an operating room team, a NASA space team, or a utility company service crew, effective decisions and outcomes can result from working together effectively. The degree of teamwork needed should be evaluated by leaders to help promote high-performance teams. Leadership should always assign tasks, evaluate outcome, and use rewards to promote safety and excellence. Measurement of team maturity is an ongoing task for leaders when building a team. A significant amount of research has been undertaken by different individuals in many industries. Researchers have made great strides in defining teams. They have identified competencies that enable and promote teams to meet their goals, and have developed techniques for capturing, measuring, and teaching those skills. Some of this research should continue to be evaluated in health care, as we continue to see negative outcomes from team failures. Evaluating team members and evaluating the teamwork consistently can help result in a safe, high-performance outcome.

Benefits of Work–Life Balance

In order for people to achieve high performance and complete any checklist required, work–life balance should be established. Workplace stress can have an effect on job or life satisfaction, physical and mental health, morale, and relationships. Long working hours, insufficient breaks, lack of resources, and unrealistic deadlines can contribute to workplace stress. Stress can definitely lead to burnout, a state of physical and emotional exhaustion. It can occur when you experience long-term stress in your job, or when you have worked in a physically or emotionally draining role for a long time. You can also experience burnout when your efforts at work or home have failed to produce the results that you expected, and you feel deeply

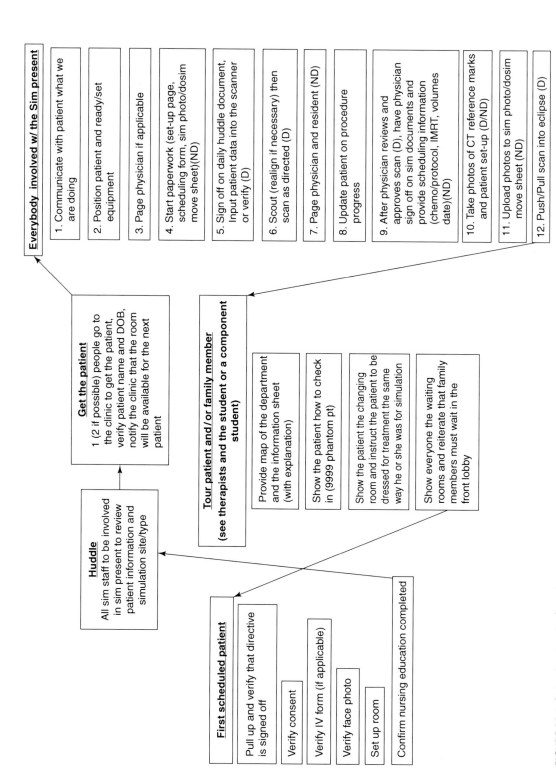

Huddle

All sim staff to be involved in sim present to review patient information and simulation site/type

Get the patient

1 (2 if possible) people go to the clinic to get the patient, verify patient name and DOB, notify the clinic that the room will be available for the next patient

First scheduled patient

Pull up and verify that directive is signed off

Verify consent

Verify IV form (if applicable)

Verify face photo

Set up room

Confirm nursing education completed

Tour patient and/or family member
(see therapists and the student or a component student)

Provide map of the department and the information sheet (with explanation)

Show the patient how to check in (9999 phantom pt)

Show the patient the changing room and instruct the patient to be dressed for treatment the same way he or she was for simulation

Show everyone the waiting rooms and reiterate that family members must wait in the front lobby

Everybody involved w/ the Sim present

1. Communicate with patient what we are doing

2. Position patient and ready/set equipment

3. Page physician if applicable

4. Start paperwork (set-up page, scheduling form, sim photo/dosim move sheet)(ND)

5. Sign off on daily huddle document, Input patient data into the scanner or verify (D)

6. Scout (realign if necessary) then scan as directed (D)

7. Page physician and resident (ND)

8. Update patient on procedure progress

9. After physician reviews and approves scan (D), have physician sign off on sim documents and provide scheduling information (chemo/protocol, IMRT, volumes date)(ND)

10. Take photos of CT reference marks and patient set-up (D/ND)

11. Upload photos to sim photo/dosim move sheet (ND)

12. Push/Pull scan into eclipse (D)

FIGURE 29.4 A step-by-step sim flow chart.

DOB, date of birth; D, driver; ND, non-driver; IMRT, Intensity-modulated radiation therapy.

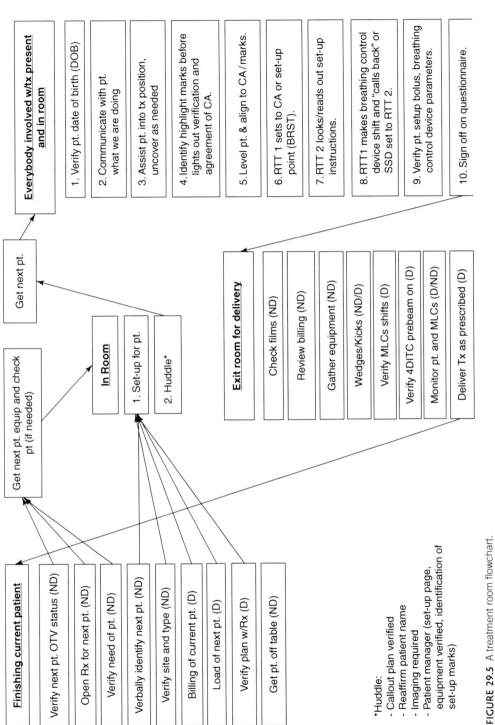

Finishing current patient

Verify next pt. OTV status (ND)

Open Rx for next pt. (ND)

Verify need of pt. (ND)

Verbally identify next pt. (ND)

Verify site and type (ND)

Billing of current pt. (D)

Load of next pt. (D)

Verify plan w/Rx (D)

Get pt. off table (ND)

Get next pt. equip and check pt (if needed)

Get next pt.

Everybody involved w/tx present and in room

1. Verify pt. date of birth (DOB)

2. Communicate with pt. what we are doing

3. Assist pt. into tx position, uncover as needed

4. Identify highlight marks before lights out verification and agreement of CA.

5. Level pt. & align to CA/marks.

6. RTT 1 sets to CA or set-up point (BRST).

7. RTT 2 looks/reads out set-up instructions.

8. RTT1 makes breathing control device shift and "calls back" or SSD set to RTT 2.

9. Verify pt. setup bolus, breathing control device parameters.

10. Sign off on questionnaire.

In Room

1. Set-up for pt.

2. Huddle*

Exit room for delivery

Check films (ND)

Review billing (ND)

Gather equipment (ND)

Wedges/Kicks (ND/D)

Verify MLCs shifts (D)

Verify 4DITC prebeam on (D)

Monitor pt. and MLCs (D/ND)

Deliver Tx as prescribed (D)

*Huddle:
- Callout plan verified
- Reaffirm patient name
- Imaging required
- Patient manager (set-up page, equipment verified, identification of set-up marks)

FIGURE 29.5 A treatment room flowchart.

BRST, breast; CA, central axis; D, driver; MLCs, multileaf collimators; ND, non-driver; OTV, On Treatment Visit; pt., patient; Rx, prescription; RTT, radiotherapy technician; tx, treatment; SSD, source to skin distance.

283

disillusioned as a result. Burnout can affect an individual's overall performance, whether at home or at work. This is why people are encouraged to find a balance between work and life duties (14).

Today, organizations continue to promote and recognize the importance of employee satisfaction and well-being. Whether a leader or an employee, everyone at some point in time will face life challenges that might cause a decreased job performance or burnout. What knowledge and tips can leaders share with each other and their staff when faced with conflicts, near misses, or variances? To accomplish this goal, professional dosimetrists and radiation therapists can continue to introduce changes in the work structure and environment, as well to pioneer new policies and practices, which can allow employees to bring more balance into their lives and avoid burnout, while also administering safe and efficient quality treatments.

Workers who experience meaningfulness in their work, and who use their knowledge and skills on the job, are more likely to be satisfied with their jobs (26). Job satisfaction and work–life balance are more likely to drive employees to remain with their current organization than benefits and salary (15). Every person has different sets of needs at different times. It is the responsibility of individuals to recognize their personal goals and evaluate their daily needs. According to a poll by the Washington-based American Psychological Association, 67% of the 1,240 full- and part-time employees surveyed cited both job satisfaction and work–life balance among the primary reasons for their decision to stay with their current employers. The poll's findings suggested a growing need among employers to foster a relationship between their employees' work environment and their lives beyond the jobsite. Today, top employers are seeking to create an environment in which employees feel connected to the organization and have a positive work experience (15).

By focusing on overall satisfaction with the way work and personal life are managed, an individual can definitely increase energy, happiness, and performance quality (29). Through life, there are many obstacles that can arise with individuals at home or at work that signify imbalance. Imbalance can decrease overall satisfaction, which in turn can decrease performance. If a person becomes imbalanced, different levels of burnout and health implications can occur (16).

According to the World Health Organization, mental health problems due to work pressure and life imbalance are expected to become the second most common cause of disability and death by 2020. No matter what profession a person is in, or how old a person is, it is never too late to reevaluate and rethink one's lifestyle (17).

There is a growing awareness in today's workplaces that employees do not give up their lives just because they work. Work and home life remain the two most important domains in the life of an employed individual. However, the challenge of balancing work and nonwork demands is one of today's central concerns for both individuals and organizations (18). Some organizations have systems that are better developed than others to address work–life balance issues. Organizations should most likely seek more flextime, job sharing, compressed hours, and work breaks. Conflicts, particularly between work and family, significantly affect the quality of family life and career attainment. If not evaluated, imbalance can cause high levels of stress and burnout (27). The continuous inability of employees to balance work and life responsibilities has significant organizational consequences, including higher rates of absenteeism and turnover, reduced productivity, and decreased job satisfaction (24). This can be seen in the dosimetrist and radiation therapist if the workload is not split or if there are no current procedures on how the workload is evaluated to give the patient the best experience. With the help of the checklist team, an organization can foster a safe atmosphere for everyone to complete their job. In simulation, planning, and at the treatment unit, there should be minimal interruptions so that a safe culture is created for the employees, together with promoting excellent patient care.

Not surprisingly, there is strong evidence to support the proposition that work–life balance benefits both the employee and the employer (25). The advantages for many organizations come from happy employees, as the latter make for improved relations between coworkers and management. Once employees' lives are balanced, their self-esteem, health, concentration, and confidence are more apt to rise. When employees become more confident, they can prove their loyalty and commitment to work and home duties (30). Employees are more likely to stay with an organization when there are opportunities for achieving work–life balance. They can better manage their tasks, and with increased motivation, the level of stress among employees is reduced, and fascinating performance improvement is observed (18).

Furthermore, benefits to the employer can maximize the available labor. Every employee will attain excellent performance at work when balanced, and this in turn will make employees feel valuable (18). Implementing work–life balance programs can prove that the organization is interested in its employees' self-development. Thus, they will feel more valuable and work harder—and better—as a result (30). The work environment will be less stressful, leading to less stress-related illness and decreased health care costs. The workforce will be more loyal and motivated, absenteeism will be reduced, and productivity will increase because of the maximized available labor (18).

However, it should also be recognized that establishing work–life balance programs in organizations is one thing; getting employees to make use of them is another (28). Thus, there remains considerable contention about the effectiveness of organizational work–life balance policies in delivering flexibility and reducing stress and job dissatisfaction in the modern workplace. The success of work–life balance depends on many factors, including the existence of a supportive family culture and the role that managers play in that context. Each individual should be held accountable in evaluating their needs so better balance can be developed. Nevertheless, some employees may not take advantage of work–life balance plans. According to Rawlings et al (18), an ambitious employee may decide to concentrate on his or her career, waiving the advantages of any work–life balance plans that may be available in the organization. Personal values of employees, for example, might discourage employees from utilizing work–life balance plans, so much so that if carried to the extreme, employee burnout may result, to the detriment of the organization.

CONCLUSION

In conclusion, in order to improve patient care, all individuals should be balanced so they can perform at their best. We can improve safety and efficiency at work by continually promoting safety. Whether you are a dosimetrist, a radiation therapist, or part of the leadership, building safety measures to ensure safe patient delivery is a requirement. Aside from having safety checks, it is important to continually meet with staff and encourage them to report any near misses or variances, creating a safety culture. To advance our policies and procedures, efforts should be directed at reviewing root causes of incidents and exploring ways to prevent them from happening. This cannot be done without a proper safety culture and work–life balance. Everyone should be encouraged to find that balance so as to make a difference in patient care.

REFERENCES

1. Kohn LT, Corrigan JM, Donaldson MS. *To Err Is Human: Building a Safer Health System*. Washington, DC: National Academy Press; 1999.

2. Baggs JG, Ryan SA, Phelps CE, et al. The association between interdisciplinary collaboration and patient outcomes in a medical intensive care unit. *Heart Lung*. 1992;21(1):18–24.

3. Cheney G, Christensen LT, Zorn TE, et al. *Organizational Communication in an Age of Globalizations: Issues, Reflections, Practices*. 2nd ed. Long Grove, IL: Waveland Press; 2011.

4. Chia C. Teamwork boon. *Malays Bus*. 2011:42.

5. Beier Y. The collaborative advantage. *Communication World*. 2014:22–25.

6. Sander AF. Lonely at the top? *Med Mark Media*. 2015;50:2.

7. Bratty CA, Barker Scott BA. *Building Smart Teams: A Roadmap to High Performance*. Thousand Oaks, CA: Sage; 2004.

8. Sohmen VS. Leadership and teamwork: two sides of the same coin. *J IT Econ Dev*. 2013;4:1–18.

9. Ladika S. The collaborative edge. *HR Magazine*. 2014;59:36–42.

10. Davenport DL, Henderson WG, Mosca CL, et al. Risk-adjusted morbidity in teaching hospitals correlates with reported levels of communication and collaboration on surgical teams but not with scale measures of teamwork climate, safety climate or working conditions. *J Am Coll Surg*. 2007;205:778–784.

11. Palanisamy R, Verville J. Factors enabling communication-based collaboration in interprofessional heath care practice: a case study. *Int J E-Collaboration*. 2015;11:8–27.

12. Fournies FF. *Coaching for Improved Work Performance*. Blue Ridge Summit, PA: Tab Books; 1987.

13. Aronson ZH, Dominick PG, Wang M. Exhibiting leadership and facilitation behaviors in NPD project-based work: does team personal style composition matter? *Eng Manag J*. 2014;26(3):25–35.

14. Leger-Hornby T, Bleed R. Work and life: achieving a reasonable balance. In: Golden C, ed. *Cultivating Careers: Professional Development for Campus IT*. Louisville, CO: EDUCAUSE; 2006: ch. 7. http://www.educause.edu/research-publications/books/cultivating-careers-professional-development-campus-it/chapter-7-work-and-life-achieving-reasonab.

15. Dunning, M. (2012). Job satisfaction, work/life balance top list of workers' retention incentives: Poll. *Busuiness Insurance Magazine*.

16. Abendroth A-K, Dulk LD. Support for the work life balance in Europe: the impact of state, workplace and family support and work-life balance satisfaction. *Work Employ Soc*. 2011;25:234–256.

17. Muna FA, Point D, Mansour N. Balancing work and personal life: the leader as acrobat. *J Manag Dev*. 2009;28:121–133.

18. Rawlings IO, Omole I, Festus I. Employee work-life balance as an HR imperative: African research review. *Int Multidiscip J*. 2012;6:109–126.

19. Baker DP, Day R, Salas E. Teamwork as an essential component of high-reliability organizations. *Health Serv Res*. 2006;41:1576–1598.

20. Dyer WG. *Team Building: Current Issues and New Alternatives*. 3rd ed. Reading, MA: Addison-Wesley; 1995.

21. Ilgen DR. Teams embedded in organizations: some implications. *Am Psychol.* 1999;54:129–139.

22. Miller PA. Nurse–physician collaboration in an intensive care unit. *Am J Crit Care.* 2001;10:341–350.

23. Paris CR, Salas E, Cannon-Bowers JA. Teamwork in multi-person system: a review and analysis. *Ergonomics.* 2000;43:1052–1075.

24. Wiegmann DA, El Bardissi AW, Dearani, JA, et al. Disruptions in surgical flow and their relationship to surgical errors: an exploratory investigation. *Surgery.* 2007;142(5):658–665.

25. Crompton R, Lyonette C. Work-life balance in Europe. *Acta Sociol J.* 2006;49:379–393.

26. Eikhof DR, Warhurst C, Haunschild A. Introduction: What work? What life? What balance? *Employee Relations J.* 2007;29:325–333.

27. Lambert CH, Kass SJ, Piotrowski C, et al. Impact factors on work-family balance: initial support for border theory. *Organ Dev J.* 2006;24:64–75.

28. Lester J. Work-life balance and cultural change: a narrative of eligibility. *Rev High Educ.* 2013;36(4):463–488.

29. Mazerolle SM, Goodman A. Fulfillment of work–life balance from the organizational perspective: a case study. *J Athl Train.* 2013;48:668–677.

30. Munn SL. Unveiling the work–life system: the influence of work–life balance on meaningful work. *Adv Dev Hum Resour.* 2013;15:401–417.

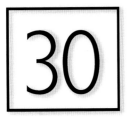

30 Quality and the Electronic Medical Record in Radiation Oncology

James Mechalakos and Sonja Dieterich

As radiation oncology clinics "go paperless" or adopt an electronic form of the chart, it is important to be prepared for the potential pitfalls in this process. Paper charts have been in existence for decades, and each clinic has developed its own method for storing information in that format over the years. Although at first sight a paper chart is a repository of information, it also serves other functions in the communication about the patient: it contains checklists (formal and informal), tracks workflow tasks (by handing the chart from one care provider to the next), and is used in essential communication that may not rise to the level of a consult note.

When a clinic is faced with the prospect of converting to electronic charting, either through the need for regulatory compliance or some other incentive such as increased efficiency or implementation of "meaningful use" criteria (1–3), the selection, design, and transition process can be daunting and initially require frequent modifications. Developers of an electronic charting system are primarily obligated to clearly communicate the patient's health status and care plan and fulfill legal and billing requirements (4). Forms must be developed, workflows must be designed, and training must be provided to those using the system so that interruptions to clinical flow are minimized during and after the transition. Doing this responsibly and safely requires cooperation from all clinical subspecialists: radiation oncologists, medical residents, nurses, physicists, dosimetrists, therapists, information technology (IT) professionals, as well as any administrative staff that is to use the new chart. Vendor training, interaction, and cooperation are also essential for a smooth transition.

In this chapter, important points concerning quality in electronic charting are discussed. The concept of electronic charting in radiation oncology is not new (5–8); however, commercial software used by most institutions today is very different from earlier home-grown systems, and because of the inherent flexibility within commercial software, the design of a chart may vary from clinic to

clinic. Quality assurance (QA) methods are still being developed by the community as electronic software becomes more sophisticated.

In this chapter, we distinguish between the radiation oncology electronic medical record/chart (RO-EMR) and the non–oncology-related or hospital EMR (H-EMR), which is often a separate system and will not be discussed here. Most examples are in the context of external beam radiation therapy, and a special section summarizing considerations for brachytherapy and other devices with limited connectivity to RO-EMR software is included.

SELECTION AND DESIGN OF THE ELECTRONIC CHARTING SYSTEM

Selection of the appropriate system requires careful planning and research, as it will fundamentally affect clinical workflow. A survey conducted by Thomas Jefferson University concerning implementation of meaningful use criteria cited unexpected difficulties in implementation and lack of adequate resources as common impediments to the implementation of an electronic health record system (9). In radiation oncology, the situation is often different because most existing record-and-verify (R&V) systems have been developed by the vendors in such a way that they can be used as the RO-EMR.

For the purposes of this chapter, we can represent the typical commercial RO-EMR as being divided into three parts, the first two of which are the primary focus of this chapter:

1. The electronic chart, which consists of forms, templates, checklists, free-text notes, and anything else in which information previously part of the "paper" chart is stored.

2. The workflow management system, which replaces handoff of the paper chart from one clinical

team member to the other and facilitates clinical workflow.

3. The treatment management system, which manages treatment delivery and communicates treatment information back to the electronic chart through a treatment history. This includes the R&V system.

As shown in Figure 30.1, the "ecosystem" with which the RO-EMR interacts can be divided into: (a) the implementation team, which designs and manages the RO-EMR, (b) users from across the clinical spectrum, and (c) other systems such as the treatment planning system and treatment delivery systems. The interaction between the treatment delivery system and other systems is beyond the scope of this chapter, and appropriate QA procedures can be found in the literature for data transfers between radiation oncology systems (10).

An implementation committee should be convened to select and, most importantly, design the electronic charting system for the clinic. It is important that representatives of each clinical subspecialty be included (11), namely,

1. Attending physicians and resident physicians

2. Physicists and dosimetrists

3. Nurses

4. Therapists

5. Hospital administration

6. Clerical staff

7. IT support-radiation oncology and hospital IT

8. A vendor representative (once a system is selected)

Important items to consider in the selection of an appropriate RO-EMR system are:

1. Connectivity to the treatment delivery system (test or "loaner" systems are helpful to evaluate this)

2. Synergy with department clinical workflow, flexibility

3. Financial considerations specific to each clinic

4. Connectivity to the H-EMR

Once the appropriate system for the clinic is selected, the process of designing the chart can begin. Major responsibilities of the implementation committee in this regard include translation of the essential elements of the paper chart to its electronic counterpart, development of general and specific workflows for each clinical subspecialty, management of rollout and training, and maintenance.

Consultation with others who have undertaken this transition can be beneficial in this process, especially through site visits that can sometimes be arranged through the vendor. It is important to allocate sufficient time to complete the process, preferably with some protected time for the members of the implementation committee, if possible. As the process can be quite extensive, it is important that the project be clearly outlined, that an achievable but firm deadline be set, and that updates are continuously provided to administrative bodies as to the progress or the transition and adherence to milestones (12).

The electronic chart as an information repository

An ideal chart should maintain the quality of patient care, enhance communication, and provide integrity in documentation (13). It should also comply with governmental and institutional regulations, be accessible to all at all times, and be HIPAA-compliant (12,13). The implementation team will be faced with many different possibilities for entering information and porting over essential documents. Settling on the format of a particular document or checklist depends on the information contained in it and the context in which it is used. In electronic charts,

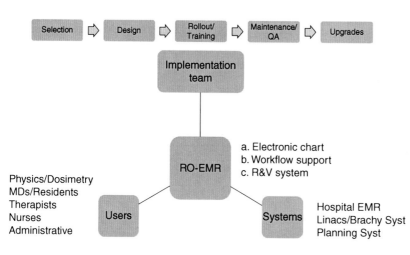

FIGURE 30.1 The RO-EMR and its "ecosystem." The system interacts with (a) the implementation team that is responsible for its design and maintenance; (b) users across the clinical spectrum; and (c) other systems, including the treatment planning system and the hospital EMR (H-EMR). (*Source*: From Ref. (24). Mechalakos J. MO-A-BRB-01: review of TG-262 internal survey of practices in EMR for external beam therapy. 2015. http://aapm.org/education/VL/vl.asp?id = 4376.)

workflow plays an intimate role in chart design, and the two must be considered together.

Table 30.1 gives an example of the types of documents that might be encountered in an electronic chart. It is by no means exhaustive, and some of these documents may exist elsewhere, such as in the H-EMR if there is one. Each document is categorized by the type of user and the context in which it is used.

Documents that are generated before treatment, such as consent, pathology reports, and orders, may reside in the H-EMR or may be created in the RO-EMR and ported to the H-EMR. The interaction between the RO-EMR and the H-EMR may be complicated in a hospital setting because of potential conflicts in policy between radiation oncology and the hospital as a whole. Radiation oncology clinics may prefer to have their entire charting system and associated documents (including consultations, consents,

etc.) in one centralized RO-EMR repository; however, the hospital may also require that documentation in its H-EMR as well. The implementation team should make sure that it allocates sufficient resources in the design phase to clear up potential issues.

The prescription can be a freestanding document or integrated into the system. When redesigning a prescription, the implementation team must consider essential elements (14), especially regulatory requirements, as well as policies for editing and approval. The electronic chart can offer some efficiency-enhancing tools, such as data tags that pull demographic data from the database, embedded macros (if allowed) that calculate total dose, and disease-site specific templates.

Electronic approval through an acceptable authentication system can be more restrictive because of the locking-down of documents upon approval (which is

Table 30.1 Documents That May Be Found in an RO-EMR, Grouped by User and by Where in the Treatment Flow They are Typically Invoked

	Pretreatment Simulation	Planning	On Treatment	Posttreatment
MD/nursing	• Consents • Initial consultation (radiation oncology) • Simulation order • Simulation note • Pathology reports • Radiology reports • Patient questionnaires	• Prescription/written directive • Special orders (not on Rx): imaging, treatment goals, etc.	• Chart rounds checklists • MD status check • Nursing status check	• MD treatment summary • Follow-up visits
Physics/ radiation therapy	• Simulation checklists and QA forms • Simulation documentation (CT-PET-MRI) • Seed inventory and calibration	• Treatment plan • Manual MU calculation forms for nonplanned cases • Treatment planning time-out • Initial chart check form • Protocol-specific dosimetry forms • Patient-specific dosimetry report • Record of previous treatment/multiple concurrent treatments • IMRT/VMAT QA • RTT initial chart check checklist	• Brachytherapy treatment delivery checklists/logs: patient-specific and room-specific • Weekly chart checks: RTT and physics • Daily treatment documentation form • SRS and SBRT QA (includes IGRT forms: onboard imaging, OSI, etc.) • Procedure-specific QA (craniospinal irradiation, respiratory gating, etc.) • EKG report • Procedure-specific dosimetry (TBI, TSEB) • In vivo dosimetry (OSL, TLD) • Set-up instructions (site/procedure specific) • Custom worksheets and QA forms (breast boost, clinical set-up, etc.) • Room surveys	• Postimplant evaluation • End of treatment check • RTT end-of-treatment check

IGRT, image-guided radiation therapy; IMRT/VMAT, intensity-modulated radiation therapy/volumetric modulated arc therapy; MU, monitor unit; OSI, optical surface imaging; OSL, optically stimulated luminescence; QA, quality assurance; RTT, radiation therapy technologist; Rx, prescription; SBRT, stereotactic body radiation therapy; SRS, stereostatic radiosurgery; TBI, total body irradiation; TLD, thermoluminescent dosimeter; TSEB, total skin electron beam.

also an important safety feature of electronic systems); thus, physicians may be called upon to reapprove the prescription in view of typographical errors and minor modifications. One possible way to reduce the number of edits is to simplify the prescription by moving non-essential items to another form. The implementation committee should consider carefully the policy on editing the prescription—that is, who can unapprove, who can edit, and who can approve—and this policy must be clearly communicated to all staff and enforced.

Formats for documentation of the treatment plan vary. Older treatment planning systems may necessitate scanning paper and importing. Treatment plan documentation can vary in depth, ranging from a more comprehensive documentation of the plan (cover sheet, treatment parameters, isodose distributions, dose volume histogram [DVH], beam's eye view, etc.) or, if the treatment planning system is linked, a scaled-down summary primarily used for chart rounds, saving a more comprehensive summary of the plan for external records requests. The plan document represents a snapshot of the approved treatment plan and should be easily connected to the approved plan through an appropriate time stamp or unique identifier (UID) in the document. Required signatures, whether electronic or scanned from paper, should be easily referenced. Ancillary documentation such as DVH reports and protocol dosimetry forms may be simplified by creating templates for each disease site and protocol with software to check that tolerance levels have been achieved. These summaries are helpful in chart rounds where a quick summary of DVH constraints may be desired and inspecting the full DVH would be impractical because of time constraints and screen size.

QA forms such as initial chart check, intensity-modulated radiation therapy/volumetric modulated arc radiotherapy (IMRT/VMAT) QA forms, and treatment planning time-out should be easily and efficiently accessed and completed. This is even more important for on-treatment forms such as checklists that are invoked in a particular clinical area and under time pressure because the patient is usually present, whether it be in the treatment room, procedure room, or status check room. Checklist accessibility and ease of use should be tested as part of the design process (15). Quality checklists are excellent tools for facilitating workflow and performing time-out processes at various points in the clinical flow, and are also available for mining to improve workflow and assess department efficiency and adherence to clinical timelines (16,17).

The implementation team should capitalize on data stored in the system whenever possible to automatically query dose-relevant information for status check reports and MD treatment summaries. Connection to the R&V system and treatment history can be a powerful tool, but must be thoroughly tested before use to ensure accuracy and detect potential failure modes.

Because the RO-EMR offers many ways to enter information, redundancy should be minimized; otherwise, confusion or error may result if redundant information is inconsistent or incomplete. As an example, specification of bolus can occur in a variety of ways: it may be inherent in the software if the planning system is linked, or it may be manually entered in any number of places. A single consistent policy for specification of this and other essential information that works for all disease sites, providers, and treatment machines should be the goal.

There will not always be a perfect solution for all types of data, and certain data elements may wind up as free text in an electronic journal or appended to an existing document such as the set-up notes, where it is not minable and may be more difficult to locate by others in the clinical team. This should be minimized to the extent possible. The implementation team should, in collaboration with the vendor, develop the electronic chart in such a way that the chart serves the clinic, not vice versa (S. Dieterich, personal communication, 2011). There will not be a perfect electronic analog for every paper document or even from one electronic system to another; therefore, the implementation team should be prepared to rethink the design of certain elements of the chart without compromising quality.

One distinct advantage of the electronic chart is the ability to structure data in such a way that it can be mined electronically. Some examples are:

1. Retrospective review of treatment data for department reports.

2. The mining of electronic workflow data for process improvement, assessment of resource allocation, and QA assessment (18).

3. Electronic chart checking, although not a substitute for human chart checking, takes over some of the more mundane functions so that the human check can focus on higher levels and more abstract parts of the check such as overall plan quality (19,20). The result is a more thorough check (21).

4. Using structured chart data for retrospective studies such as comparative effectiveness research (22).

Workflow considerations

The team should anticipate that fundamental clinical workflow will change appreciably; therefore, the importance of well-designed workflows to the smooth functioning of the clinic cannot be overestimated. Electronic workflows replace handoff of the paper chart from one member of the clinical team to another. Workflow management tools can facilitate robust QA through standardization of processes such as simulation and treatment planning. They allow users to more easily introduce forcing functions and to track work. Data can be mined from the system to evaluate efficiency and suggest improvements. Input of each subspecialty is just as important in workflow design as in the design of electronic forms and checklists.

An efficient workflow requires sufficient space. Dual monitors or extra-large single monitors are highly recommended to avoid having to constantly maximize and minimize portions of the chart. Certain workflows may require two instances of the application to be run in parallel by one user. A physicist performing the initial physics check of a treatment plan may need to have multiple windows open at the same time: the PDF of the plan, the prescription, the treatment planning system, a previous treatment summary form, and so on; therefore, the more electronic space available, the more efficient the workflow. Therapists may likewise need to move between different documents during a treatment. Physicians and nurses will require access to treatment summaries and perhaps the treatment plan during status check appointments. Forethought should be given to the amount of electronic desktop space required for safe and efficient workflow in all areas of the clinic. Inadequate space to complete one's work may not only encourage unsafe workarounds, but will also affect the overall reception of the new system by clinical staff.

A quality workflow should be able to handle ad hoc events, such as changes to treatment plans initiated by chart rounds review, which require proper notification of involved parties. These events are particularly at risk of "falling through the cracks" in an electronic task–based system, because a paper chart is no longer acting as a trigger by changing hands.

Adequate hardware for the various types of input to the system should be available and commissioned. This includes scanners for paper and for film, portable workstations for therapists to open and interact with set-up instructions or QA forms from within the treatment room, and adequate computing resources for supporting the full clinical workload. Remote access options (for example, through Citrix) are also increasingly important, and an adequate allocation of servers is essential to a cloud-based system. There should be vendor recommendations for the appropriate allocation of hardware to meet anticipated clinical usage in order to avoid system slowdowns due to inadequate computing resources. Potential system expansion due to increased usage should be considered in yearly budgeting.

The electronic chart opens up more channels of communication, and inconsistent communication can cause confusion and delays. For example, a physician may receive electronic tasks alerting him or her to sign a plan from some personnel and emails from others, or some physicians may prefer one form of communication over another, resulting in a mix of communication channels that is inefficient. It is best for the group as a whole to decide on the best form of communication and use it consistently. As much as possible, communication and workflow should be standardized across providers to maximize efficiency and clarity in the process, and thus minimize confusion.

TRAINING AND IMPLEMENTATION IN THE CLINIC

The clinic should be adequately prepared for a temporary reduction in clinical efficiency as the new process is assimilated. This is true both for the initial rollout and for major upgrades (23). The transition period varies greatly in length, depending on the size of the clinic and availability of training and support resources. Several systems for rollout can be used:

1. Gradual rollout, in which one component of the paper chart is replaced at a time

2. Complete rollout by a target date (e.g., similar to the rollout of the euro)

3. Sectional rollout, in which one physician, disease site, or treatment machine leads the way

When the electronic chart is initially released, there is in some cases a period in which a hybrid chart is in place or both paper and paperless charts are used in parallel. The length of time during which this hybrid chart exists can vary depending on the type of rollout. In addition, some clinics may choose to maintain a scaled-down paper chart for convenience, the contents of which depend on the needs of the clinic (23). In addition, for sites with multiple centers, the rollout may occur center by center; therefore, there is not only the possibility of a hybrid paper/electronic chart, but also the possibility that more than one charting system is being used at the same time. Proper training is important to ensure that all stakeholders are familiar with the different types of charts, and the length of time required for proper training should not be underestimated. The sooner consistency in practice can be achieved and everyone is using the same charting system, the better.

With the release of an entirely new system of charting, there will be resistance to change. Therefore, care should be taken to educate the clinical staff about the positive aspects of transitioning to an electronic system, such as increased accessibility and efficiency, as well as the unique and powerful safety features of an electronic system. A champion in each of the clinical subspecialties, especially a physician champion, is necessary for a smooth transition to the new process. It may be beneficial to begin with those least resistant to change, especially in the physician group, and progress to those who are most resistant, in order to give them more time to adapt to and accept the new process (24). Once those who are more resistant are reached, the transition would have for the most part been completed and improvements developed.

The team responsible for training should carefully consider the amount and type of training that each clinical subspecialty will require. Different subspecialties interact with the chart in different ways, and training should be tailored with that in mind. For example, nursing staff will need up-to-date prescription and dose-to-date data, clerical staff will often be asked to provide treatment data to other institutions, and physicians will need quick access to data for treatment summaries. Both vendor training and training from the clinical team should be utilized. It is beneficial to provide some measure of formal competency assessment, where possible, within each of the clinical subspecialties in order to solidify training and smooth the initial rollout. Periodic competency assessment after upgrades or major changes in procedure should also be considered.

ACCEPTANCE TESTING AND ONGOING QUALITY ASSURANCE

Acceptance testing varies from clinic to clinic and typically involves a combination of local IT and the vendor. In addition to the prescribed tests from the vendor, users should develop their own acceptance tests appropriate for their clinic. If the vendor is able to provide one, it is helpful to have a test system before release. It is important to test connectivity with all systems in the clinic that the system touches, especially treatment machines.

Ongoing QA of the electronic chart is an evolving process. It can consist simply of periodic reviews of the forms used in the electronic chart and the workflow to determine whether those items continue to meet the needs of the clinic, and/or involve more systematic methods, including failure mode and effects analysis (25–30). The process by which changes are made to the chart should be agreed to ahead of time. Smaller ad hoc changes may be allowable by certain individuals, but larger changes to the process should first be discussed with the implementation team. There should be periodic communication between the implementation team and the appropriate QA committees; recorded events and near-miss data are important sources of feedback regarding the effectiveness of the charting system.

Upgrades can be intensive processes that require preplanning; therefore, preparation for upgrades should begin as early as possible, often months ahead of time for major changes as opposed to incremental upgrades. Major changes in the software, especially those accompanied by database migrations, can fundamentally affect the clinical process, unlike the consistency of a paper chart. Upgrades may also involve multiple vendors; for example, if an RO-EMR receives treatment plan information via digital imaging and communications in medicine (DICOM) from a third-party planning system, it is essential that the connectivity be confirmed ahead of time; this process usually involves both vendors, possibly both on site during the upgrade period. Availability of the third-party vendor(s) should be confirmed before the upgrade. It is important to do the following before a major upgrade of the RO-EMR:

1. Provide directed training on the changes in workflow.

2. Confirm availability of representatives for all vendors involved, especially those connecting to the RO-EMR.

3. Confirm connectivity of third-party systems with the new version.

4. Confirm availability of clinical staff for the upgrade, which typically happens during off hours or weekends.

5. Plan carefully the events of the upgrade weekend, because a large amount of validation/verification is done in a short time and with minimal clinical disruption. This will involve cooperation between IT, physics, and radiation therapy. Discuss how workflow tools can be used to manage the handoff that will occur during the upgrade period (see following section on events of the upgrade weekend).

6. If there is a database migration, it will take time, and therefore it may be necessary to manually transfer patient data to the new system for any changes that occur after the database snapshot is obtained. These treatments must be carefully tracked, and a system should be established ahead of time for tracking them.

7. Plan for emergency treatments that may be necessary during the upgrade period.

8. Create test patients for spot checks of basic clinical functionality such as IMRT delivery, imaging, and the like.

9. Major upgrades to RO-EMR systems connected to treatment planning systems will also require QA and acceptance of the upgraded planning system.

During the upgrade period, which is always under time pressure, the following QA checks should be performed:

1. Verify basic clinical functionality on the machines using previously created test patients.

2. Mode up existing patients, and investigate any errors or warnings.

3. If there is a database migration,

   a. Accept the new database—this can be done by choosing a subset of existing patients across the clinical range and checking that information has been transferred correctly to the new database. This includes all documents, treatment parameters, and images.

   b. Once the new database is accepted, verify transfer of patient information to the new database for all patients on treatment. Some clinics have software that can query and compare the old and new databases on a patient-specific basis. This greatly accelerates the validation process (31).

c. Enter information on changes that occurred after the database snapshot was obtained, and check independently. It is important to check these manual entries carefully.

d. It may be helpful to take advantage of workflow tools in the system, such as using tasks to alert the therapists that physics has finished checking the data transfer for patient A so the therapist can proceed with the test mode-up.

4. Check synchronization of software from third-party vendors touching the system using test patients.

IT CONSIDERATIONS

Support for the system is typically provided by a combination of IT representatives and members of the implementation team. It is important that physicists be involved in the IT support of the system, especially in cases where there is no dedicated radiation oncology IT administrator who is familiar with radiation oncology practices. IT support for the hospital (outside the radiation oncology clinic) may not be familiar enough with the practices of radiation oncology electronic charting to properly support the system, and may make changes that disrupt clinical workflow. The medical physicist should collaborate with hospital IT staff, clinical IT staff, radiation oncology IT staff, service engineers, and vendors (32). Discussion with radiation oncology IT and physics should always precede any changes to server configurations, IP addresses, and the like that affect the radiation oncology clinic.

Hospital IT and dedicated radiation oncology IT, if it exists, will be intimately involved in the process of setting up an oncology information system (OIS) or changing from one OIS to another. The support system should be established and communicated to all, including guaranteed response times. Oftentimes, hospital IT services require a "ticket" for service, which may not be suitable for issues when a patient is on the table; this may require intervention by the medical physicist as the front line of defense in the absence of dedicated radiation oncology IT personnel who are familiar with RO IT systems (11). As recommended by the American Association of Physicists in Medicine (AAPM) working group on information technology, clear lines of collaboration and communication must be established between administrators, medical physicists, IT staff, equipment service engineers, and vendors, especially in an era of increasing sophistication of radiation oncology technology and the associated increase in volume of data (32).

An adequate disaster recovery (DR) infrastructure is essential to the smooth flow of the clinic. The option to "fall back on paper" will no longer be feasible, and adequate resources must be allocated to DR because extended outages of the OIS can have serious consequences for clinical operations and patient care. Periodic testing of the disaster recovery system is essential, and there should be a clear protocol for rollover to the DR system requiring discussion and consensus by essential personnel.

Access control and protection of private health information is another major consideration. The system will have many access points, whether through a thick client, a thin client, web-based or cloud access, and the system must meet all the requirements of the institution for safeguarding protected health information. Also, the types of access should be considered in the context of the tasks being performed; for example, what kinds of access are available for image review, and are they appropriate? Access via smartphone or tablet may not be suitable for certain tasks requiring a full desktop system with adequate screen size.

CONSIDERATIONS IN BRACHYTHERAPY AND NONSTANDARD DELIVERY DEVICES

Because RO-EMR software is often built on the existing R&V system, full delivery device connectivity for treatment delivery is usually assumed in electronic chart design. However, older RO techniques such as brachytherapy and Gamma Knife, as well as newer technology developments such as CyberKnife, Tomotherapy, and Viewray, pose specific challenges for electronic charting. See Table 30.2. Stand-alone devices are devices that do not offer any connecting modules to the RO-EMR system, or cannot be connected by design (seed implants, eye plaques, nuclear medicine applications). Devices with R&V connectivity capabilities are those that offer limited connectivity to the RO-OIS. Examples are single-vendor high dose rate (HDR) brachytherapy solutions, or CyberKnife/Tomotherapy. In general, the current design of the connectivity software requires patient scheduling in the RO-EMR, which then makes patient treatment plans available to the machine to deliver. After each delivery, the treated dose is automatically recorded back to the RO-EMR, but not other data such as imaging.

The chart design for limited-connectivity devices usually mimics the full electronic chart very closely. The two major differences are (a) the device R&V is kept separate from the RO-EMR, and (b) the safety features of the RO-EMR (such as electronic interlocks for lacking plan signatures etc.) are not functional. As a result, the workflow will likely be managed as a hybrid paper–electronic chart, or be fully electronic with the intermediate step of keeping selected aspects of the chart on paper and later scanning and discarding the paper records.

Table 30.2 A Survey of Brachytherapy and Nonstandard Delivery Devices in the Context of the RO-EMR

	Written Directive	Stand Alone	R&V Connectivity	Full Connectivity
Prostate seed implant	x	x		
LDR	x	x		
HDR	x	x	x	x (selected vendors)
CyberKnife		x	x	
Gamma Knife		x	x	
Tomotherapy	x	x	x	
Vero		x		
Viewray	x	x		

The workflow for stand-alone devices and procedures will deviate the most from the fully electronic workflow. Certain aspects of the chart that are not directly connected to the treatment itself, such as history and physical (H&P) documents, patient vitals, appointment scheduling, and so on, will be electronic, whereas the treatment itself will be documented on paper, which can later be scanned into the RO-EMR as an electronic repository.

Devices and procedures using by-product material (brachytherapy, Gamma Knife) are a special case in the electronic chart transition, because the use of nuclear by-product materials carries with it special requirements for documentation. Depending on whether the state in which the clinic is located is an agreement state or not (in the United States), requirements may differ. Specifically, the use of electronic signatures in the written directive may or may not be accepted as valid by local regulatory bodies. The authors advise initiating communication about electronic charting for brachytherapy with local regulatory agencies for the purpose of pre-empting any legal questions.

CONCLUSION

The electronic chart introduces to the clinic new ways of storing information, new ways of communicating, and new ways of managing workflow. It replaces a system that has been in use for decades, and requires careful planning and forethought and a dedicated team of champions to maximize its potential. This new environment can provide powerful QA tools and substantially improve accessibility and efficiency in the clinic. It can also greatly facilitate access to data for reporting and review. In this chapter, the authors attempted to educate users on essential elements to consider when implementing and maintaining an electronic charting system. Electronic charting systems will continue to expand and to mature, and it is the responsibility of the users to continue to maintain high standards of quality and safety as these changes come, and the obligation of administration to provide adequate support for maintenance of the system.

REFERENCES

1. Classen DC, Bates DW. Finding the meaning in meaningful use. *N Engl J Med.* 2011;365:855–858.

2. Dick RS, Steen EB, eds. *The Computer-Based Patient Record—An Essential Technology for Health Care (Summary)*. Washington DC: National Academy Press; 1997.

3. U.S. Congress. American Recovery and Reinvestment Act of 2009, Division B, Title IV. 2009. https://en.wikisource.org/wiki/American_Recovery_and_Reinvestment_Act_of_2009/Division_B/Title_IV.

4. Schiff GD, Bates DW. Can electronic clinical documentation help prevent diagnostic errors? *N Engl J Med.* 2010;362(12):1066–1069.

5. Fraass BA, McShan DL, Matrone GM, et al. A computer-controlled conformal radiotherapy system: Part IV: electronic chart. *Int J Radiat Oncol Biol Phys.* 1995;33(5):1181–1194.

6. Salenius SA, Margolese-Malin L, Tepper JE, et al. An electronic medical record system with direct data-entry and research capabilities. *Int J Radiat Oncol Biol Phys.* 1992;24(2):369–376.

7. Sailer SL, Tepper JE, Margolese-Malin L, et al. RAPID: an electronic medical records system for radiation oncology. *Semin Radiat Oncol.* 1997;7(1):4–10.

8. Ragan DP. Radiotherapy departmental automation. *Comput Med Imaging Graph.* 1989;13(3):295–305.

9. Shen X, Dicker AP, Doyle L, et al. Pilot study of meaningful use of electronic health records in radiation oncology. *J Oncol Pract.* 2012;8(4):219–223.

10. Siochi RA, Balter P, Bloch CD, et al. A rapid communication from the AAPM Task Group 201: recommendations for the QA of external beam radiotherapy data transfer: AAPM TG 201: quality assurance of external beam radiotherapy data transfer. *J Appl Clin Med Phys.* 2011;12(1):3479.

11. Benedetti L. Clinical implementation of electronic charting. 2013. https://vimeo.com/90160027.

12. Kirkpatrick JP, Light KL, Walker RM, et al. Implementing and integrating a clinically driven electronic medical record for radiation oncology in a large medical enterprise. *Front Oncol.* 2013;3:69.

13. Martin LA. Essentials of radiation oncology chart design. *Med Dosim.* 1999;24(1):39–41.

14. American College of Radiology. ACR-ASTRO practice parameter for radiation oncology. 2014. www.acr.org/~/media/ACR/Documents/PGTS/guidelines/Radiation_Oncology.pdf.

15. Fong de los Santos LE, Evans S, Ford EC, et al. Medical Physics Practice Guideline 4.a: development, implementation, use and maintenance of safety checklists. *J Appl Clin Med Phys.* 2015;16(3):5431.

16. Potters L, Kapur A. Implementation of a "no fly" safety culture in a multicenter radiation medicine department. *Pract Radiat Oncol.* 2012;2(1):18–26.

17. Colonias A, Parda DS, Karlovits SM, et al. A radiation oncology based electronic health record in an integrated radiation oncology network. *J Radiat Oncol Inform.* 2011;3(1):3–11.

18. Kapur A, Potters L. Six Sigma tools for a patient safety-oriented, quality-checklist driven radiation medicine department. *Pract Radiat Oncol.* 2012;2(2):86–96.

19. Yang D, Wu Y, Brame RS, et al. Technical note: electronic chart checks in a paperless radiation therapy clinic. *Med Phys.* 2012;39(8):4726–4732.

20. Covington E, Younge K, Chen X, et al. SU-D-BRD-03: improving plan quality with automation of treatment plan checks. *Med Phys.* 2015;42(6):3210–3210.

21. Siochi RA, Pennington EC, Waldron TJ, et al. Radiation therapy plan checks in a paperless clinic. *J Appl Clin Med Phys.* 2009;10(1):2905.

22. Miriovsky BJ, Shulman LN, Abernethy AP. Importance of health information technology, electronic health records, and continuously aggregating data to comparative effectiveness research and learning health care. *J Clin Oncol.* 2012;30(34):4243–4248.

23. Nowlan AW, Sutter AI, Fox TH, et al. The electronification of the radiation oncology treatment cycle: the promises and pitfalls of a digital department. *J Am Coll Radiol.* 2004;1(4):270–276.

24. Mechalakos J. MO-A-BRB-01: review of TG-262 internal survey of practices in EMR for external beam therapy. 2015. http://aapm.org/education/VL/vl.asp?id=4376.

25. Fong de los Santos LE, Herman MG. Radiation oncology information systems and clinical practice compatibility: workflow evaluation and comprehensive assessment. *Pract Radiat Oncol.* 2012;2(4):e155–e164.

26. Ford EC, Gaudette R, Myers L, et al. Evaluation of safety in a radiation oncology setting using failure mode and effects analysis. *Int J Radiat Oncol Biol Phys.* 2009;74(3):852–858.

27. Ford EC, Smith K, Terezakis S, et al. A streamlined failure mode and effects analysis. *Med Phys.* 2014;41(6):061709.

28. Kapur A, Goode G, Riehl C, et al. Incident learning and failure-mode-and-effects-analysis guided safety initiatives in radiation medicine. *Front Oncol.* 2013;3:305.

29. Scorsetti M, Signori C, Lattuada P, et al. Applying failure mode effects and criticality analysis in radiotherapy: lessons learned and perspectives of enhancement. *Radiother Oncol.* 2010;94(3):367–374.

30. Kovalchuk NN. Optimizing efficiency and safety in a radiation oncology department through the use of ARIA 11 visual care path. *Pract Radiat Oncol.* 2015;5(5):295–303.

31. Hadley SW, White D, Chen X, et al. Migration check tool: automatic plan verification following treatment management systems upgrade and database migration. *J Appl Clin Med Phys.* 2013;14(6):4394.

32. Siochi RA, Balter P, Bloch CD, et al. Information technology resource management in radiation oncology. *J Appl Clin Med Phys.* 2009;10(4):3116.

31 | Quality and the Third-Party Payer

Heather A. Curry

"Simply put, health care quality is getting the right care to the right patient at the right time – every time."

—Carolyn M. Clancy, MD (1)

Third-party payers (TPPs) are the insurers, private or public, that reimburse health care organizations and are the main source of revenue for most providers. The rise of the TPP structure has resulted in specific pressures and pitfalls in the U.S. health care system. TPPs have become major stakeholders in health care policy and agendas, informing key issues such as which services, procedures, and therapeutics are covered and how such services are reimbursed, resulting in an often unanticipated impact on the quality and cost of health care. This chapter examines key concepts related to insurance; ways in which TPPs influence access to care and services, and, ultimately, the quality of care delivered; and examples of how TPPs measure and use the concept of quality in their coverage determinations.

THIRD-PARTY PAYERS

Third-party payment systems traditionally involve the interaction of three self-interested stakeholder groups: a first party who is in need (or may require services in the near future), a second party who is willing to sell or give products or services that might meet those needs, and a third party who is willing and able to pay the second party on behalf of the first party. In the health care system, the term *third-party payer* is used to refer to any organization, public or private, that pays or insures health or medical expenses on behalf of beneficiaries or recipients. This includes not-for-profit and for-profit private insurance companies and government-run programs such as Medicare and Medicaid. In the United States, where a majority of Americans (more than 150 million) receive insurance coverage through their employer, the concept of a fourth-party payer, which purchases health insurance on behalf of the first party, also exists (2).

The Centers for Medicare and Medicaid Services (CMS) estimates that national health spending, which includes all health expenditures by private companies, public programs, and individuals, will reach a total of $3.4 trillion by the end of 2016 and continue to increase at an average of 5.8% per year through 2024, eventually rising to a total of $5.4 trillion, or 19.6% of gross domestic product (GDP) (3). The major source of funds for payment of these costs comes from TPPs. In 2013, CMS programs (which include Medicare, Medicaid, and Children's Health Insurance Program [CHIP]) accounted for 35.9% of spending, private health insurance companies funded 32.9% of spending, and other TPPs contributed 8.1%. Out-of-pocket spending by individuals accounted for only 11.6% of all health expenditures (4). Owing to their considerable financial impact, TPPs are thus key stakeholders in the health care system.

A MANDATE FOR QUALITY

In 2002, the Institute of Medicine (IOM) published *Crossing the Quality Chasm,* a landmark book that has shaped subsequent discussions regarding quality in health care (5). The book charged all stakeholders in the health care system to actively engage in improving the quality of health care, and was released to offer solutions to serious safety and quality issues outlined in a *Journal of the American Medical Association* report and a prior IOM publication, *To Err Is Human* (6,7).

Crossing outlined six specific aims that the health care system must meet to deliver quality care:

1. *Safe:* Health care facilities should ensure the safety of patients and procedures

2. *Effective:* Evidence-based practices should be applied and mark the standard for delivery of care

3. *Efficient:* Care and services should be cost-effective and without waste

4. *Timely:* Patients should receive prompt care and services

5. *Patient-centered:* The system should focus on the patient, respect patient preferences, and recognize patient autonomy

6. *Equitable:* Disparities in care should be eliminated

The report highlighted the need for changes in American health care at four distinct and hierarchical levels: the experience of patients; the functioning of small units of care delivery ("microsystems"); the functioning of the organizations that house or otherwise support microsystems; and the environment of policy, payment, regulation, accreditation, and other such factors that shape the behavior, interests, and opportunities of the organizations at the other levels. The model asserts that the quality of actions ought to be defined as the effects of those actions at the level of the patient (8). All stakeholders in the health care system are thus accountable to ensure the quality of health care. However, the interests of the various stakeholders may be aligned or at odds with one another, depending upon which aspect of quality is prioritized and which quality defect is targeted for remediation.

The concept of quality may vary depending upon the needs and interests of the stakeholder in question. For the patient, quality may refer to the ease of access to the services and providers of their choice, along with improvements in overall health and symptoms. For providers, quality may be based on balancing evidence-based practices with unique patient factors to optimize individual clinical outcomes. To payers, quality is based on providing coverage for care that is evidence based, results in good health outcomes for a given population of patients, and is cost-effective. TPPs seek to ensure that each insured within a specific health plan has similar access to safe, effective, timely care and therapies. However, access to every possible therapy for every patient is not financially sustainable. Payers must determine which services will be covered in a given plan, and price the plan accordingly.

QUALITY MEASURES TO ASSESS PAYERS

Clinical quality measures are tools that measure and track the quality of health care services provided by professionals, hospitals, or health care systems. These measures are used to evaluate various aspects of patient care, including individual health outcomes, clinical processes, patient safety, efficient use of health care resources, care coordination, patient engagement, population and public health, and adherence to clinical guidelines. Common uses of quality measurements include accreditation and/or certification of providers and health plans, public reporting, and design of provider incentive and reimbursement programs.

Private and public payers must meet certain quality parameters in order to comply with state and federal regulations. Organizations that work to set standards and measures for health care quality include government health

systems, accreditation programs, philanthropic foundations, and health research institutions. These organizations seek to define the concept of quality in health care, establish processes to measure that quality, and promote ongoing measurement of quality so as to provide evidence that health interventions are effective (9). Quality measures inform the standards that are used by organizations such as the National Committee for Quality Assurance (NCQA), URAC, and the Joint Commission on Accreditation of Health Care Organizations (JCAHO) in their accreditation and/or certification of providers, facilities, and health plans. Accreditation and certification status are viewed as important symbols of quality and consumer protection and are components of insurance laws and mandates (10).

For example, the Affordable Care Act (ACA) requires all qualified health plans that are sold in the state health insurance marketplace and the federally facilitated marketplace to be accredited, to ensure that the company's policies and practices are consistent with standards set forth by the ACA (11). The Department of Health and Human Services (HHS) recognized the NCQA and URAC as accrediting entities. Both are established, independent organizations that audit and certify various health care stakeholders, including health plans, case management organizations, accountable care organizations, and pharmacies. The accreditation processes involve measuring and benchmarking the payer's performance against clinical quality measures such as those required to be reported under the Healthcare Effectiveness Data and Information Set (HEDIS), Hospital Consumer Assessment of Healthcare Providers and Systems (HCAPS), and Agency for Healthcare Research and Quality (AHRQ) metrics, consumer satisfaction scores, and evaluation of payers' organizational processes. Specific dimensions of payer and plan performance assessed by the accreditation process include corporate quality management activities, regulatory compliance, patient access to services, credentialing of health care providers and facilities, utilization of evidence-based guidelines in coverage determinations, and transparency of company policies (12,13).

The quality of a given health plan may also be determined by federal and state statutes regarding health care services and benefits that must be offered by the plan. *Mandated benefits* are those that require coverage of the treatment of specific health conditions, certain types of health care providers, and some categories of dependents, such as adopted children. A number of health care benefits are mandated by either state law, federal law, or, in some cases, both. Before the passage of the Patient Protection and Affordable Care Act (PPACA), there were more than 1,900 such statutes among all 50 states; another analysis tallied more than 2,200 individual statute provisions, adopted over a period of more than 30 years (14).

In addition to defining specific quality measures that health plans must meet, the ACA mandated an assessment of the quality impact of endorsed measures and required the development of a National Quality Strategy

(NQS). The strategy set national goals to (a) improve the quality of health care to make care more accessible, safe, and patient-centered; (b) address environmental, social, and behavioral influences on health and health care; and (c) make care more affordable. The NQS was first published in 2011, and outlined six priorities that are mapped to measure health care domains similar to the IOM's definition of quality, including Patient Safety (Safety), Patient and Family Engagement (Patient Engagement), Care Coordination, Clinical Process/Effectiveness (Effective Treatment), Population/Public Health (Healthy Communities), and Efficient Use of Healthcare Resources (Affordable Care). The strategy outlined comprehensive processes to set clinical performance standards, publicly report quality measures, provide technical assistance to frontline providers, promote adoption of evidence-based national coverage determinations, and establish survey and certification processes for quality assurance and quality improvement initiatives (15).

Consequently, the CMS designs quality evaluations and disseminates quality reports as part of its oversight of the central government Medicare and Medicaid programs. Medicare uses a "Star Rating System" to measure how well Medicare Advantage and prescription drug (Part D) plans perform. Medicare reviews plan performances annually and releases star ratings each fall. Scores are based upon how well plans perform with regard to access to preventive services, meeting specified quality indicators related to chronic disease management, customer satisfaction scores, complaints and customer attrition, accuracy of drug pricing, and the plan's appeals process. Plans receive an overall rating of 1 (lowest) to 5 (highest) stars; separate star ratings are also given in each individual category reviewed. The scoring system provides a way for patients to compare performance among several plans (16). Similar consumer-facing comparison tools, also developed by CMS, include information regarding hospitals, nursing homes, home health care agencies, and dialysis facilities.

Measuring the quality of care and quality initiatives

CMS quality measures have a broad impact beyond the Medicare population, with more than 40% of the measures used in CMS quality reporting programs being applied to Medicaid recipients and more than 30% applied to individuals covered by other payer sources (17). Quality measurement is a key component to improve care under the various CMS quality initiatives. The first set of CMS standardized quality measures was developed in 1997 for managed care plans, and results was publicly reported in 1999. CMS has since developed and implemented numerous additional quality measures and programs that have shaped the health care system in the United States with regard to the process of care and reimbursement.

For example, under the Tax Relief and Health Care Act of 2006 (TRHCA), CMS implemented the Physician Quality Reporting Initiative (PQRI), now called the Physician Quality Reporting System, or PQRS, to facilitate reporting of quality measures for Medicare recipients (18). A major goal of the program was to collect and disseminate information that would improve delivery and coordination of care, and ultimately support the transition to novel payment systems. In its almost decade-long existence, the PQRS program has gradually shifted from payment incentives to penalties, with CMS and the federal government using legislative power to shape the program and tie the reporting of quality measures under PQRS to other quality and reimbursement initiatives. Eligible providers and groups have multiple options for reporting quality information about their patients, including submission of claims data, participation in a qualified PQRS registry, direct electronic health record (EHR) submission, and EHR submission through a data submission vendor. Initially, participation was voluntary and incentivized providers for successful participation with lump-sum bonus payments based on the estimated total allowed charges for all covered services during the reporting period; incentive rates were 1.5% for 2007 and 2008, and 2% for 2009 and 2010. Under the Medicare Improvement for Patients and Providers Act of 2008 (MIPPA), the PQRS program became permanent and required that names of eligible providers and groups who have satisfactorily reported under the PQRS, along with additional measure performance information, be posted on the Medicare Physician Compare website. In 2010, the ACA required that CMS furnish providers with timely feedback and a mechanism for appeal regarding PQRS performance and implemented PQRS payment penalties starting in 2015. The Act authorized incentive payments through 2014 with a 1% rate in 2011 and 0.5% rate for 2012, 2013, and 2014. CMS used the annual Medicare Physician Fee Schedule (MPFS) final rule to delineate provider penalties for unsatisfactory PQRS participation. Under the 2012 MPFS rule, physicians electing not to participate, or found unsuccessful during the 2013 program year, became subject to a 1.5% payment penalty in 2015 and 2% thereafter in years when they fail to meet reporting requirements during the specified reporting period; the 2014 and 2015 MPFS rules maintained the 2% penalty rate for 2016 and 2017 payments, respectively. PQRS reporting is also used as the initial basis for determining payment incentives under the Value-Based Payment Modifier program (19). In this way, CMS hopes to shape the transition from paying for the volume of services rendered to the quality of care delivered.

Initial uptake of PQRS by providers was slow, particularly for oncology specialists. A variety of factors contributed to this phenomenon, including lack of awareness and lack of knowledge about how to participate during the early phases of the initiative, as well as provider perception that the program was of low value owing to lack of measures relevant to oncology, and insufficient financial gain to offset the administrative burden of reporting (20). Over time, provider participation has increased because the financial impact has switched from the incentive to the penalty phase; engagement of professional societies with CMS has yielded introduction of specialty-specific measures, such as the Oncology Measure set; and additional reporting mechanisms, such as use of qualified clinical data registries (QCDRs), have been established that are viewed as less onerous than claims-based reporting. In addition, CMS's push for increasing data transparency has resulted in publishing of participating providers and the reported measures on the Physician Compare website; this places provider data in the public domain subject to access by consumers and private TPPs.

The absolute number and proportion of eligible radiation oncologists participating in PQRS have increased over time, with 995 participants (22.4% of eligible radiation oncology providers) in 2010, 1,291 (28.7%) in 2011, 2,215 (43.8%) in 2012, and 3,134 (60.9%) in 2013 (21). In 2013, most radiation oncologists participated in PQRS via claims reporting (32.8% of those eligible) compared with 21.9% who participated via a registry mechanism (individual or group measure reporting) and 0.1% who participated via EHR report. A total of $218,930,348 in PQRS incentives was earned in the 2013 program year, representing a 31% increase in payments compared with those in 2012. The average incentive was $443 per provider. Of the 3,134 radiation oncologists who participated in 2013, 77.5% (2,428) earned incentives totaling $4,703,458 and accounting for 2.1% of the national total of PQRS incentive payments; the average incentive for radiation oncology providers was $1,937. Just over 60% of eligible professionals avoided the 1.5% reduction to their 2015 payments; 98% of those subject to the penalty incurred the reduction because of failure to participate. Nearly 25% (1,282) of eligible radiation oncology providers did not avoid the 2015 rate reduction. Possible factors contributing to the increased participation and successful incentive earnings rates for radiation oncologists in the 2013 reporting period include greater provider awareness of the looming penalty phase of the program and reduced burden of participation through registry reporting due to the implementation of the Oncology Measures Group in 2013 and the specialty-specific American Society for Radiation Oncology (ASTRO) PQRSwizard reporting tool.

TPPs have worked to develop intelligible and reliable information on patient outcomes and provider performance, to improve quality and help consumers make informed choices. Payers develop and use quality metrics to share with providers to identify gaps in care and formulate best practices to achieve improved health outcomes. In addition, public reporting of provider performance data can help patients become more educated consumers and make more informed choices about which providers and sites of care will best suit their needs. Some of the earliest quality improvement programs implemented by payers have included incentivizing providers and hospitals for meeting national benchmarks, demonstrating outstanding performance, and making measurable improvements over time. Payers also designate Centers of Excellence based upon review of nationally reported data and results from internal analyses to establish networks of facilities and providers with strong records of providing quality care, improving health outcomes, and meeting patient satisfaction goals. Targeted quality improvement programs encourage physicians and hospitals to improve health outcomes by meeting specific quality or safety goals such as prevention of nosocomial infections or development of disease management programs to reduce admissions.

In a 2009 survey of commercial and Medicare Advantage plans, covering a total of over 95,000,000 lives, the American's Health Insurance Plans (AHIP) found that 95% of payers were engaged in processes to measure and improve quality: 91% of plans prepared "report cards" for physicians, practices, and medical groups; 92% had physician recognition programs to highlight quality performance; 92% utilized a pay-for-performance program to incentivize physicians to meet quality targets; 81% identified Centers of Excellence to report on quality, safety, and cost (22).

QUALITY AND COVERAGE DETERMINATIONS

TPPs use various aspects of quality to inform medical policy and coverage determinations and establish provider networks, quality initiatives, and reimbursement strategies. These functions are often interrelated and complementary. Payers must decide how best to allocate financial resources, and thus TPPs are also engaged in evaluating the quality of care they reimburse for. Inherent in the notion of most payers' definition of medical necessity are underlying issues pertaining to quality. Coverage policies, and thus decisions regarding which services and therapies will be reimbursed by insurers, are meant to be applied uniformly across groups rather than to individual patients.

As the insurer of more than 52.3 million Americans, Medicare's coverage decisions impact patterns of care across the United States (23,24). The Medicare coverage determination process is viewed by policymakers as a tool to improve the quality of health care through promotion of evidence-based practices, reduction in geographic variations in care, and reduction of spending on unnecessary or unproven care (25). Medicare's policies also exert significant influence on the commercial insurance market, as many private payers consider Medicare's coverage decisions when determining medical policy (26).

In determining coverage, CMS evaluates medical and scientific evidence in accordance with a standardized hierarchy of evidence, ranking the most authoritative first (27):

1. Controlled clinical trials published in peer-reviewed medical or scientific journals

2. Controlled clinical trials completed and accepted for publication in peer-reviewed medical or scientific journals

3. Assessments initiated by CMS

4. Evaluations or studies initiated by Medicare contractors

5. Case studies published in peer-reviewed medical or scientific journals that present treatment protocols

Medicare coverage is restricted to items and services that are considered "reasonable and necessary" for the diagnosis or treatment of an illness or injury and fall within the scope of one of the defined Medicare benefit categories. National coverage determinations (NCDs) are made through an extensive process consisting of a thorough review of the evidence base along with opportunities for public participation and comment. CMS may supplement its own analysis with outside technology assessments and/or consultation with the Medicare Evidence Development & Coverage Advisory Committee (MEDCAC) (28). In the absence of a national coverage policy, an item or service may be covered at the discretion of the Medicare Administrative Contractor (MAC), the designated fiscal intermediary/carrier under part A or part B, as outlined by local coverage determinations (LCDs). LCDs can strongly influence patterns of care and, ultimately, cost. A claims analysis by Smith et al (29) found that billing for intensity-modulated radiation therapy (IMRT) for breast cancer increased nearly 10-fold from 2001 to 2005. Rates of IMRT billing were more than fivefold higher in regions with coverage policies favorable toward breast IMRT than in regions with coverage unfavorable toward breast IMRT. The mean cost of radiation per patient within the first year of diagnosis was 28% higher in regions with coverage favorable toward breast IMRT than in regions with coverage unfavorable toward breast IMRT.

Historically, the dividing line between covered and noncovered interventions for private insurers is whether interventions are deemed "medically necessary." The concept of *medical necessity* is broadly understood as health care services or supplies needed to prevent, diagnose, or treat an illness, injury, condition, disease, or its symptoms and that meet accepted standards of medicine (30). While each payer establishes its own rules and methods for coverage determination, in general, an intervention must fall within generally accepted standards of medical practice, be considered clinically appropriate in terms of type and frequency, and not be utilized primarily for the convenience of the patient in order to be covered under a specific health plan's medical policy. Payers base decisions regarding medical necessity upon a wide variety of sources, including clinical data from peer-reviewed published medical journals, review of available studies

on a given topic, evidence-based consensus statements, expert opinions of health care professionals, guidelines from nationally recognized health care organizations, and available technology assessments conducted by payers, health policy analysts, and/or governmental agencies. Therapies and services that are of unproven benefit, or experimental, or are for cosmetic purposes are not considered medically necessary, and are typically excluded from coverage, unless specified within the terms of an individual's insurance contract.

Like CMS, private payers evaluate the quality of the evidence in support of a given technology. While each payer ultimately defines its own processes and policies, under URAC and NCQA accreditation standards, payers are required to clearly outline and provide access to such policies and procedures. The established criteria developed by the Blue Cross and Blue Shield Association's Technology Evaluation Center for evaluating whether a medical technology warrants clinical coverage illustrate how private payers make such coverage determinations (31):

1. The test or treatment must have final approval from appropriate governmental regulatory bodies, where required.

2. Scientific evidence must permit conclusions about its effect on medical outcomes.

3. The technology must improve net health outcomes.

4. The technology must provide as much health benefit as established alternatives.

5. The improvement in health must be attainable outside investigational settings.

Thus, the quality of the data supporting the efficacy of a given intervention and whether the intervention meets standards as defined by professional societies or subject matter experts are key factors in determining whether a therapy meets criteria to be covered under the concept of medical necessity.

Payers may also seek input from providers when developing coverage policies. One example of an effective collaborative program for determining medical necessity is the pilot study between radiation oncologists and Blue Cross Blue Shield of Massachusetts (BCBSMA) to develop an evidence-based policy for coverage determinations regarding IMRT (32). Concern developed in the BCBSMA community regarding the increased use of IMRT, and the resulting increased costs, without demonstrable improvements in outcomes. BCBSMA leadership and members of the radiation oncology treatment community in Massachusetts (Massachusetts Radiation Oncology Physician Advisory Committee [PAC]) convened to address these issues and develop a strategy to better define the use of IMRT for oncology patients in Massachusetts. The pilot aimed to create a clear and consistent process for approval of IMRT that minimized administrative burden and focused on medical decision making in the context of clinical evidence, best practices, and patient-specific factors.

The program outlined and agreed upon a list of diagnoses for which IMRT could be viewed as the standard of care and thus did not require preauthorization for treatment with IMRT; these included head and neck cancers, anal cancer, and prostate cancer. Using a framework for agreed-upon dose volume constraints as defined by the Quantitative Analyses of Normal Tissue Effects in the Clinic (QUANTEC), the group developed guidelines for each organ at risk, and specified parameters for the use of IMRT for all disease sites and body regions, including revised constraints for patients with contributing medical comorbidities (33). A clear process for application of the guidelines, escalation to peer-to-peer discussion with a radiation oncologist, and formal appeal was established. The process resulted in a 17% decrease in the use of IMRT and a 6% increase in the use of less costly 3D-CRT treatment for BCBSM subscribers compared with the reference period prior to implementation of the intervention. Assuming a median cost of $1,266 per IMRT encounter rate and applying the observed reduction encounter rates, the investigators estimated that application of the IMRT policy across the state would result in an annual saving of $4.7 million. In addition to the projected cost savings, the program improved quality through reduction of unwarranted use of IMRT and provision of a transparent process for equitable and more rapid approval for radiation treatments, reducing delays in therapy.

QUALITY AND VALUE

The earliest quality initiatives began as metrics, benchmarking with incentivizing providers and hospitals that met the benchmarks. But merely rewarding systems or physician groups with additional incentives does not address the core quality problems that can result from fee-for-service (FFS) payment structures: namely, perverse incentives for overuse of more favorably reimbursed technologies resulting in underuse of necessary or beneficial services that may be underreimbursed or not reimbursed at all. To that end, payers have begun a shift away from traditional FFS models to focus on value-based health care initiatives. The shift to value-based payment structures seeks to address current or potential quality defects.

As described by Chassin and Galvin (34), defects of quality fall into three broad categories:

- Underuse, which refers to scientific practices not being used as often as they should be

- Overuse, which refers to procedures and therapies being prescribed though unlikely to be of benefit

- Misuse, which refers to a proper procedure that is not administered correctly

To the payers, the concepts of quality and value have become essentially related. Absent a universally agreed

upon set of standards and benchmarks to measure quality and/or prioritize one aspect of quality over another, payers have developed a variety of new payment models that link reimbursement to quality. The most successful of these have focused on collaborative efforts between various stakeholders, particularly robust engagement of providers by payers to ensure subscriber access to preferred providers and networks. Payers' attempts to reduce health care costs by limiting patient access to health care resources through elimination of contracts with hospitals or providers with higher reimbursement rates have met with antipathy and resistance from patients and providers, as well as criticism from professional medical societies; implementation of strict preauthorization requirements has also garnered ire.

Payers must balance the various dimensions of quality to provide reimbursement for safe, effective care that meets the needs of individuals, yet is uniformly accessible across the subscriber base. Payers and providers are experimenting with a variety of innovative care delivery systems and payment models to improve health care outcomes, increase use of evidence-based practices, and lower overall health care costs. According to an American Society of Clinical Oncology report, 72% of practices reported that they continued to work in a fee-for-service environment. However, new payment models are increasingly being tested: with 8% of practices reporting participation in capitation agreements, 9% involved in use of bundling/ episodes of care arrangements, and 11% engaged in use of other alternative payment models. Among practices already using or considering novel models of care delivery, 36% reported that they had implemented or were considering a pathway-adherence program, and 30% were considering medical home programs emphasizing care coordination (35). Numerous models of value-based care and payment structures have been applied to oncology services in general, and radiation oncology specifically.

Oncology accountable care organizations (ACOs)

ACOs are alliances of doctors, hospitals, and other health care providers that deliver and coordinate care. In an ACO, providers are responsible for improving the quality of patient care and health outcomes, at equal or lower costs, through better coordination and preventive care. Doctors and health systems that successfully improve quality and control the cost of care share in savings with the payer; however, if they do not, they accept financial liability.

In May 2012, Blue Cross and Blue Shield of Florida (Florida Blue) partnered with Baptist Health South Florida and Advanced Medical Specialists (AMS), a multispecialty physician group focused on cancer care, to build the Miami-Dade Accountable Oncology Program. Florida Blue identified oncology as a top disease category, accounting for 80% of the company's medical spending. In the population identification process, the three organizations chose active cancer patients attributed to AMS during the prior year, and calculated the average per-member, per-year expense within the population. They established financial targets to reach the medical Consumer Price Index and specified shared savings percentages between the payer and the ACO. The program maintained an FFS pricing structure, with any realized savings of 2% or more to be shared between the parties, provided the ACO had also met specific quality metrics, including Quality Oncology Practice Initiative (QOPI) certification (36).

The ACO initially enrolled 226 patients and targeted six types of cancer: breast, digestive system, leukemia and lymphoma, female reproductive, male reproductive, and respiratory. The total cost of care in its baseline year was $23 million, or about $102,300 per member. Spending analysis revealed that injectable drugs and hospital admissions were the largest expense categories, each constituting 25% to 30% of the total spend. The ACO developed specific programs to contain drug costs, including a tightly managed approval process for chemotherapy and supportive care drug administration using pathways to prioritize use of the most cost-efficient therapies and minimize care delivery in the higher-cost hospital setting. In addition, the ACO refined its efforts to improve patient education, decrease emergency department visits, and improve end-of-life planning. A nurse practitioner was utilized to manage all chemotherapy education and coordinate transitions between inpatient and outpatient settings. The ACO developed a robust outpatient palliative care program to provide patients and families with ongoing education and discussion to establish and refine goals of care throughout the disease course, improve symptom management during active treatment, and reduce inappropriate therapies at end of life. Efforts to reduce inpatient costs focused on reducing avoidable admissions and length of stay through increased use of an after-hours triage system to handle calls and direct patients to nonemergency department settings for care if needed, use of an oncology nurse practitioner with access to patient medical records to support ED physicians in determining whether admission is necessary, development of a sophisticated case management program using predictive modeling software to identify and engage patients at risk for admission to prevent or limit symptoms or toxicities that could lead to hospitalization, and use of an advanced practice provider in the inpatient setting to coordinate among the hospitalist, oncologist, and floor personnel to ensure that care remains focused on the goals of admission and thus limit the length of stay (37).

In the first year, the program was able to reduce Florida Blue's cancer care costs, which had been increasing at a rate of 10% annually, to achieve $250,000 in savings; however, this did not meet the threshold for shared savings. In the second and third years, the ACO was able to sufficiently reduce costs and earn shared savings. Quality

targets were met each year by the ACO. The success of the program prompted the ACO to renew participation in the program for an additional 3 years and Florida Blue to launch another oncology-specific ACO with Moffit Cancer Center and utilize the model as a basis for four additional single-specialty ACOs.

Shared savings programs and oncology ACOs

Medicare's Physician Group Practice Demonstration (PGPD) was a shared savings program, not specific to oncology, that included 10 physician practices (38). The program collected data on cost and quality from 2005 to 2010. Subsequent analysis shows that the PGPD resulted in a 3.9% reduction in spending on 104,766 cancer patients' care. Savings were derived entirely from reductions in acute care payments for inpatient stays, due, at least in part, to a reduction in inpatient utilization. The PGPD was also associated with a reduction in mortality among cancer patients.

Pathways

Oncology clinical pathways are decision support tools that consider evidence from clinical guidelines and the medical literature to determine the most efficient, least toxic, and least costly treatment course for a given cancer diagnosis. Additional program components include measuring and enforcing physician adherence rates, which are typically set between 65% and 80%; developing a reporting structure to share physician performance metrics as well as patient outcomes; and realigning payment to reward providers for pathway adherence and meeting clinical performance metrics. A key tenet of the pathways approach is that quality of care will be improved by reducing unwarranted variability in care through clinical pathways. On-pathway treatment has been linked to decreased costs in patients with breast, lung, and colon cancer; improved survival in colon cancer; and reduced cost. Ultimately, improved quality, efficiency, and outcomes along with reductions in cost achieved through the use of pathways can provide leverage for provider groups and health systems in negotiations with payers (39–42).

Use of radiation oncology–specific pathways has been linked to decreased variation in care, increased adherence to evidence-based practices, and cost savings. The University of Pittsburgh Medical Center Cancer Center (UPMC) created a clinical pathways program (Via Pathways) to ensure quality and consistency of care across a network of 37 academic and community oncology and radiation oncology practices. Radiation treatment pathways for more than 90% of cancers were developed by committees of UPMC community and academic radiation oncologists and national subject matter experts. The available medical literature was reviewed to delineate the most effective and least toxic therapy for specific disease presentations, including detailed recommendations for simulations, contouring, treatment planning, and treatment delivery. Through an interface with the electronic medical record, the pathways were presented to physicians on a patient-specific basis as part of the clinical workflow. Over a period of 1 year, 31 radiation oncologists used the pathways in their daily practice. A pathway status was recorded for 98% of patient consults ($n = 10,178$). Of the 6,239 treatment decisions, 95% were on-pathway. All off-pathway decisions were approved before treatment through a designated peer-review process utilizing disease experts within the UPMC radiation oncology department. The study demonstrated the feasibility of implementing pathways across multiple clinical sites and numerous providers to obtain high adherence rates to evidence-based practices and increased consistency in care (43).

As part of the pathway review process, the breast cancer pathway was modified in January 2011 to reflect the long-term results regarding the efficacy of hypofractionated whole breast irradiation (HF-WBI) in early stage breast cancer. Within the UPMC network, consensus was reached that HF-WBI should be recommended as the first option for adjuvant breast radiation for women aged 70 years and above. Review of the system's electronic medical records (EMR) database identified a total of 2,426 patients treated between April 2002 and July 2013 meeting inclusion criteria for HF-WBI. Overall utilization of HF-WBI increased significantly, from 6.5% before pathway modification to 33.8% afterward (44). Among community physicians, the relative risk of HF-WBI use did not significantly change following publication of the Whalen article, but was 21.0 following pathway modification ($P < .001$). For academic physicians, the relative risk of HF-WBI utilization was 3.8 following publication of the landmark Canadian trial, and 10.6 following pathway modification ($P < .001$). The authors estimated that increased adoption of HF-WBI saved approximately $154,000 of health care spending annually within the network; assuming an idealized utilization of HF-WBI (normalized to the 2013 academic practice utilization rate of 70.8%), an estimated $347,000 would have been saved within the institution as a result of pathways.

Oncology medical home (OMH)

Under the OMH model, an oncologist leads a clinical team to oversee the care of each patient in a practice. Financial incentives are tied to shared savings realized through performance of specific quality measures that improve access, coordination, and outcomes. The first report on the use of this model for oncology patients was detailed by Consultants in Medical Oncology and Hematology, in Pennsylvania. The practice contracted with two regional plans and implemented care coordination and evidence-based care measures that reduced emergency department visits by 51%, decreased inpatient admissions

by 68%, and resulted in savings to payers of $1 million per physician per year (45). Funded by a 3-year Center for Medicare and Medicaid Innovation (CMMI) grant, the COME-HOME initiative implemented care pathways and elements of care coordination to transform seven oncology practices into OMHs; CMMI projects savings of $33.5 million (46). The Priority Health's Michigan Oncology Medical Home Demonstration Project entailed partnership between a regional payer and a group of oncology practices to funded transition to an OMH with an enhanced payment model. The drug margin was replaced with a per-member-per-month care management payment and yielded reductions in inpatient admissions and department visits and generated first-year savings of $550 per patient (47). Aetna has worked with multiple providers and institutions, including Moffitt Cancer Center, and now has 14 OMH projects in 10 states. The payer plans to increase the number of payments tied to value-based reimbursement structures from 30% in 2015 to 50% by 2018 and 75% by 2020 (48).

Episode of care/bundled payments

An *episode payment* is a single price for all of the services needed by a patient for an entire episode of care. Under such bundled arrangements, payment rates are determined on the basis of the costs expected for a particular treatment or course of therapy ("episode"), as well as costs for any preventable complications that may arise. Theoretically, the incentive to overuse unnecessary services within the episode is removed, and health care providers have the flexibility to decide what services should be delivered, rather than being constrained by fee codes and amounts.

The first phase of UnitedHealthcare's episode-based payment for medical oncology ran from 2009 to 2012 and included five independent oncology practices. An episode fee was calculated on the basis of prior data paid immediately. All services were billed to UnitedHealthcare using a fee-for-service format. The initial pilot reported a total net savings of $33,361,272, representing a 34% reduction in total costs of care, in spite of an observed 179% increase in chemotherapy spending. Subset analysis demonstrated a statistically valid decrease in hospitalization and therapeutic radiology usage for the episode arm. The pilot has entered its second phase (49). Other payers are developing payments associated with episodes or courses of care in which providers are incentivized with payments in addition to fee-for-service reimbursements to utilize more cost-effective drug regimens that payers have designated as "preferred" therapies. Anthem has implemented a Cancer Care Quality Program in which providers receive additional payment of $350 per month for treatment planning and care coordination when they select a preferred treatment regimen (50).

In December 2014, the University of Texas MD Anderson Cancer Center and UnitedHealthcare began a 3-year pilot to evaluate a bundled payment strategy for the multidisciplinary care of patients treated at MD Anderson's Head and Neck Center. Up to 150 patients with newly diagnosed primary head and neck tumors enrolled in employer-sponsored health plans insured or administered by UnitedHealthcare will be managed under the program. Episodes under the bundle include all cancer care provided at MD Anderson for the patient in 1 year. Under the pilot, patients will receive the same care, approach, treatment, and diagnostics for their disease as those who are not part of the program. Head and neck cancer treatment was selected for the pilot for two key reasons: (a) low patient volume compared with other cancer types posed less financial risk to the cancer center from shifts in reimbursement; and (b) necessary resources and services were already concentrated in a single location where existing multidisciplinary teams centered on care coordination, health care costs, and patient outcomes. Through the process of time-driven activity-based costing, the careful mapping of a clinical condition on the basis of its granular components, assessing the time and the cost of each part of the clinical process, MD Anderson sought to develop bundled payment prices for eight of the most common head and neck cancer diagnoses. Initial efforts structured the bundles according to type and stage of tumor, but cost analysis showed that those two factors were poor predictors of cost. Patient comorbidities and the type of care required with regard to number and complexity of treatment modalities (for example, surgery versus surgery and reconstruction or definitive surgery versus surgery plus adjuvant chemotherapy or radiation) were more accurate cost indicators. Four treatment-based payment bundles were developed, along with extra payment for patients with two or more comorbidities. A multidisciplinary team decides upon the appropriate treatment course for the patient, and then the patient is assigned to a bundle. United also included a stop-loss provision for cases in which the patient has a catastrophic event that does not relate to the quality of care. Clinical outcome measures were developed in collaboration with Harvard Business School on the basis of physician input and subsequent validation within patient groups. In addition, MD Anderson enhanced its clinical information technology systems to collect and share patient-reported and physician-reported outcomes with payers as part of the quality measures associated with the pilot (51).

Bundled payment models pertaining specifically to radiation oncology continue to evolve, with most current models involving negotiations with large groups or health systems contracting directly with payers for specific clinical scenarios. In August 2012, 21st Century Oncology and Humana initiated the first agreement between a provider and a major payer to reimburse external beam radiation therapy services on an episodic basis for almost all cancer cases. An *episode* was defined as beginning at consultation and ending 90 days after treatment. Each bundled cancer diagnosis was assigned a fixed payment to cover all direct radiation therapy expenses, both technical and professional. Indirect treatment expenses such as medications, laboratory tests, and diagnostic imaging were excluded. Payment is triggered and processed in full immediately upon consultation with the radiation oncologist. Although the first phase of episodic payments did not require reporting of quality metrics, several benefits were realized. The episodic payment agreement reduced the administrative burden for both parties. Resource utilization and physician prescribing habits remained greater than 98% compliant with regard to type and frequency of services modeled for each diagnosis group. Utilization of clinically appropriate hypofractionation increased, particularly for breast cancer patients. Patient satisfaction as measured by Press Ganey survey was high before and after implementation, with a statistically significant increase in perceived ease of insurance approval (52).

ASTRO initiated work on the development of payment reform models for radiation oncology treatment; the initial focus has been on revising the Current Procedural Terminology (CPT) codes related to radiation therapy, implementing the APEx accreditation program, and development of new payment models specific to radiation oncology. In the spring of 2015, CMS announced plans for 30% of all Medicare reimbursement to be tied to quality or value through alternative payment models by the end of 2016, increasing to 50% by 2018. ASTRO began collaboration for two potential payment bundles, one for treatment of bone metastases and another for treatment of early stage breast cancer, that if successful could be replicated for use with other large payers. As initially proposed, the ASTRO bundles would include the costs associated with delivery of radiation, with the fee representing the weighted average of the aggregate of appropriate fee-for-service charges as determined by Surveillance, Epidemiology and End Results (SEER) claims analysis. Ninety-five percent of the fee would be paid up front, with an additional 5% paid at the end of treatment based on demonstration of specified quality measures. An incentive of 5% would be paid just over 1 month from the end of treatment based on the documentation of appropriate clinical follow-up. Quality metrics could be met through APEx accreditation status or documentation of disease-specific process quality measures. ASTRO has set a target of fall 2016 to launch these pilots (53).

CONCLUSION

While TPPs exert considerable influence over the quality of health care with regard to coverage determinations and reimbursement policies, payers themselves are subject to quality evaluation with regard to their business processes, adherence to federal and state mandates, and customer satisfaction concerning access to care and variety of services covered. As health care costs continue to rise, payers seek to ensure that reimbursement occurs for care that delivers the best outcomes at the most effective price, to optimize value. Transition from traditional fee-for-service models, under which payment is based on volume and intensity of care, toward value-based systems, in which payment is tied to dimensions of quality, is a key strategy for cost containment. Within oncology, a variety of value-based reimbursement strategies have emerged and continue to evolve. Alternative

payment models specific to radiation are also under development. Ongoing evaluation of the impact of such programs on cost, utilization of resources, and correlation with patient outcomes will be needed to determine the optimal delivery strategies. It is likely that no single model will emerge as the paradigm for reimbursement, as payers and providers seek to find balance between efficacy, safety, accessibility, patient-centeredness, and cost.

REFERENCES

1. Transcript of remarks by Carolyn Clancy. In: *Measuring Health Care Quality*. Washington, DC: Kaiser Family Foundation; 2008. http://kff.org/archived-kaiseredu-org-tutorials.
2. Congressional Budget Office. *Updated Budget Projections: 2015–2025*. Washington, DC: CBO; 2015. https://www.cbo.gov/publication/49973.
3. Fleming C. *Health Affairs* Web First: health spending growth to remain moderate compared to pre-recession highs. http://healthaffairs.org/blog/2015/07/28/health-affairs-web-first-health-spending-growth-to-remain-moderate-compared-to-pre-recession-highs.
4. Peterson-Kaiser Health System Tracker: interactive tool. 2016. www.healthsystemtracker.org.
5. Institute of Medicine. *Crossing the Quality Chasm: A New Health System for the Twenty-first Century*. Washington, DC: National Academy Press; 2001.
6. Chassin MR, Galvin RW; National Roundtable on Health Care Quality. The urgent need to improve health care quality. *JAMA*. 1998;280(11):1000–1005.
7. Kohn LT, Corrigan JM, Donaldson MS, eds. *To Err Is Human: Building a Safer Health System*. Washington, DC: National Academy Press; 1999.
8. Berwick DM. User's manual for the IOM's "Quality Chasm" report. *Health Aff*. 2002;21(3):80–90.
9. Cleary PD. Health care quality—incorporating consumer perspectives. *JAMA*. 1997;278(19):1608–1612.
10. National Committee for Quality Assurance. *The Essential Guide to Health Care Quality*. Washington, DC: National Committee for Quality Assurance; 2012. www.ncqa.org/Portals/0/Publications/Resource%20Library/NCQA_Primer_web.pdf.
11. Patient Protection and Affordable Care Act. Pub. L. No. 111-148 (March 23, 2010), as modified by the Health Care and Education Reconciliation Act of 2010, Pub. L. No. 111-152 (March 30, 2010), Title 1, Subtitle D, Section 1311. www.gpo.gov/fdsys/pkg/FR-2013-02-25/pdf/2013-04084.pdf.
12. National Committee for Quality Assurance. NCQA health plan accreditation requirements. 2016. www.ncqa.org/Portals/0/Programs/Accreditation/2016_HPA_SGs.pdf.
13. URAC. Health plan accreditation standards. Version 7.3. 2016. www.urac.org/wp-content/uploads/STDGlance_HealthPlan3.pdf.
14. Bunce VC, Wieske JP. 2011. Council for Affordable Health Insurance: health insurance mandates in the States 2011. https://lintvwpri.files.wordpress.com/2013/10/mandatesinthestates2011execsumm.pdf.
15. Centers for Medicare and Medicaid Services. *CMS Quality Strategy —2013—Beyond*. Baltimore, MD: Centers for Medicare and Medicaid Services; 2013. http://www.ahrq.gov/workingforquality/agency-plans/cms-quality-strategy.pdf.
16. Medicare. Star ratings. www.medicare.gov/find-a-plan/staticpages/rating/planrating-help.aspx.
17. Centers for Medicare and Medicaid Services. *National Impact Assessment of the Centers for Medicare & Medicaid Services (CMS) Quality Measures Report*. Baltimore, MA: Centers for Medicare and Medicaid Services; 2015. www.cms.gov/Medicare/Quality-Initiatives-Patient-Assessment-Instruments/QualityMeasures/QualityMeasurementImpactReports.html.
18. Centers for Medicare and Medicaid Services. Physician quality reporting system. 2012. www.cms.gov/Medicare/Quality-Initiatives-Patient-Assessment-Instruments/PQRS/index.html?redirect=/pqri/.
19. Centers for Medicare and Medicaid Services. Detailed methodology for the 2016 value modifier and the 2014 quality and resource use report. 2015. https://www.cms.gov/Medicare/Medicare-Fee-for-Service-Payment/PhysicianFeedbackProgram/Downloads/2014QRUR-2016VM-DetailedMethodology.pdf.
20. Hendricks CB. PQRS reporting for medical oncologists. 2015. http://am.asco.org/pqrs-reporting-medical-oncologists.
21. Centers for Medicare and Medicaid Services. Reporting experience including trends (2007–2013): physician quality reporting system and electronic

prescribing (eRx) incentive program. *Radiation Therapy Alliance*. 2014. www.radiationtherapyalliance.com/newsletter/files/2014-05-experience-report.pdf.

22. AHIP. Health insurance plans making a difference: driving quality improvement and accountability. 2009. http://www.healthymemphis.org/assets/docs/2009%20Health%20Plans%20Making%20Difference.pdf.

23. NCPSSM. Fast facts about Medicare. www.ncpssm.org/Medicare/MedicareFastFacts.

24. Foote SB, Virnig BA, Town RJ, et al. The impact of Medicare coverage policies on health care utilization. *Health Serv Res*. 2008;43(4):1285–1301.

25. Foote SB, Town RJ. Implementing evidence-based medicine through Medicare coverage decisions. *Health Aff*. 2007;26(6):1634–1642.

26. Foote SB, Wholey D, Halpern R. Rules for medical markets: the impact of Medicare contractors on coverage policies. *Health Serv Res*. 2006;41(3, Pt 1):721–742.

27. Medicare Payment Advisory Commission. *An Introduction to How Medicare Makes Coverage Decisions*. Report to the Congress: Medicare Payment Policy. Washington, DC: MedPAC; 2003.

28. Centers for Medicare and Medicaid Services. Procedure for producing guidance documents describing Medicare's coverage process [CMS–3141–N]. *Federal Register*. 2004;69(185).

29. Smith BD, Pan IW, Shih YC, et al. Adoption of intensity-modulated radiation therapy for breast cancer in the United States. *J Natl Cancer Inst*. 2011;103(10):798–809. doi:10.1093/jnci/djr100.

30. Uniform Glossary of Coverage and Medical Terms. https://www.dol.gov/ebsa/pdf/SBC-Uniform-Glossary-final.pdf.

31. Blue Cross Blue Shield. www.bcbs.com/blueresources/tec.

32. Steingesser L, Acker B, Berman S, et al. Bending the cost curve: a unique collaboration between radiation oncologists and Blue Cross Blue Shield of Massachusetts to optimize the use of advanced technology. *J Oncol Pract*. 2014;10(5):e321– e327.

33. Marks LB, Yorke ED, Jackson A, et al. Use of normal tissue complication probability models in the clinic. *Int J Radiat Oncol Biol Phys*. 2010;76:S10–S19.

34. Chassin MR, Galvin RW. The urgent need to improve health care quality. Institute of Medicine National Roundtable on Health Care Quality. *JAMA*. 1998;280(11):1000–1005.

35. American Society of Clinical Oncology. The state of cancer care in America, 2015: a report by the American Society of Clinical Oncology.

J Oncol Pract. 2015;11(2):79–113. doi:10.1200/JOP.2015.003772.

36. Kalman LA. Advanced medical specialties during the 2013 Cancer Center Business Summit "Transforming Oncology through Innovation" meeting October [2013] in Chicago, IL. www.onclive.com/news/First-Year-Savings-of-an-Oncology-Accountable-Care-Organization.

37. Aston G. Exploring cancer care and payment models. 2015. www.hhnmag.com/articles/3066-health-cares-3-cs-collaboration-coordination-continuum.

38. Colla CH, Lewis VA, Gottlieb DJ, et al. Cancer spending and accountable care organizations: evidence from the Physician Group Practice Demonstration. *Healthcare*. 2013;1(3–4):100–107.

39. Neubauer MA, Hoverman JR, Kolodziej M, et al. Cost effectiveness of evidence-based treatment guidelines for the treatment of non-small-cell lung cancer in the community setting. *J Oncol Pract*. 2010;6:12–18.

40. Hoverman JR, Cartwright TH, Patt DA, et al. Pathways, outcomes, and costs in colon cancer: retrospective evaluations in two distinct databases. *J Oncol Pract*. 2011;7(Suppl):52s–59s.

41. Kreys ED, Koeller JM. Documenting the benefits and cost savings of a large multistate cancer pathway program from a payer's perspective. *J Oncol Pract*. 2013;9(5):e241–e247. doi:10.1200/JOP.2012.000871.

42. Feinberg BA, Lang J, Grzegorczyk H, et al. Implementation of cancer clinical care pathways: a successful model of collaboration between payers and providers. *J Oncol Pract*. 2012;8(3)(Suppl):e38s–e43s. doi:10.1200/JOP.2012.000564.

43. Lokay K, Heron DE. Reducing unwarranted variability in care in radiation oncology through clinical pathways. 2014 ASCO Quality Care Symposium [abstract 171]. *J Clin Oncol*. 2014;32(suppl 30).

44. Sprandio JD. Oncology patient–centered medical home. *J Oncol Pract*. 2012;8(3)(Suppl):47s–49s. doi:10.1200/JOP.2012.000590.

45. Rajagopalan MS, Flickinger JC, Heron DE, et al. Changing practice patterns for breast cancer radiation therapy with clinical pathways: an analysis of hypofractionation in a large, integrated cancer center network. *Pract Radiat Oncol*. 2015;5(2):63–69.

46. Sanghavi D, Samuels K, George M, et al. Case study: transforming cancer care at a community oncology practice. *Healthcare (Amst)*. 2014;3(3):160–168.

47. Kuntz G, Tozer J, Snegosky J, et al. Michigan oncology medical home demonstration project: first-year results. *J Oncol Pract*. 2014;10:104.

48. Brino A. Aetna sees promise in medical oncology home. 2015. http://www.healthcarefinancenews.com/news/aetna-sees-promise-oncology-medical-home.

49. Newcomer LN, Gould B, Page RD, et al. Changing physician incentives for affordable, quality cancer care: results of an episode payment model. *J Oncol Pract.* 2014;10(5):322–326. doi:10.1200/JOP.2014.001488.

50. Doyle C. Anthem's Clinical Pathways Demonstrate Value: The Payer Perspective. American Health & Drug Benefits. 2015;8(Spec Issue):28. http://www.ncbi.nlm.nih.gov/pmc/articles/PMC4570054/

51. Ellis LD. Leading cancer center pilots extensive value-based payment plan. 2015. http://strategichcmarketing.com/leadingcancer-centerpilots-extensivevalue-based-payment-plan/.

52. Falit BP, Chernew ME, Mantz CA. Design and implementation of bundled payment systems for cancer care and radiation therapy. *Int J Radiat Oncol.* 2014;89:950–953.

53. Kavanaugh B, Patel S, Chen A. Payment reform initiatives in radiation oncology. Educational Session presented at 57th American Society of Radiation Oncology Meeting; October 18–21, 2015; San Antonio, TX.

Appendix: Quality Assurance and Patient Safety Checklists

CHECKLIST FOR PEER REVIEW PAPER

Chart audit

Name: _____ M.R. #:
Physician: _____ Treatment Start Date: _____ End Date: _____

INTAKE CHART AUDIT
- ❏ Patient history and documentation
- ❏ Imaging   ❏ N/A
- ❏ Pathology
- ❏ Prior radiation records
- ❏ Urgency of treatment _____
- ❏ Physician review for appropriateness of consult
- ❏ Special instructions for consults/simulation

CONTOUR REVIEW
- ❏ Physician contours—targets, relevant OARs
- ❏ Dose prescription
- ❏ Diagnostic image fusion

- ❏ Clinical history for chart rounds
- ❏ Special instructions for planning _____
- ❏ Standard planning constraints   ❏ N/A
- ❏ Special instructions _____
- ❏ Timeline for starting _____

PLAN REVIEW
- ❏ Review plan and DVH
- ❏ Special setup instructions _____
- ❏ Treatment start and schedule
- ❏ Schedule for resimulation   ❏ N/A
- ❏ OTV schedule

EXTERNAL BEAM PLAN CHECKLIST

Checklists should highlight items frequently forgotten without being inclusive.	Dosimetry Initial Plan Check	Physics Second Check
Date		
Plan name		
Site		
1 PRESCRIPTION		
Approved by attending?		
Is it complete and internally consistent? Consider: • IGRT structure • Specification of laterality • Beam energy • Breathing status (BH or FB)		
Is laterality confirmed?		
Is prior treatment noted?		
COMMENTS/ACTION NEEDED		
2 PLAN		
Is the plan consistent with the prescription?		
Is there a plan sum and/or is prior treatment considered in this course?		
Are the treatment parameters appropriate? Consider: • Energy • Machine choice • Field labeling (incl. BH or FB if applicable) • Dose rate • Tolerance tables • Field size and alignment • Calculation algorithm (grid 2.5 mm, AAA_11031, hetero:ON)		
Is the technique appropriate? Consider: • Wedges • IMRT/VMAT		
Is the use of bolus appropriate?		
Is the localization information appropriate? Consider: • Communication of shifts • Tabletop distance calculation • Isocenter selected correctly • Set-up information		
Is the segmentation/dose distribution appropriate? Consider: • Target coverage • PTV generation and margin • OAR doses • Segmentation of organs in field at risk or pacemaker		
Implanted devices handled well? Consider: • Handling of high Z materials • Pacemaker beam energy <10 MV • Physics consult for pacemaker		
Independent MU Check Complete?		
COMMENTS/ACTION NEEDED		

3 TRANSFER TO TREATMENT MANAGEMENT SYSTEM		
Did transfer happen correctly? Consider: • Treatment parameters • MLC presence • Motion of MLCs		
DRR generation? Consider: • Structure outline needed for matching • DRR quality • Would field projection on skin be helpful to therapy?		
Are dose limits appropriate? Consider: • Daily dose • Total dose • Fractions/day		
Is the plan schedule appropriate? Consider: • Number of fractions • IGRT		
Is the plan approved for delivery?		
Has charge capture happened?		
COMMENTS/ACTION NEEDED		

PLAN CHECKS AND PRETREATMENT PHYSICS QUALITY ASSURANCE CHECKS

1	Patient name and ID on plan match EMR	
2	Confirm correct CT scan used for planning	
3	Plan name is confirmed	
4	Plan is associated with prescription in EMR	
5	Plan Number of Fractions = Prescription Fractionation	
6	Plan is confirmed with RX: a. Site and side b. energy	
7	If requested in Rx, Special Physics Consult completed	
8	Density corrections are appropriate	
9	Plan normalization is verified	
10	Blocking tray factors or immobilization is confirmed	
11	Isocenter/weight point validated	
12	DVH reviewed for coverage and OARs	
13	Planned fields match EMR fields	
14	Setup directions and imaging verified to plan	
15	Images are associated appropriate for positioning checks	
16	Dose tracking for prescription and OARs verified	
17	Radcalc/Second dose calculation complete and associated	
18	Associate IMRT/VMAT QA face sheet	
19	Physics/Dosimetry comments:	

This assessment/quality checklist lives in our EMR and uses a click-box completion of each item. When complete, the physicist approves the assessment and locks the quality checklist. Our therapists review this list prior to treatment and have their own assessment/quality checklist to complete pretreatment. There are additional physics quality checklists for after first treatment, weekly, and end of treatment.

CHECKLIST FOR STEREOTACTIC BODY RADIATION THERAPY TREATMENT

Date: _____
Fx #: _____ of _____ fraction
Dose: _____Gy

			INITIALS
PATIENT SETUP PRE-CBCT			
	1.	Site confirmed with patient/physician disease location: _____	/
	2.	Bionix frame on indexer bars	/
	3.	Patient aligned to marks on the sides of the bag	/
	4.	Patient tattoos aligned with lasers	/
	5.	Isocenter position confirmed and patient marked (using ceiling laser)	/
	6.	Compression belt indexed	/
	7.	Motion view approved by physician and physicist	/
POST-CBCT CHECKS			
	1.	CBCT approved by physician	
	2.	Isocenter remarked if move indicated on CBCT (using ceiling laser)	/
	3.	Couch parameters captured on first day of treatment	/
	4.	Table readings: Long _____ Lat: _____ Vert: _____ Confirmed	/
	5.	Procedural pause (Physician or physicist must initial)	
POST-SECOND CBCT CHECKS			
	1.	CBCT approved by physician	
	2.	Isocenter remarked if move indicated on CBCT	/
	3.	Table readings: Long _____ Lat: _____ Vert: _____ Confirmed	/
TREATMENT			
	1.	Isocenter marks on patient confirmed after manual couch movement	/
	2.	Isocenter marks on patient confirmed at end of treatment	/

TIME OUT CHECKLIST

Type: Procedural	**Date:**	**Time:**
Verified Patient's Name		
☐ Yes ☐ No		
Verified Patient's Birth Date		
☐ Yes ☐ No		
Verified Patient's Face Photo		
☐ Yes ☐ No		
Verified Correct Treatment Site(s)		
☐ Yes ☐ No		
Verified Correct Plan		
☐ Yes ☐ No		
RT Team Huddle Pretx		
☐ Yes ☐ No		

Therapist Initials

Date:

Approve   OK   Cancel

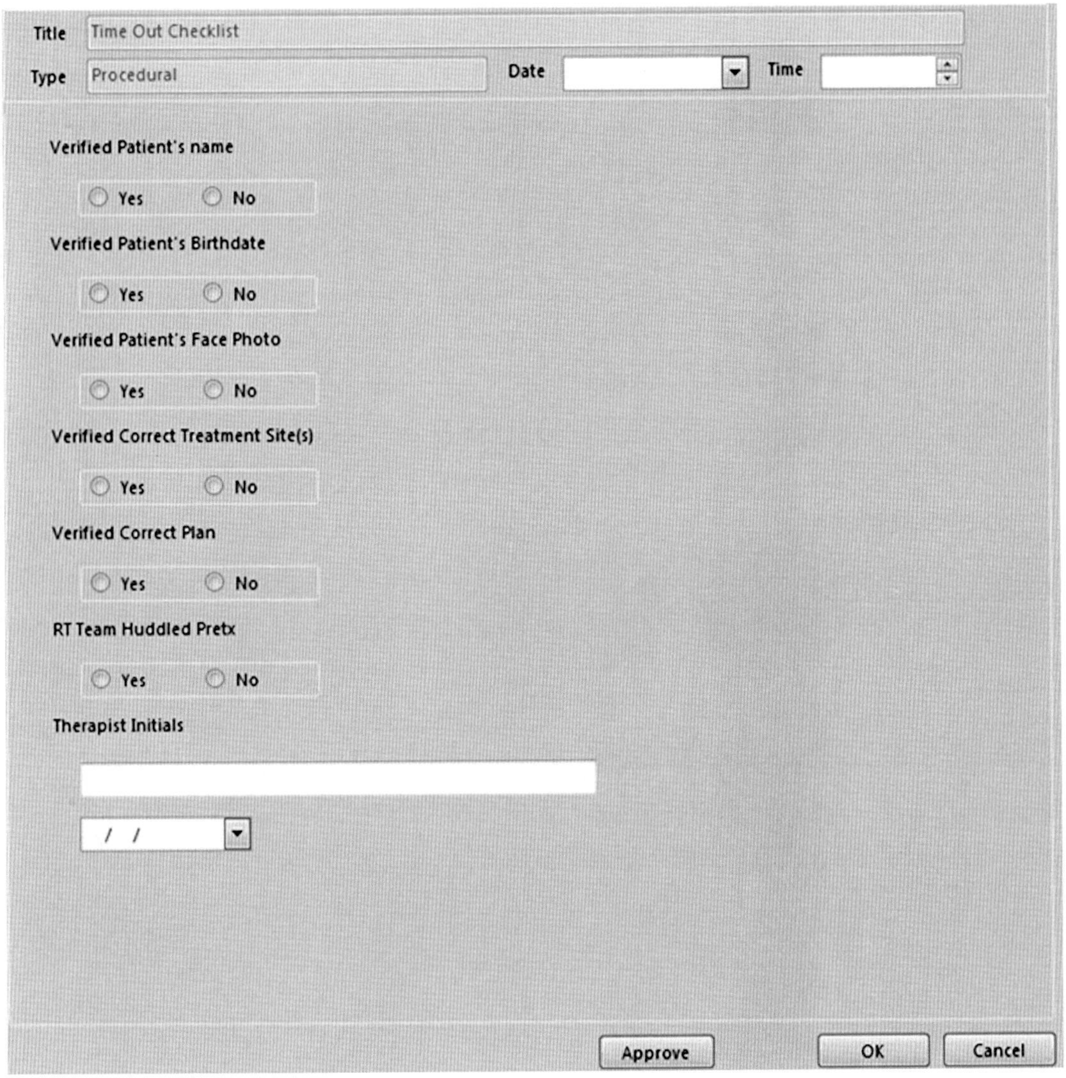

Title	Time Out Checklist				
Type	Procedural		Date		Time

Verified Patient's name

◯ Yes   ◯ No

Verified Patient's Birthdate

◯ Yes   ◯ No

Verified Patient's Face Photo

◯ Yes   ◯ No

Verified Correct Treatment Site(s)

◯ Yes   ◯ No

Verified Correct Plan

◯ Yes   ◯ No

RT Team Huddled Pretx

◯ Yes   ◯ No

Therapist Initials

[   ]

[/ / ▾]

[Approve]   [OK]   [Cancel]

FIGURE A.1 Time Out Checklist in Aria.

CHECKLIST OF A GAMMA KNIFE PERFEXION DAILY QUALITY ASSURANCE EXAMPLE

Item	Tolerance
Survey meter	Functional
In-room area monitor	Functional
Frame-to-couch adaptor	Functional
Radiation indicator lights	Functional
Frame adaptor gamma angles (70°, 90°, 120°)	Functional
Emergency alarm	Functional
Interlocks	
Couch clutches	Functional
Couch side rails	Functional
Vault door	Functional
Couch-isocenter precision	Max dose at (100, 100, 100) coordinates ± 1 mm
Treatment Console Tests	
Pause button	Functional
Emergency stop button	Functional
Audio/visual	Functional
Treatment Plan Printout	
Standard daily QA plan printout date & time	Accurate
Standard daily QA plan printout daily dose rate	±2%
Standard daily QA plan printout treatment time	±2%

CHECKLIST FOR TREATMENT DAY QUALITY ASSURANCE OF PERFEXION

Date: _____   Tests performed by: _____

1.	Turn unit power ON (with key)	
2.	Turn video monitors ON, and verify proper function of video monitors.	
3.	Clear couch top. Clear areas around GK for emergency access.	
4.	Diode tested passed – deviations (mm): X: Y: Z:	
5.	Alarm test.	
6.	Two-shot plan created, plan downloads to treatment console correctly.	
7.	Co-60 decay by hand matches planning system to within ± 1%.	
8.	Side rail interlock, left and right.	
9.	Frame adapter interlock is working, two angles of two-shot run clear, the other interlocks	
10.	During test run, confirm: • Primalert radiation monitor in the room and the slave at console are flashing. • In-room source exposure indicator light. • Perfexion warning lamp and beam on light at Perfexion room door functional.	
11.	Check door interlock.	
12.	Check functionality of "Pause" button.	
13.	Time for second shot of two-shot run is accurate to ± 2 seconds.	
14.	Check that "emergency interrupt" stops all movement.	
15.	Confirm that movement resumes after "emergency interrupt" released.	
16.	Ensure that audio equipment is working.	
17.	Confirm that the Notice to Employees, Emergency Instruction, and Operating Instruction are posted at or near the control console.	
18.	Emergency handles facilitate free movement of couch (X and Z).	
19.	Survey meter response checked by holding the meter against the shutters.	

Turn video monitoring off after treatment day ends, power down the Perfexion unit, and secure the keys.

In the case of a malfunction/emergency, the Perfexion will be locked and posted to show that it is out of clinical use. The keys for the treatment console will be given to clinical engineering for them to pass on to the manufacturer to repair the unit.

CHECKLIST FOR GAMMA KNIFE PERFEXION PRETREATMENT

GAMMA KNIFE TREATMENT PLAN CHECKLIST	
Daily QA approved	
CT image has low fiducial error	
MR image has low fiducial error (or registered to CT)	
Fusions checked by RO/NS	
Contours checked by RO/NS	
Matrix size is reasonable (per matrix)	
Prescription confirmed (per matrix)	
70%, 50%, 25% Isodose lines are reasonable	
DVHs are reasonable	
Conformity index is reasonable	
Gradient index	
All shots are within targets (MP + RO + NS)	
Low (<10%) or zero-weighted shots removed	
Gamma angles checked (use 70°/120° only if necessary)	
Treatment plan signed (MP + RO + NS)	
Secondary time check	
Therapists/RO shot check	
Time out	

CHECKLIST FOR TREATMENT DELIVERY QUALITY ASSURANCE OF PERFEXION PATIENTS

Patient Name: _____ ID #: _____ Date: _____

MR#: ☐ ☐ ☐ ☐ ☐ ☐ ☐

I.		PATIENT IDENTIFICATION (Check by at least two means)	
	a.	Photo identification	
	b.	Medical records #	
	c.	Birth date	
	d.	Name	

II.		PLANNING	
	a.	Fiducial markers detected with acceptable accuracy	
	b.	Image dimensions are within limits	
	c.	Plan approved by the neurosurgeon and radiation oncologist	
	d.	Plan downloaded to treatment console	
	e.	Frame adapter fits on patient frame	
	f.	Prescription in MOSAIQ is approved by the radiation oncologist	
	g.	Prescription in MOSAIQ and on GK plan are the same Signatures of three responsible personnel: A: _____ B: _____ C: _____	

III.		PATIENT SETUP AND TREATMENT	
	a.	Double-check treatment parameter(s) for each shot according to section L3d of license (at start of treatment for APS) Names of responsible personnel A: _____ B: _____	A____ B____
	b.	Treatment site verification by physician	
	c.	Confirm radiation oncologist, neurosurgeon, physicist are GK-trained users	
	d.	Procedural pause at time (_____)	
	e.	Staff member responsible for monitoring treatment delivery	

CHECKLIST FOR GAMMAMED HDR TREATMENT

MEDICAL CENTER
ANYTOWN, USA

Name of Patient:
Date of Birth:
Place Label Here

Initial all lines

Treatment date:
Plan name:

Therapist	Pretreatment General Checks	
	Intercom and CCTV functional	
	Pretreatment survey:_____mR/hr	Tolerance <1 mR/hr
	Survey meter #:_____	Cal due date: _____
	***If radiation level is > 1 mR/hr, give explanation: _____	
	Confirm radiation oncologist and physicist are authorized for HDR	

Therapist	Physicist	Treatment Plan Checks	
		Patient name correct	
		Date and time correct	
		Source strength correct	
		Total scaled Curie-seconds are correct	on Planned Treatment Report
		Dwell position and times correct	
		Signatures of RadOnc, physicist and RTT	
		RadOnc approved prescription	in MOSAIQ
		RadOnc and physicist approved plan pdf	

Therapist	Physicist	Patient Checks	
		Patient identified by two methods	
		Guide tube integrity	
		Guide tube/applicator length	
		Connection to indexer channel correct	
		SAVI pretreatment check sheet complete	For SAVI only
		SAVI expansion tool in place	
		Probe extension ____cm Tolerance 9.25 ± 0.1 cm	Cylinder only, use 250 mm transfer tube
		Procedural pause at time:	

Therapist	Posttreatment Checks
	Treatment delivered as planned
	Posttreatment survey: _____ **mR/Hr** *** If post-Tx reading > pre-Tx reading, confirm reading, then implement emergency procedures ***
	SAVI expansion tool removed
	Treatment delivery report printed
	Treatment recorded and charged in MOSAIQ

In case of error or treatment emergency, document error(s) and total treatment interruption time:

CHECKLIST FOR COMMISSIONING

1. Do not start commissioning till ATP is fully completed, verified, and signed satisfactorily within the limit of operation.

2. Check water phantom operation and software.

3. Check TPS requirements, e.g., depth dose, TMR, field size diagonal scans, absolute dose, etc.

4. Create a spreadsheet for scanning data collection as well as nonscanned data.

5. Set up tank properly and in correct orientation. Do not rush. Spend fair amount of time for initial setup.

6. Verify that tank alignments and arm movements are orthogonal and there is no hysteresis in motion.

7. Select low or intermediate dose rate for scanning to avoid overheating of machine.

8. Choose proper detector for type of scan.

9. Use proper voltage on detector (ion chambers typically 300–400 V; most diodes, diamonds, and plastic scintillators use zero volts).

10. Check leakage and zero readings of the system.

11. Frequently ensure that SSD is correct, as water evaporates over time.

12. Pay attention to data quality. If too much noise, check scanning speed.

13. Always save data if saves are not done automatically.

14. Analyze data before changing parameters, detectors, or protocol.

15. Make clear and elaborate note in comment section that may be useful later.

Index